Rorschachiana 42

Rorschachiana

Journal of the International
Society for the Rorschach

Volume 42 / Issues 1&2 / 2021

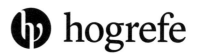

Rorschachiana, Volume 42, 2021 (Book)

Publishing Offices	USA: Hogrefe Publishing Corporation, 361 Newbury Street, 5th Floor, Boston, MA 02115 Phone (857) 880-2002; E-mail customerservice@hogrefe.com EUROPE: Hogrefe Publishing GmbH, Merkelstr. 3, 37085 Göttingen, Germany Phone +49 551 99950-0, Fax +49 551 99950-111; E-mail publishing@hogrefe.com
Sales and Distribution	USA: Hogrefe Publishing, Customer Services Department, 30 Amberwood Parkway, Ashland, OH 44805, Phone (800) 228-3749, Fax (419) 281-6883; E-mail customerservice@hogrefe.com UK: Hogrefe Publishing, c/o Marston Book Services Ltd., 160 Eastern Ave., Milton Park, Abingdon, OX14 4SB, Phone +44 1235 465577, Fax +44 1235 465556; E-mail direct.orders@marston.co.uk EUROPE: Hogrefe Publishing, Merkelstr. 3, 37085 Göttingen, Germany Phone +49 551 99950-0, Fax +49 551 99950-111; E-mail publishing@hogrefe.com
Other Offices	CANADA: Hogrefe Publishing, 82 Laird Drive, East York, Ontario, M4G 3V1 SWITZERLAND: Hogrefe Publishing, Länggass-Strasse 76, 3012 Bern Hogrefe Publishing Incorporated and registered in the Commonwealth of Massachusetts, USA, and in Göttingen, Lower Saxony, Germany Printed and bound in Germany
ISBN	978-0-88937-614-4

Rorschachiana: Journal of the International Society for the Rorschach

Publisher	Hogrefe Publishing GmbH, Merkelstr. 3, 37085 Göttingen, Germany, Phone +49 551 99950-0, Fax +49 551 99950-111, publishing@hogrefe.com USA: Hogrefe Publishing Corporation, 361 Newbury Street, 5th Floor, Boston, MA 02115, USA, Phone (857) 880-2002, customerservice@hogrefe.com
Production	Juliane Munson, Hogrefe Publishing, Merkelstr. 3, 37085 Göttingen, Germany, Phone +49 551 99950-422, Fax +49 551 99950-111, production@hogrefe.com
Subscriptions	Hogrefe Publishing, Herbert-Quandt-Str. 4, 37081 Göttingen, Germany, Phone +49 551 99950-900, Fax +49 551 99950-998
Advertising / Inserts	Hogrefe Publishing, Merkelstr. 3, 37085 Göttingen, Germany, Phone +49 551 99950-423, Fax +49 551 99950-111, marketing@hogrefe.com
ISSN	1192-5604
Publication	Published in two online issues and a print compendium per annual volume.
Subscription Prices	Calendar year subscriptions only. Rates for 2022: Institutions - from US $259.00/ €221.00 (detailed pricing can be found in the journals catalog at hgf.io/journals catalog); Individuals - US $132.00/€98.00 (print & online). Single issue (online only) - US $135.00/€118.00
Payment	Payment may be made by check, international money order, or credit card, to Hogrefe Publishing, Merkelstr. 3, 37085 Göttingen, Germany. US and Canadian subscriptions can also be ordered from Hogrefe Publishing, 361 Newbury Street, 5th Floor, Boston, MA 02115, USA
Electronic Full Text	The full text of *Rorschachiana* is available online at www.econtent.hogrefe.com
Abstracting Services	Abstracted/indexed in PsycINFO, PSYNDEX, Scopus, EMCare, and Cinahl Information Systems.

The Rorschach® Test has probably generated more subsequent literature in the field of psychology than any other work. Due to its universal applicability, timeless appeal to clinicians, and proven track record, this particular instrument has been utilized many millions of times throughout the world.

For more than 60 years, the International Society of the Rorschach and Projective Methods has played an important role in promoting the research and application of the Rorschach and other projective techniques. The first Congress of the Society took place in Zurich in August 1949. Subsequent meetings have been held periodically through the years, in a variety of locations: Rome [1956], Brussels [1958], Freiburg [1961], Paris [1965], London [1968], Zaragosa [1971], Fribourg [1977], Washington [1981], Barcelona [1984], Guarujá, São Paulo [1987], Paris [1990], Lisbon [1993], Boston [1996], Amsterdam [1999], Rome [2002], Barcelona [2005], Leuven / Louvain [2008], Tokyo [2011], Istanbul [2014], and Paris [2017]. The ISR judged that conditions in 2021 were not safe and therefore postponed the Centenary Congress in Switzerland to 2022.

To contribute to *Rorschachiana,* authors are welcome to submit papers:

1) Targeting the metrics and the validity of any of the Rorschach systems available in literature with the goal of providing users with more reliable, sensitive, and useful procedures to administer and interpret the test;
2) Focusing on the understanding of the client's perception of projective measures within online testing practices;
3) That provide visibility to all projective measures, especially those with demonstrated reliability and validity, and show their clinical utility to understand and help clients;
4) On new tests, or new coding systems for traditional tests, providing scientifically sound literature reviews of these measures, illustrating the psychometric properties of their coding systems, demonstrating their clinical utility, and informing readers about the training procedures available to become proficient in their use.

Contents

Volume 42, Issue 1, 2021

Volume 42, Issue 2, 2021

Special Issue: The Rorschach Test Today: An Update on the Research

Research Article

Teaching the Rorschach Comprehensive System

Students' Difficulties With the Administration Process

Damien Fouques[1], Dana Castro[1], Marion Mouret[3], and Tristan Le Chevanton[2]

[1]Laboratory EVACLISPY, Department of Clinical Psychology, Paris Nanterre University, Nanterre, France
[2]Laboratory VCR, École de Psychologues Praticiens, Paris, France
[3]Private Practice, Paris, France

Abstract: The administration process of the Rorschach test is of utmost importance as it influences both the coding and the interpretative procedures. Performing it appropriately requires complex skills, knowledge, and solid training. The aim of the study is to describe students' interests in and difficulties with administering the Rorschach (Comprehensive System) for the first time. A two-phase methodology, including an analysis of questionnaire responses followed by a study of students' written narratives, using Iramuteq textual analysis software, was implemented with two different samples of third-year undergraduates (including 63 and 253 participants, respectively), recruited from a French psychology school. Our results show that students have a strong interest in understanding the test and wish to use it in their future practice. When administering the Rorschach for the first time, students find it difficult to cope with the complexity of the procedures at a technical, emotional, and relational level.

Keywords: administration process, emotional control, inquiry, relational dynamics, Rorschach test

The Rorschach Comprehensive System (CS; Exner, 1974, 2003) can be controversial but is still a frequently used evaluation method in clinical practice (Wright et al., 2017). It also continues to be refined in the research context (Smith et al., 2018).

Despite a decrease in the number of hours devoted to teaching projective methods in the training of clinical psychologists in faculty curricula (Evans & Finn, 2017), the Rorschach test is still appreciated by the directors of internships and is frequently a part of clinicians' assessment batteries (Ready et al., 2016). Currently, the Rorschach test ranks eight in the top 10 of the assessment measures used by practicing psychologists (Ready et al., 2016; Wright et al., 2017).

The Rorschach (CS) remains present in more than half of the training programs and, "In general...is the most popular non-self-report test of psychopathology" (Mihura et al., 2017, p. 10). The Rorschach test continues to be effectively used in psychopathology, forensic, inpatient and outpatient practices for diagnosis and treatment recommendations (Erdberg, 2019; Wright et al., 2017). There is also interest in new applications, for example, Finn's model of therapeutic assessment in psychotherapy (2020), the differential diagnosis of unipolar versus bipolar depression (Le Chevanton et al., 2020), or the application to disabilities such as autistic disorders (Frigaux et al., 2020).

Thus, despite criticism, a reduction in the hours of training, or the influence of other measurement tools, the Rorschach test remains resilient, possibly due to its perceived clinical utility. Clinical psychologists report that the Rorschach test usefully enlightens their patients' personality dynamics and diagnosis (Norcross & Rogan, 2013), and reveals the holistic dimensions of the individual (Frigaux et al., 2020).

Psychology students report being attracted to the Rorschach training experience as they appreciate the emphasis on authentic case studies in the training (Mouret, 2017) and expect the Rorschach to become a significant tool in their professional careers (Mihura & Weinle, 2002).

Mastering the use of the Rorschach test (CS) in the assessment process is difficult as it is a demanding, time-consuming, and multifaceted technique (Grønnerød & Hartmann, 2010). Appropriate care must be taken regarding factors such as administration, instructions, recording responses, and inquiry (Exner 1974, 2003; Weiner, 2004). Furthermore, coding and interpreting the Rorschach test require careful, disciplined behavior and thinking (Andronikof, 2004) to obtain valid protocols. Coding and interpreting the Rorschach test are strongly linked to the administration procedures (Exner, 1974, 2003), which, according to our teaching experience, seem to be the cornerstone of the Rorschach training.

Yet, in the international literature on Rorschach training, little has been reported about students' perspective on administering the Rorschach test. The international literature focuses on three main themes related to: (1) the difficulties students experience when coding, especially with determinants, special scores, and FQ (Fouques et al., 2017; Hilsenroth et al., 2007; Viglione et al., 2017); (2) the place of the Rorschach training in faculty curricula (Lewey et al., 2019; Mihura et al., 2017) since the Rorschach training is generally offered in graduate programs; (3) the conditions required for efficient training, particularly number of hours and coding responses (respectively 21–35 hours of training and 50 coding responses according to Hilsenroth et al., 2007), supervision (Viglione et al., 2017), and teaching techniques, such as videorecording (Hilsenroth et al., 2007). The goal of this research is to ascertain students' interests and impediments in administering the RCS

(Exner, 1974, 2003), thereby understanding their perceived difficulties with the process and improving the teaching of the test.

To fully achieve the research goal and broaden the understanding of the multi-faceted dimensions of the Rorschach learning process, we have selected a two-phase methodology including both quantitative and qualitative elements and have formulated the following research question: What are the typologies of the Rorschach administration difficulties and their prevalence among a population of undergraduate psychology students running the test for the first time? The first phase of the research aims to answer the research question through a survey, built upon an exploratory questionnaire, which is analyzed quantitatively. The second phase consists in exploring the students' narratives of their experiences of their first Rorschach (C.S.) administration. The study, as a whole, was approved by the Research Evaluation Committee of the Research Department of the Ecole de Psychologues Praticiens.

The First Phase: Analysis of the Questionnaire

Context of the Study: Teaching of the Rorschach

In our private school, the teaching of the Rorschach is progressive, starting in the third year with a study of the history of the test, from Hermann Rorschach to the CS (Exner, 1974, 2003), including epistemological issues (11 hr) and the coding techniques and structural summary completion (36 hr). In the fourth year, a structural summary interpretation is completed (36 hr) and advanced case studies are offered in the fifth and last year before graduation (24 hr).

At the end of the third year, as part of the students' professional education, they were asked, as a mandatory assignment, to administer a Rorschach test to a non-consulting adult participant, to score the protocol, and to carry out a critical analysis of their work. Students were asked to recruit a participant over the age of 18, whom they had never met before, who was neither a patient nor a student in psychology and who agreed to sign a participation consent form. They received a handout summarizing the procedures for administering the test in accordance with Exner's recommendations after classroom training (Exner, 1974, 2003).

For those students who agreed to participate, an anonymous questionnaire was independently proposed (there was no link made between the questionnaire and the mandatory work) and a consent form was signed. The survey respondents are therefore students in their third year of psychology studies.

Participants

The study was offered to 200 students. The participation rate was 31.5%. The research sample comprised 64 third-year volunteer students from a French private professional psychology school recruited from 2013 to 2015. The average age of the sample was 21.5 years (*SD* = 2.4), 84% of whom were women.

The attendance rate for the course was of 92%. Students were evaluated through two examinations: a theoretical one consisting of a multiple-choice questionnaire about the history of the test, and about the CS basis, as well as a coding one, in which students' ability to code a given protocol was evaluated. A score of "overall performance" was calculated (test theory: 30% + coding: 70%). The mean obtained was 11.8/20 (*SD* = 2.7), min = 8, max = 15, equivalent to "B minus" in Anglo-Saxon countries. The performance on the coding evaluation resulted in a mean of 11.9/20 (*SD* = 2.6; min = 7, max = 17) or "B minus."

Measures

An exploratory questionnaire was developed, informed by a literature review and our relevant teaching experience. The thematic fields were acknowledged after a deductive–inductive qualitative analysis. Deductively, authors identified themes based on the framework of Ritzler and Gaudio (1976) and of Ritzler and Alter (1986); inductively they developed new themes through an iterative process based on a reading and analysis of the notes and observations of three Rorschach teachers. Themes were further grouped into categories to construct the questionnaire.

Questions were divided into four categories:

(1) The administration process including perceived general technical skill (e.g., "I could write everything down").
(2) Interpersonal dynamics including perceived relational skill (e.g., "I managed to maintain the framework").
(3) Emotional experience including the management of emotions (e.g., "I was tense").
(4) Professional stance including the perception of the test as a possible tool in professional practice (e.g., "I want to continue administering Rorschach tests").

The questionnaire comprised 36 items covering the four categories, randomly distributed, rated on a 6-point Likert scale (from *not at all* to *totally*) without the possibility of a neutral response and allowing for a continuous and dichotomous treatment of the items (*yes/no*). A total of 19 items were reversed. Reliability analysis revealed a Cronbach's α of .84, which demonstrates good internal consistency.

In order to assess the administration quality, two teachers (first and last authors) conducted a consensual evaluation of the protocols. They identified the lack of prompting after the first response, possible problems of sequencing of the responses, which both led to erroneous numbers of protocol responses (R); and the quality of the enquiry: correct questions asked, misformulated ones, or lack of questions.

Data Analysis
Statistical Analysis
For each item, distributions were analyzed and a categorial classification was made. When participants rated a 0, 1, or 2, a "no" score was coded. When 3, 4, or 5 were chosen, a "yes" was coded. In this way, we were able to analyze proportion tendencies for each question and compute percentages. Since each question is independent and mandatory, the sum of the "yes" percentages obtained for each question may exceed 100.

Bivariate Analysis
To test possible links between continuous variables, correlation coefficients (Pearson) were performed. To test possible links between categorial variables, a chi-square analysis was used. Statistical analyses were performed with Jamovi software.

Results

The complete results of the questionnaire are available in the table in Electronic Supplementary Material 1 (ESM 1).

The Administration Process – Technical Aspects
In general, 75% declared that the task was difficult but 92% estimated that they had managed the situation well. Overall, 73% overestimated their performance since they perceived their collected protocols as valid according to the administration instructions, but according to their teachers few were valid, because of administration and enquiry mistakes. Of the sample, 33% needed to refer to their documents during the administration and 20% encountered difficulties in notetaking.

During the response phase, only 5% of the sample declared that it was difficult to master the task and 41% experienced difficulties in separating responses. Moreover, 20% of the whole sample made a mistake on R (according to first and fourth authors' evaluations) and among these, more than one-third (8% of the whole sample) did not seem to recognize the mistake as they did not find it difficult to separate responses even though they obviously had trouble in doing so.

The inquiry phase task was perceived as more difficult than the first one, with 45% declaring not having mastered it. Overall, 67% of the sample acknowledged not having asked enough questions; 42% declared having worded the questions poorly (e.g., using "why" instead of "how" or forgetting to question keywords). Of the sample, 70% believed they had made mistakes during this phase.

Thus, fewer than half of the sample declared having less control during the inquiry phase than during the response phase. A comparison of these opinions with the teachers' evaluation of the protocols reveals that 30% were not fully aware of their shortcomings. Difficulties included: not asking enough questions, formulating them poorly, or, more importantly, forgetting to question keywords.

Interpersonal Dynamics – Relationship With the Participants

The interpersonal aspects of the task were experienced as difficult for 36% of our sample. Although 27% felt too close to the subject and 8% too distant, 94% declared that they were at the right distance. The most surprising results were that 98% of the whole sample declared they were able to set a framework, and 91% believed that they were able to maintain it.

We further analyzed this result and found that among the 94% of the students who considered themselves proficient, none of them felt they were too distant. Of the respondents, 73% felt that they were too close. Reasons for this might include: The testers were young and inexperienced; they were not working in an institution; the assessment was not done for clinical reasons, or requested by the participants (who were informed that they would not receive any feedback).

The Emotional Experience – Management of Emotions

Of the respondents, 61% declared they were sometimes anxious during the exercise, 41% felt like laughing and 20% were embarrassed by some of the participants' responses. Despite that, emotional reactions did not alter the level of overall satisfaction, as 92% enjoyed the exercise.

Another result emerged when we compared the responses for two items: "I felt comfortable" and "I was tense during the exercise." Coherent answers were given by 48.4%, indicating that they were comfortable, without tension, while 51.6% gave ambivalent responses, indicating they were at ease and tense or not tense but not at ease. None of the participants provided the "tense and uncomfortable" response. However, after dividing the sample into two groups – "at ease" versus "ambivalent" – no significant differences were found in the rest of our data (according to the chi-square analysis).

The Professional Stance – The Use of the Rorschach in Professional Settings

All the respondents declared they wished to improve their mastery of the Rorschach test. Of these, 95% wish to carry on with the Rorschach test administration and training and 92% reported that they would probably use it in their future practice.

Rorschach Technical Mastery – Theoretical and Technical Learning

Academic performances are positively linked to the feeling of comfort during administration and to the perceived technical mastery during the inquiry phase. Correspondingly, feelings of embarrassment are negatively linked to academic performance (as shown in the table in ESM 2). We observed that better performance in coding is linked to mastery of the inquiry, and vice versa.

To summarize the findings of the questionnaire, we can assert that:

The Rorschach test is of interest to undergraduate psychology students, who imagine using it as a clinical tool in their professional practice. However, unless students thoroughly understand the real clinical value of the test, one cannot exclude the possibility that a desirability bias has inflated this result.

The administration process is flawed by the lack of mastery of the inquiry process and by the interpersonal dynamics. We speculate that in the "at ease group," some students must have felt too self-confident considering the quality of the protocols. In the "ambivalent group," some students probably had to deal with contradictory emotions, which may have restricted their learning progress or resulted in an indication of too little self-confidence.

Improving the test training of students in administration of the Rorschach is vital to help them evaluate their performance correctly, progress in their inquiry methods, improve their coding skills, and better manage their relationship with the participants.

The Second Phase: Exploring Students' Perceptions

On the basis of the analysis of the questionnaire, from a theoretical, ontological position (Zou et al., 2014), we implemented a second phase. Our aim was to comprehensively explore the subjective perceptions of a population of psychology undergraduates regarding their difficulties in learning the administration of the Rorschach test.

Method

Participants

The participants were 301 undergraduate students in their third year of psychology, enrolled in the same private professional psychology school as the questionnaire respondents of the first phase. They were asked, as a mandatory exercise at the end of their first Rorschach course, to proceed with a Rorschach test administration (CS) in non-consulting settings (as in the first phase). To diminish potential "desirability bias," the design was modified. This exercise did not involve any coding or work on the protocols collected at this stage. Students were instructed to answer the following question in writing: "What are the difficulties I met during this clinical sequence?" The word "clinical" might come as a surprise in a non-consulting environment. But students were instructed to understand it as a professional act that was to meet the ethical requirements of any professional encounter. A total of 235 narratives were collected from 2015 to 2017.

Because of the complete anonymity of the narratives, the average age or sex ratio of this sample could not be computed. However, thanks to an excellent participation rate (78%), we can assume that the demographics are very close to those of the third-year student population in this French psychology school (between 21 and 23 years old; 89% were women).

Data Analysis

The collected narratives were processed using Iramuteq lexicometric software (Ratinaud, 2012) based on the Reinert method (1983, 2008). The Iramuteq textual analysis aims to ascertain how participants talk about their difficulties when administering the Rorschach test. The algorithm used by the Iramuteq program is based on a hierarchical bottom–up classification and the calculation, through the χ^2, of word occurrence in a text. The Reinert method consists of four steps (for a detailed description of the four steps of the lexicometric analysis, see Reinert, 1983, 2008).

Ethics

All narratives were anonymous. The students previously gave their written consent for the use of their written feedbacks for research purposes.

Results

The lexicometric analysis revealed five word-classes as shown in Figure 1 (85.86% of classified text segments that were identified by the Iramuteq software). For each word class, the words to be interpreted were those whose χ^2 of association with the class was greater than 10. Tool words (prepositions, articles, adverbs)

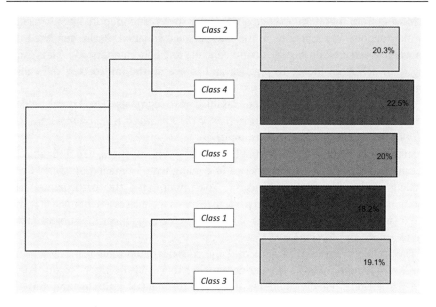

Figure 1. Lexicometric analysis: Classificatory analysis dendrogram of the corpus. Dendrogram representing the distribution of the corpus.

and 210 polysemic words (that cannot be clearly interpreted, used in different contexts, such as "to go," "to take," etc.) were excluded from the interpretation of the results. The size of the class is indicated by the percentage of the classified corpus (e.g., Class 2 represents 20.3% of the entire corpus).

A description of the words in the five classes and the χ^2 of association with the classes are provided in the tables in ESM 3.

Class 1 included 18.25% of the classified text segments. The lexical field of Class 1 is associated with the *description of the administration of the Rorschach* test from a technical point of view.

Students described the test administration process as an interesting and instructive exercise, allowing them to understand the real value of the test. They perceived their experience as an additional preparation for their degree and for their self-confidence. For example: "The administration exercise is interesting, enriching, and positive and requires a lot of training."

The administration situation could make them feel anxious or intimidated. They mentioned their lack of experience and practice but were optimistic, declaring that difficulties would decrease with experience and training: "The administration process is somehow anxiety inducing but to do it was really good."

Moving from theory to practice allowed the students to identify hitches related to their actions and reactions in the interpersonal situation. It also rendered the knowledge acquired during the course concrete and better understood: "It is exciting to switch from theory to practice and to see all the unexpected difficulties emerge."

Class 2 included 20.26% of the classified text segments. The lexical field of Class 2 is associated with the *description of the Rorschach test and more precisely with the cards and the participants' answers.*

Students were concerned with the number of given responses, had difficulties in getting the participant to verbalize or in dealing with a detailed answer: "I was anxious to have enough responses." They interpreted the participants' long moments of silence as a refusal to participate or as the expression of unease within the relationship: "When moments of silence are too long, I fear the subject's refusal to go on, and feel uneasy."

The students expressed doubts over the administration rules (e.g., turning the card, removing the card), wondering whether they had the right "to do that to the participant." Finally, students discussed the neutral attitude that must be adopted during the test and the need to master their own thoughts, urges to laugh, or interventions: "When the participant's responses are like those studied in class, I cannot prevent myself from interpreting or laughing."

Class 3 included 19.07% of the classified text segments. The lexical field of Class 3 is associated with the description of the relationship between the student and the participant.

Students described the role of the future psychologist that they tried to embrace, sometimes with difficulty, as being uncomfortable. Their goal was to investigate the psychological functioning of the participants through a relationship within which they strive to embody benevolent neutrality by making sure that their emotions are not manifest and by finding the right posture and emotional distance in order to reassure the participant. This exercise allowed them to gain confidence, regulate their nervousness, and control the situation, even if amusing or unexpected responses made this attitude difficult to maintain.

Sometimes students had difficulties in establishing a framework of trust with the participant, as they had to manage their requests, account for everything they said and did, and, ultimately, manage their own emotions. The students felt the weight of the relationship dynamics and their difficulties in controlling the feelings shared by the participants: "I feared like opening a door in the participant's life that must not be opened."

The students experienced a conflict between the need for interaction with the participant (for the sake of the relationship) and the need for recording all the given responses verbatim (for the sake of the protocol validity). As such, they emphasized the necessity for intensive test administration training to experience different participant reactions and to learn how to avoid being overwhelmed by the participant's emotional state: "It is the training that will empower us and enable us to control over all the parameters of the communication situation, the reactions we ourselves might have, and the way they might influence the participant."

Class 4 included 22.46% of the classified text segments. The lexical scope of Class 4 is associated with *the questions asked by students during the enquiry.*

Students seemed to be reassured by not having to score the collected protocols because of the large number of difficulties encountered during the administration process. They acknowledged that awkwardness could lead to invalid or incomplete protocols (e.g., asking too few or too many questions). Students expressed doubts over the right determinants to be scored (especially shadings but also form, movement, and color), over the keywords to be asked, to clarify a response, and over the need to question the participant when all the information had already been given in the response phase: "I am sure that I missed a lot during the inquiry phase and did not further investigate other aspects."

Class 5 included 19.96% of the classified text segments. The lexical field of Class 5 is associated with *notetaking during the Rorschach test.*

Students stated that they were tense when taking notes to record all the answers and that this exercise required a high degree of concentration. The difficulty stemmed from the need to be quick, and at the same time, write what the participant was saying, the response location, and think about words that require more explanation. The difficulties were also linked to the difficulty of finding the right balance between observing, listening, and writing and the risk of missing or forgetting important aspects of the process. A student summarized most of the difficulties encountered as follows: "It is difficult to observe the participant's gestures and attitudes at the same time, to refocus on their discourse about the card when a digression becomes too important and to appear as relaxed as possible, despite a hand cramp."

To summarize the findings of the qualitative phase we can assert that: The results obtained in the second phase (five lexicometric classes) overlap the four categories described in the first phase. Thus, from the analysis of students' narratives, the following difficulties in the Rorschach administration process can be discerned:

(1) Technical aspects of the administration process including management of practicalities (Class 1 and 2), the inquiry process (Class 4), and comprehensive notetaking (Class 5). The administration process was perceived to be difficult because of its complexity: From the practicalities of notetaking

or time control to the subtleties of the inquiry, the undergraduates were lost in the middle of the simultaneous management of all these tasks.

(2) Relational dynamics (Class 3) were dominated by students' difficulties in regulating emotions, in building a working frame, and in setting limits with the participant. As a coping strategy, some avoided being overwhelmed emotionally by not paying attention to the participant but focusing on note-taking and on their inner world (Class 5).

(3) Emotional experience (class 2) includes anxiety in coping with one's own emotions and avoiding any negative bias or sharing emotions with the participant.

(4) Professional stance (Class 2) comprises the struggle that students experience to maintain the assessment frame within a professional interaction. The correct professional stance is difficult to achieve at this level of training, but students were aware of their shortcomings and willing to improve through more training.

Overall, the Rorschach test aroused great interest in students, who found it enriching for their professional development (Class 1) and experienced the administration process as a "step into real life!"

General Discussion: Synthesizing Findings From Phase 1 and Phase 2

The two surveys yielded similar findings: All the respondents in both phases held positive views of the Rorschach and considered using it in their future clinical practice, which is a trend that has not faded through the decades (Mihura & Weinle, 2002).

The Rorschach administration process was appreciated as it provides an initial authentic professional experience, despite generating some anxiety and trepidation (Miller, 2009). Most of our sample students felt that their classes had prepared them well for the administration process, but this was contradicted by their initial practices, as their ability to structure the administration process was not yet mastered and their proficiency either under- or overestimated. The feeling of being well prepared might stem from the clarity of the administration instructions. The latter do not require much decision-making and are not difficult to learn, thus allowing students to focus on their proficiency in coding (Exner 1974, 2003).

The main difficulty expressed by our students was coping with the complexity of these procedures at a technical and interpersonal level. Students were required to juggle: mastery of the system's practicalities; the appropriateness of inquiry interventions; the uniqueness of the professional relationship; and the regulation of their emotional state while being alone in an unknown context. It was evident that when confusion or anxiety arose during the Rorschach administration process, students focused on notetaking, for the sake of the protocol validity, and thus tried to cope by avoiding the relationship with the participant. Avoidance helped students to complete the whole administration process but probably hindered viewing the Rorschach administration as an interactive process (Handler, 2013). On the contrary, students who are better prepared theoretically were more aware of their attitudes and relational difficulties during the Rorschach administration process.

We can compare the difficulties encountered within the Rorschach administration process with those involving coding Cognitive Special Scores, Determinants, and coding Form Quality for objects that were not listed (Viglione et al., 2017), because these tasks are intimately linked and require observation, logical thinking, organization, knowledge, and cognitive flexibility in adjusting concepts to the uniqueness of the participant's perceptions.

We can reasonably assume that feelings of mastery and ease with the Rorschach administration will improve as competency in coding develops along with the clinical experience, continuing education, and supervision (Viglione et al., 2017).

Strengths and Limitations of the Study

One of the strengths of the study is the focus on a relatively under-researched topic, which draws attention to the difficulties arising during the Rorschach administration process. Another is the combined quantitative and qualitative elements of the methodology that facilitate the exploration of a complexity of experiences.

This study had some limitations. First, the samples: our participants were not randomly selected, and the samples were not of the same size. The timing for the two phases was not designed to be simultaneous, and thus the same subjects did not respond to the same research design. Our sample is context-bound (a private French school of psychology); therefore, the findings might not represent a wider population of Rorschach students and cannot be generalized. The sample also has a gender imbalance; however, the predominance of women studying psychology in this group is consistent with the distribution in the general French population (Schneider & Mondière, 2017). Second: The survey questionnaire did not undergo a strict psychometric validation. Third: Despite the anonymization procedure, a possible desirability bias may have influenced some results because the researchers were also the teachers of the students.

Conclusion

The Rorschach test must continue to develop at a professional and academic level. On a professional level, internship training directors (as well as numerous interns) confirm that competency in projective assessment is a desired skill for professional practice (Joy, 2020) as it harbors unique clinical value in providing rich data that can foster potential working hypotheses for psychotherapy (Piotrowski, 2015).

Proficiency in the test is most likely the key to resilience and viability. For that purpose, teachers and clinical instructors must take the time to explain procedures and answer questions, to enable students to acquire more didactic and practical experience (Mihura & Weinle, 2002) and develop interpretive skills that will serve them well in standard clinical practice (Joy, 2020). For this reason, we believe that starting to learn the Rorschach in the undergraduate years is an opportunity to prepare *readiness internship competency* (American Psychological Association, n.d.) by developing: First, an awareness of the strengths and limitations of administration, scoring, and interpretation is created (the basic foundations of the test are acquired through at least 2 years of intensive courses of 36 hr/year). Second, self-awareness and reflexivity in clinical practice are reinforced by the ongoing training and theoretical recall in the following years. Third, interpersonal skills in establishing professional relationships and frame-keeping are developed. The learning is progressive and includes technical skills, reflectivity, and mindfulness.

In our curricula, the third year of the undergraduate psychology studies corresponds to a transition from theoretical courses to more applied ones like psychometrics, Wechsler's scales, the Thematic Apperception Test (TAT), the helping relationships, and an introduction to research methodology. The third year is also the beginning of the professional path, because students must complete 300 hr of observational internship under the supervision of a senior psychologist. The Rorschach test might be part of those observational assignments.

To reach this goal it might be useful to adapt the test-teaching methods to the students' needs and faculty constraints. We suggest addressing the concern that students under- or overestimate their skills, by providing a systematic presentation of the administration process and coding, along with practical exercises including modeling and recorded role playing with instructors' feedback (Hilsenroth et al., 2007; Mihura et al., 2017). For example, the teacher could play the role of a participant and the student do the inquiry and code. The coding can then be discussed and evaluated. As progress is made with practicalities, interpersonal difficulties could be introduced into the role play. Alternatively, peer role-play, under the teachers' supervision, can be organized where students alternate, playing the roles of interviewer and participant, to gain insight into both experiences.

The provision of a role model by a teacher is an important component of efficient Rorschach training (Hilsenroth et al., 2007). Students need identificatory models on which to project themselves in the future (Mouret, 2017). In our private school, Rorschach teachers (CS) are appropriately trained by a certified clinician, undergo supervision for at least 3 years (in coding and interpreting), and are required to update their knowledge regularly through continuing education. As such, they can fulfill three important functions: practice, research, and student supervision. They are able to introduce their students to the significance and use of the test while motivating and encouraging them to improve.

In addition, we believe that the same Rorschach teacher must be able to link the content of their teaching to other courses, essential to the comprehension and use of the test, namely, psychometry, psychopathology, and psychotherapy, which comprehensively introduce students to the complexity of the clinical work.

The supervision of Rorschach administration process and coding is necessary to:

(1) Empower students in the management of clinical relationships with diverse clients (consultants or non-consultants) and understand the fundamentals of clinical helping relationships;

(2) Adjust students' self-evaluation as Rorschach users, to balance inappropriate feelings of anxiety or over evaluation and build self confidence in testing skills; and

(3) Help them to integrate the complexity of the Rorschach test, which contains in all its aspects the quintessence of the clinical work – a form of "clinical psychology in a nutshell."

All these steps will lead students to be, "Good examiners who exercise good judgment in the process of administering the test, and deal with their subjects in a tactful, sensitive and very human manner" (Exner & Erdberg, 2005, p. 82).

Electronic Supplementary Materials

The electronic supplementary material is available with the online version of the article at https://doi.org/10.1027/1192-5604/a000138

ESM 1. Table showing the questionnaire (French and English version) and the results of Phase 1

ESM 2. Table showing the correlations between theoretical test knowledge, coding mastery, and administration process self-evaluation

ESM 3. Tables showing the words of the five classes of the lexicometric analysis

References

American Psychological Association (n.d.). *Competency benchmarks in professional psychology*. https://apa.org/ed/graduate/competency

Andronikof, A. (2004). Le Rorschach en système intégré: Introduction [The Rorschach as an integrated system: Introduction]. *Psychologie Française, 49*(1), 1–5. https://doi.org/10.1016/j.psfr.2003.11.005

Erdberg, P. (2019). The Rorschach. In G. Goldstein, D. N. Allen, & J. DeLuca (Eds.), *Handbook of psychological assessment* (4th ed., pp. 419–432). Academic Press. https://doi.org/10.1016/B978-0-12-802203-0.00014-6

Evans, F. B., & Finn, S. E. (2017). Training and consultation in psychological assessment with professional psychologists: Suggestions for enhancing the profession and individual practices. *Journal of Personality Assessment, 99*(2), 175–185. https://doi.org/10.1080/00223891.2016.1187156

Exner, J. E. Jr. (1974). *The Rorschach test: A comprehensive system*. Wiley.

Exner, J. E. Jr. (2003). *The Rorschach: A comprehensive system, Basic foundations and principles of interpretation, Vol. 1* (4th ed.). John Wiley & Sons.

Exner, J. E. Jr., & Erdberg, P. (2005). *The Rorschach: A comprehensive system, Advanced interpretation, Vol. 2* (3rd ed.). John Wiley & Sons.

Finn, S. E. (2020). *In our clients' shoes: Theory and techniques of therapeutic assessment* (2nd ed.). Routledge.

Fouques, D., Le Chevanton, T., Pons, E., Constantin-Kuntz, M., & Castro, D. (2017, July 18–21). Perception of difficulties met by students when using the Rorschach comprehensive System for the first time. In D. Castro (Ed.), *Teaching projective methods*. [Symposium]. 22nd Congress of the International Rorschach Society, Paris, France. Abstract 304.

Frigaux, A., Evrard, R., & Lighezzolo-Alnot, J. (2020). L'intérêt du test de Rorschach dans l'évaluation diagnostique des troubles du spectre autistiquex [The interest of the Rorschach test in the diagnostic evaluation of autism spectrum disorders]. *L'Évolution Psychiatrique, 85*(1), 133–154. https://doi.org/10.1016/j.evopsy.2019.11.002

Grønnerød, C., & Hartmann, E. (2010). Moving Rorschach coding forward: The RN-Rorschach coding system as an exemplar of simplified coding. *Rorschachiana, 31*(1), 22–42. https://doi.org/10.1027/1192-5604/a000003

Handler, L. (2013). The importance of teaching and learning personality assessment. In M. J. Hilsenroth, D. L. Segal, & M. Hersen (Eds.), *Teaching and learning personality assessment* (pp. 35–62). Routledge.

Hilsenroth, M. J., Charnas, J. W., Zodan, J., & Streiner, D. L. (2007). Criterion-based training for Rorschach scoring. *Training and Education in Professional Psychology, 1*(2), 125–134. https://doi.org/10.1037/1931-3918.1.2.125.

Joy, S. (2020). Why teach future psychotherapists to administer and interpret projective tests? Well, why teach future physicians and surgeons to perform dissections? *SIS Journal of Projective Psychology & Mental Health, 27*(1), 6–11.

Le Chevanton, T., Fouques, D., Julien-Sweerts, S., Petot, D., & Polosan, M. (2020). Differentiating unipolar and bipolar depression: Contribution of the Rorschach test (Comprehensive System). *Journal of Clinical Psychology, 76*(4), 769–777. https://doi.org/10.1002/jclp.22912

Lewey, J. H., Kivisalu, T. M., & Giromini, L. (2019). Coding with R-PAS: Does prior training with the Exner comprehensive system impact interrater reliability compared to those examiners with only R-PAS-based training? *Journal of Personality Assessment, 101*(4), 393–401. https://doi.org/10.1080/00223891.2018.1476361

Mihura, J. L., Roy, M., & Graceffo, R. A. (2017). Psychological assessment training in clinical psychology doctoral programs. *Journal of Personality Assessment, 99*(2), 153–164. https://doi.org/10.1080/00223891.2016.1201978

Mihura, J. L., & Weinle, C. A. (2002). Rorschach training: doctoral students' experiences and preferences. *Journal of Personality Assessment, 79*(1), 39–52. https://doi.org/10.1207/S15327752JPA7901_03

Miller, A. (2009). *Teaching the Rorschach backwards, forwards, and upside down: Creative ideas to engage students in the learning process* [Conference session abstract]. 8th Conference on Best Practices in Teaching Controversial Issues in Psychology, Atlanta, GA. https://doi.org/10.1037/e522282013-053

Mouret, M. (2017). L'enseignement de la psychologie: Point de vue des étudiants en France [The teaching of psychology: Students' point of view in France]. *Pratiques Psychologiques, 23*(3), 325–344. https://doi.org/10.1016/j.prps.2017.04.001

Norcross, J. C., & Rogan, J. D. (2013). Psychologists conducting psychotherapy in 2012: Current practices and historical trends among Division 29 members. *Psychotherapy, 50*(4), 490–495. https://doi.org/10.1037/a0033512

Piotrowski, C. (2015). Clinical instruction on projective techniques in the USA: A review of academic training settings 1995–2014. *SIS Journal of Projective Psychology & Mental Health, 22*(2), 83–92.

Ratinaud, P. (2012). *Iramuteq* [Computer software]. http://www.iramuteq.org/

Ready, R. E., Santorelli, G. D., & Romano, F. M. (2016). Psychology internship directors' perceptions of pre-internship training preparation in assessment. *North American Journal of Psychology, 18*(2), 317–334.

Reinert, A. (1983). Une méthode de classification descendante hiérarchique: Application à l'analyse lexicale par contexte [A method of hierarchical classification: application to lexical analysis by context]. *Cahiers de l'analyse des données, 8*(2), 187–198.

Reinert, M. (2008). Mondes lexicaux stabilisés et analyses statistiques de discours [Stabilized lexical worlds and statistical analysis of discourse] In Mondes lexicaux stabilisés et analyses statistiques de discours. In S. Heiden & B. Pincemin (Eds.), *Actes des 9èmes Journées internationales d'Analyses Statistiques des Données Textuelles* (pp. 579–590). Presses Universitaires de Lyon.

Ritzler, B., & Alter, B. (1986). Rorschach teaching in APA-approved clinical graduate programs: Ten years later. *Journal of Personality Assessment, 50*(1), 44–49. https://doi.org/10.1207/s15327752jpa5001_6

Ritzler, B. A., & Gaudio, A. C. D. (1976). A survey of Rorschach teaching in APA-approved clinical graduate programs. *Journal of Personality Assessment, 40*(5), 451–453. https://doi.org/10.1207/s15327752jpa4005_1

Schneider, B., & Mondière, G. (2017, April). Les Psychologues en France: nombre et activités, des données actualisées et inédites [Psychologists in France: Number and activities, updated and unpublished data]. *Fédérer, 87*, 16–21.

Smith, J. M., Gacono, C. B., Fontan, P., Taylor, E. E., Cunliffe, T. B., & Andronikof, A. (2018). A scientific critique of Rorschach research: Revisiting Exner's issues and methods in Rorschach research (1995). *Rorschachiana, 39*(2), 180–203. https://doi.org/10.1027/1192-5604/a000102

Viglione, D. J., Meyer, G. J., Resende, A. C., & Pignolo, C. (2017). A survey of challenges experienced by new learners coding the Rorschach. *Journal of Personality Assessment, 99*(3), 315–323. https://doi.org/10.1080/00223891.2016.1233559

Weiner, I. B. (2004). Rorschach assessment: Current status. In M. J. Hilsenroth & D. L. Segal (Eds.), *Comprehensive handbook of psychological assessment: Vol. 2: Personality assessment* (pp. 343–355). John Wiley & Sons.

Wright, C. V., Beattie, S. G., Galper, D. I., Church, A. S., Bufka, L. F., Brabender, V. M., & Smith, B. L. (2017). Assessment practices of professional psychologists: Results of a national survey. *Professional Psychology: Research and Practice, 48*(2), 73–78. https://doi.org/10.1037/pro0000086

Zou, P. X. W., Sunindijo, R. Y., & Dainty, A. R. J. (2014). A mixed methods research design for bridging the gap between research and practice in construction safety. *Safety Science, 70*, 316–326. https://doi.org/10.1016/j.ssci.2014.07.005

History
Received June 29, 2020
Revision received November 29, 2020
Accepted December 15, 2020
Published online March 18, 2021

ORCID
Damien Fouques
 https://orcid.org/0000-0002-9850-5896

Damien Fouques
Laboratory EVACLISPY
Department of Clinical Psychology
Paris Nanterre University
200 avenue de la République
92001 Nanterre Cedex
France
dfouques@parisnanterre.fr

Summary

Qualified psychologists and students appreciate the Rorschach Test for its originality and the insights it can offer. To be effective, this test must be understood theoretically and mastered clinically. This begins with the integration of the administration process, on which its validity and interpretability depend. The administration process involves subtle and complex procedures on a technical, cognitive, and emotional level. The objective of this study was to describe and analyze the difficulties experienced by psychology students during their first administration of the Rorschach. Suggestions are offered to adjust the teaching to the specific needs of students. The methodology consisted of two distinct phases: first, the analysis of a questionnaire constructed for the purpose of the research, aimed at identifying and classifying the students' difficulties. It was based on the answers of 64 participants, 18–24 years old, mostly women, in their third year in a

French school of psychology. The second phase aimed to deepen the understanding of the results obtained from the questionnaire. Written responses were collected from 235 third-year students, recruited from the same school, in answer to the question: "What difficulties did I encounter in taking the Rorschach test for the first time?" Data analysis was carried out using Iramuteq software, based on the Reinert method. The results highlighted four main classes of difficulties related to the administration of the Rorschach, which include: (1) technical management aspects, (2) management of the relational dynamics with the participant, (3) control of students' emotions, and (4) maintenance of the professional framework with the participant. Despite these difficulties, all respondents stated that they appreciated the exercise of administering the Rorschach test, which they perceived as a first step toward clinical practice. Based on these results, pedagogical suggestions are formulated to help students learning the Rorschach test to overcome them as quickly as possible and to invest themselves with pleasure and interest in the test administration process.

Résumé

Les psychologues cliniciens et les étudiants en psychologie apprécient le test de Rorschach pour son originalité et les pistes de réflexion qu'il peut offrir. Pour donner toute sa mesure, ce test doit être compris théoriquement et maîtrisé cliniquement. Cela commence par l'intégration du processus d'administration, dont dépendent sa validité et son interprétabilité. Le processus d'administration comporte des procédures subtiles et complexes au niveau technique, cognitif et émotionnel. L'objectif de cette étude est de décrire et d'analyser les difficultés et intérêts rencontrés par les étudiants en psychologie lors de leur première administration du Rorschach en Système Intégré. Des suggestions sont proposées pour adapter l'enseignement aux besoins spécifiques des étudiants. La méthodologie se compose de deux phases distinctes : premièrement, l'analyse d'un questionnaire construit pour les besoins de la recherche, visant à identifier et classer les difficultés des étudiants. L'analyse est basée sur les réponses de 64 sujets, âgés de 18 à 24 ans, majoritairement des femmes, en troisième année dans une école française de psychologie. La deuxième phase vise à approfondir la compréhension des résultats obtenus à partir du questionnaire. Des réponses écrites sont recueillies auprès de 235 élèves de troisième année, recrutés dans la même école, en réponse à la question : « Quelles difficultés ai-je rencontrées en passant le test de Rorschach pour la première fois? » . L'analyse des données a été réalisée à l'aide du logiciel Iramuteq, basée sur la méthode Reinert. Les résultats ont mis en évidence quatre grandes classes de difficultés liées à l'administration du Rorschach qui comprennent : (1) les aspects de gestion technique (2) la gestion de la dynamique relationnelle avec le participant (3) le contrôle des émotions des étudiants et (4) le maintien du cadre professionnel avec le participant. Malgré ces difficultés, tous les répondants ont déclaré apprécier l'exercice d'administration du test de Rorschach, qu'ils ont perçu comme un premier pas vers la pratique clinique. Sur la base de ces résultats, des suggestions pédagogiques sont formulées pour aider les étudiants apprenant le test de Rorschach à les surmonter le plus rapidement possible et à s'investir avec plaisir et intérêt dans le processus d'administration du test.

Resumen

Los psicólogos y estudiantes aprecian la prueba de Rorschach por su originalidad y la información que puede ofrecer. Para ser eficaz, esta prueba debe entenderse teóricamente y dominarse clínicamente. Esto comienza con la integración del proceso de administración, del cual dependen su validez e interpretabilidad. El proceso de administración implica procedimientos sutiles y complejos a nivel técnico, cognitivo y emocional.

El objetivo de este estudio es describir y analizar las dificultades experimentadas por los estudiantes de psicología durante su primera administración del Rorschach. Se presentan sugerencias para ajustar la enseñanza a las necesidades específicas de los estudiantes. La metodología consta de dos fases diferenciadas: en primer lugar, el análisis de un cuestionario construido con el objetivo de la investigación, dirigido a identificar y clasificar las dificultades de los estudiantes. Se basa en las respuestas de 64 sujetos, de 18 a 24 años, en su mayoría mujeres, en su tercer año en una escuela francesa de psicología.

La segunda fase tiene como objetivo profundizar en la comprensión de los resultados obtenidos en el cuestionario. Se recopilan respuestas escritas de 235 estudiantes de tercer año, reclutados en la misma escuela, en respuesta a la pregunta: "¿Qué dificultades encontré en la utilización de la prueba de Rorschach por primera vez?"

El análisis de datos se realizó mediante el software Iramuteq, basado en el método Reinert. Los resultados destacaron cuatro clases principales de dificultades relacionadas con la administración del Rorschach que incluyen: (1) aspectos técnicos de gestión (2) gestión de la dinámica relacional con el participante (3) control de las emociones de los estudiantes y (4) mantenimiento del contexto profesional con el participante. A pesar de estas dificultades, todos los encuestados manifestaron que aprecian el ejercicio de administrar la prueba de Rorschach, que perciben como un primer paso hacia la práctica clínica. Con base en estos resultados, se formulan sugerencias pedagógicas para ayudar a los estudiantes que están aprendiendo la prueba de Rorschach a superarlos lo más rápido posible y a participar con placer e interés en el proceso de administración del examen.

要約

資格を持った心理学者や学生ロールシャッハ・テストの独創性とそこから得られる洞察を高く評価している。このテストが理論的に理解され、臨床的に習得されなければ、それは効果的ではなくなってします。これは、その有効性と解釈可能性に依存する手続き過程を統合することから始まる。手続き過程には、技術的、認知的、感情的なレベルでの微妙で複雑な手順が含まれている。この研究の目的は、心理学を専攻する学生が初めてロールシャッハを受けた時に経験した困難を示し、分析することであった。学生の特定のニーズに合わせて指導を調整するための提案が提供されている。方法論は、2つの異なる段階から構成されている。1つ目は、調査の目的で作成されたアンケートの分析で、学生の困難を特定して分類することを目的としている。これはフランスの心理学部の3年生で、18歳から24歳の女性を中心とした64名の参加者の回答に基づいている。2つ目は、アンケートから得られた結果の理解を深めることを目的とした。同じ学校から募集した3年生235名から、「ロールシャッハを初めて受ける際に、どのような困難に直面しましたか」という質問に対する回答を書面で回収した。データ分析は、Reinert法に基づいて、Iramuteq ソフトウエアを用いて行われた。その結果、ロールシャッハ実施に関連した4つの主要な困難が浮き彫りになった。(1) 技術的な管理、(2) 参加者との関係力動の管理、(3) 学生の感情コントロール、(4) 参加者との専門的な枠組みの維持、である。これらの困難にも関わらず、すべての回答者は、ロールシャッハ・テストを実施したことを評価しており、臨床実習への第一歩であると認識していた。これらの結果に基づいて、ロールシャッハ・テストを学習する学生が、できるだけ早くこの困難を克服し、テストの実施過程に喜びと興味を持って研鑽を積むことができるような教育的な提案を行った。

Research Article

How Reliably Can Examiners Make Form Quality (FQ) Judgments in the Absence of the Form Quality (FQ) Tables?

Claudia Pignolo[1] ⓘ, Donald J. Viglione[2],
and Luciano Giromini[1]ⓘ

[1]Department of Psychology, University of Turin, Italy
[2]California School of Professional Psychology, Alliant International University, San Diego, CA, USA

Abstract: Form Quality (FQ) scores are well-validated measures of the accuracy of perceptive processes, of reality testing, and of the severity of psychological disturbance. Research studies reveal that inter-rater reliability of FQ scoring is good when visualized objects are available in the FQ tables. However, many visualized objects are not found in the FQ tables so that scoring must rely on one's individual judgment. Thus, a major question remains unsolved: How reliably can examiners make FQ judgments in the absence of the FQ tables? To address this question, we used the Rorschach Performance Assessment System (R-PAS) method. We asked 21 graduate students from our research labs to rate Form Accuracy (FA) and FQ for 86 objects from a subset of four Rorschach card (I, III, VI, and VIII). The results clearly reveal that FQ judgments made by individual examiners without using the FQ tables are not reliable. When scoring FQ, one should carefully scrutinize the empirically supported FQ tables and base the FQ score on these rather than personal judgments.

Keywords: Form Accuracy (FA), Form Quality (FQ), R-PAS, Rorschach

Form Quality (FQ) is an essential variable that has been recognized for its importance since the development of the Rorschach Inkblot test (Rorschach, 1921) and refers to the "goodness of fit" of objects[1] involved in a response to the area of the blot used by the examinee. In other words, whether the object or image seen by the respondent looks like the area where it is seen in the blot. Exner (1974, 2003), while developing the Comprehensive System (CS), identified four types of FQ: (1) *Superior-overelaborated (+)*, unusually well-articulated form responses; (2) *Ordinary (o)*, a high frequency response in which an object fits the blot contours; (3) *Unusual (u)*, an uncommon response in which the blot contours are appropriate; (4) *Minus (−)*, are of two types: Responses reported usually with low frequencies that are not congruent with the contours of the blot, and those which involve

---

1   In this article we use the word "object" to refer to images seen by respondents and the word "entry" to refer to the words listed in the table.

Rorschachiana (2021), *42*(1), 21–34
https://doi.org/10.1027/1192-5604/a000135

creating contours that do not exist in the blot, often called "arbitrary lines." FQ was not assigned to responses without any structure. To establish the thresholds between FQo and FQu, Exner utilized the frequency distribution of 7,500 protocols (162,427 responses), so that objects that were reported in at least 2% (150 or more) of the records in whole (W) or detail (D) areas or by at least 50 subjects in unusual detail (Dd) areas were coded as FQo, and objects with lower frequencies were coded as FQu.

Subsequently, the authors of the Rorschach Performance Assessment System (R-PAS; Meyer et al., 2011), by using a specific algorithm, combined three different sources of data to determine the R-PAS FQ codes: (1) fit, which refers to the degree to which objects reported in a specific area fit to the blot contours; (2) frequency, which refers to how often objects have been spontaneously reported by examinees at that location; and (3) the FQ coding retrieved from the most recent CS tables. Thus, FQ is operationally defined as the degree to which the reported objects are common and fit the blot area. Moreover, objects were classified as ordinary (FQo), unusual (FQu), and distorted (FQ–), and responses without any structure were classified as "none" (FQn). Overall, the R-PAS FQ tables have approximately 34.3% of minus (FQ–), 45.2% of unusual (FQu), and 20.5% of ordinary (FQo) objects.

FQ scores are a well-validated measure of perception accuracy, reality testing, and severity of psychological disturbance (e.g., Meyer et al. 2011; Mihura et al., 2013; Su et al., 2015). Evaluating FQ validity in the CS, Mihura et al. (2013) reported that Conventional (X + %) and Distorted (X–%) Form variables were significantly related to external criteria such as DSM diagnoses or observer ratings (respectively, $r = .48$, $p < .001$, and $r = .49$, $p < .001$) and that X–% appropriately differentiated patients with psychosis from other patients with distorted perceptions (e.g., borderline and schizotypal PD). As for the R-PAS FQ scores, Su and colleagues (2015) reported on the incremental validity of the R-PAS FQ–% and variables to which the FQ codes are crucial subcomponents (i.e., TP-Comp and EII-3) over the CS counterpart (i.e., X–%, PTI, and EII-2), suggesting that improvements in the R-PAS FQ tables have enhanced the interpretive validity of the FQ codings.

Despite the good-to-excellent support for FQo and FQ–, different studies have shown lower inter-rater reliabilities for FQu codes compared with the other codes. Considering CS variables, Acklin et al. (2000) reported moderate reliabilities at response level for nonpatient ($\kappa = .521$) and clinical ($\kappa = .585$) protocols, respectively, whereas kappa values for FQo and FQ– were higher than .70 for both nonclinical and clinical protocols. Moreover, at a protocol level of analysis, intraclass correlation coefficients (ICC) for Xu% were poor (ICC = .156) for nonpatient protocols and fair (ICC = .483) for clinical protocols. Meyer et al. (2002) also reported lower, although excellent, reliability values for FQu (ICC = .93) compared with FQo (ICC = .98) and FQ– (ICC = .96). Considering R-PAS variables at protocol level, Viglione et al. (2012) found that R-PAS FQu% showed good reliability (ICC = .64) but lower than reliabilities of FQo% (ICC = .84) and FQ–% (ICC = .81). Recently, Pignolo et al. (2017) reported an excellent reliability for the FQo% (ICC = .82), and fair reliability values for both the FQu% (ICC = .59) and FQ–% (ICC = .53). As for response-level reliabilities, Kivisalu and colleagues (2016, 2017) reported the same pattern, with a lower value for FQu (κ = .59) than reliabilities of FQo (κ = .77) and FQ– (κ = .62). Consistently, Lewey et al. (2019), examining response-level, inter-rater reliability values between coders who had only R-PAS training and coders who had both CS and R-PAS training, found that the poorest inter-rater reliability coefficients were for FQu (R-PAS group: AC = .63, κ = .53; CS and R-PAS group: AC = .72, κ = .62). Thus, it seems that higher inter-rater reliabilities have been reached for FQo codes, followed by FQ– codes, and that raters had more difficulties to code FQu objects reliably.

From teaching experience and from previous studies, one of the difficulties with which students struggle the most is coding FQ when objects are not listed in the FQ tables (Viglione et al., 2017). To reduce examiner errors, the R-PAS manual (Meyer et al., 2011) provides a step-by-step method to code FQ. The *Preliminary Step* involves reviewing the response location in the FQ tables to match the response object in its entirety. If the object is not found, examiners should extrapolate the object's FQ going through the following steps. First, examiners should search objects with *Like Shapes* in the same area (*Step 1*) or the same object in *Like Areas* (*Step 2*), and then examiners should look at subcomponents of objects (*Step 3*). In *Step 4* examiners should *Review the Accumulated Information to Make an FQ Judgment*. Although the R-PAS manual strongly suggests giving more weight to evidence from the aforementioned steps, the examiner's judgments may be made carelessly or with errors.

Although many studies have investigated the validity and inter-rater reliability of FQ codings from both response- and protocol-level perspectives, a major question remains unsolved: How reliably can individuals make FQ judgments in the absence of the FQ tables? The answer to this question has implications for the individual examiner's ratings of FQ with individual records. As such, the aim of the present study was to shed light on the ability of Rorschach examiners to code FQ in the absence of the FQ tables and to evaluate the extent to which they agree with each other in evaluating the FQ and FA of response objects, in the absence of the FQ tables. The results of this study may help explain how examiners would code the FQ when objects are not listed in the FQ tables.

Method

Raters

Because our aim was to evaluate the extent to which examiners could code FQ correctly in the absence of the FQ tables, 21 graduate students in the authors' research laboratories (i.e., research collaborators) from the United States and Italy served as raters. All raters were trained in R-PAS coding and had completed at least one semester of Rorschach instruction. Thus, they were well-acquainted with FQ determination and because they had not been exposed to CS coding, were not affected by previous scoring systems or systematic errors in the coding of FQ. All ratings were completed in English. This manuscript should be considered to be an inter-rater reliability lab exercise among researchers in training. Because objects rated by the raters were listed in the FQ tables and were not taken from responses given by human participants, there are no ethical aspects to disclose.

The Survey

The survey was developed to investigate how raters rated both the FA and FQ of objects without using the FQ tables. As for the FA ratings, we replicated the procedure used by R-PAS authors in developing the R-PAS FQ tables. Raters examined the fit and provided FA ratings for a list of objects and gave an evaluation based on a 5-point Likert scale, that is: 1 = *No. I can't see it at all. Clearly, it's a distortion*; 2 = *Not really. I don't really see that. Overall, it does not match the blot area*; 3 = *A little. If I work at it, I can sort of see that*; 4 = *Yes. I can see that. It matches the blot pretty well*; 5 = *Definitely. I think it looks exactly or almost exactly like that.* To identify the thresholds to divide FA values in categories that reflected the traditional FQ categories (i.e., –, u, and o), we applied the same cut scores as reported in the R-PAS manual, so that objects with a mean rating of 2.4 or less were evaluated as FA–; objects with a mean rating between 2.5 and 3.4 were evaluated as FAu; objects with a mean rating of 3.5 or more were evaluated as FAo. Moreover, among the three categories of FQ (i.e., FQ–, FQu, and FQo), some objects seem to be more easily classified into each FQ categories than others, so that it is possible to distinguish prototype objects from objects that are considered on the threshold between two categories (Meyer et al., 2011). The division between prototype and threshold objects was made by referring to FA values. FA values lower than 1.75 indicate FQ– prototypes, FA values between 2.85 and 3.05 indicate FQu prototypes, and FA values higher than 4.15 indicate FQo prototypes. As for the thresholds, FA values between 1.90 and 2.20 indicate threshold objects between FQ– and FQu, whereas FA values between 2.55 and 2.75 indicate threshold objects between FQu and FQo.

For the Rorschach, one administers five black and gray cards, two black, gray, and red cards, and three multi-colored cards. Consistent with this relative frequency, we selected two black and gray cards (I and VI), one black and red card (III), and one multi-colored card (VIII) for our survey. Within each card, we selected commonly used, individual locations because they provide enough FQ table entries to populate the prototype and threshold FA values noted in the paragraph above. Indeed, variability in the number of FQ entries across cards for prototypes and thresholds is due to fluctuations in frequencies across locations in the FQ tables. Accordingly, uncommon details (Dd) were not used. Since the frequency per record of whole (W, mean = 9.6) and common details (D, mean = 10.7) are about equal, we included two W and two D locations.

Thus, we selected four locations from four different cards: W Location for Cards I and VIII, D1 for Card VI, and D2 for Card III. In selecting the entries from the FQ tables, we divided them into prototypes and thresholds according to the R-PAS Manual (Meyer et al., 2011). Prototypes had FA < 1.75 for FQ− (e.g., Card I, W, Bear, FA = 1.55), FA between 2.85 and 3.05 for FQu (e.g., Card III, D2, Hook, FA = 2.95), and FA > 4.15 for FQo (e.g., Card I, W, Insect or Bug (Winged), FA = 4.17). We established two different thresholds between FQ− and FQu: The first threshold for FQ− had FA values between 1.90 and 2.20 (e.g., Card VIII, W, Jacket, FA = 1.98), whereas the second threshold for FQu had FA values between 2.55 and 2.75 (e.g., Card VI, D1, Urn, FA = 2.61). Then, we randomly selected 86 entries that fell within the ranges indicated from the R-PAS manual (Table 1): 23 response objects for both Card I (W) and Card VIII (W), and 20 objects for both Card III (D2) and Card VI (D1).

Raters were asked to look at the relevant Rorschach card and response location and rate the fit of each object according to the 5-point FA scale used by the authors of R-PAS in developing the FQ tables, knowing that, generally, FA values of 1 and 2 represent FQ− codes, an FA value of 3 corresponds to FQu codes, whereas FA values of 4 and 5 are considered FQo. They were also asked to decide on whether they would code FQo, FQu, or FQ−, knowing that 10% of the objects should be coded FQo, about 45% FQu, and about 45% FQ−. The raters could not use the FQ tables, so they rated each entry relying only on their ability to see the objects.

Data Analysis

In the first step, we considered the FQ classifications made by the raters without looking at the FQ tables in the manual. Because we selected entries from the FQ

Table 1. Form Quality (FQ) entries listed in the survey

	Card				
	I	III	VI	VIII	Total
FQo	4	2	0	2	8
Prototypes	4	2	0	2	8
FQu	10	9	10	11	40
Prototypes	6	5	5	6	22
Thresholds	4	4	5	5	18
FQ−	9	9	10	10	38
Prototypes	3	5	5	4	17
Thresholds	6	4	5	6	21
Total	23	20	20	23	86
Prototypes	13	12	10	12	47
Thresholds	10	8	10	11	39

Note. FQo = Form Quality Ordinary; FQu = Form Quality Unusual; FQ − = Form Quality Minus.

tables, we were able to determine the degree of convergence between raters' classifications and the R-PAS FQ tables. In other words, we examined how individual examiners would code a specific entry when left to rely only on their ability to see the objects. Thus, to evaluate whether the raters coded each entry listed in the survey correctly, we computed correct classification and Cohen's kappa values comparing the codes of the raters with those reported in the R-PAS FQ tables. For Cohen's kappa values, we considered the following cut-offs: kappa values between .20 and .40 = fair, kappa values between .41 and .60 = moderate, kappa values between .61 and .80 = good, and kappa values above .80 = very good (Altman, 1991; Landis & Koch, 1977).

Second, given that in the development of the FQ tables FA ratings were used to evaluate the degree to which each object fits with the contour of the inkblot, we examined average FA ratings produced by the raters. We were particularly interested in evaluating whether raters would be able to agree with each other on the degree of fit to the inkblot of the selected entries. To do that, we computed two-way random Intraclass Correlations (ICC) between average FA values by the raters and those used by R-PAS authors in developing the R-PAS FQ tables. For ICC values, we considered the following cut-offs: ICCs < .40 = poor reliability, ICCs between .40 and .59 = fair reliability, ICCs between .60 and .74 = good reliability, and ICCs of .75 or above = excellent reliability (Cicchetti, 1994; Shrout & Fleiss, 1979).

Table 2. FQ correct classifications and Cohen's kappa between raters and R-PAS manual

	# of ratings	Overall CC%	κ	Card I CC%	κ	Card III CC%	κ	Card VI CC%	κ	Card VIII CC%	κ
FQ−	798	68.1		71.3		69.8		60.4		71.3	
FQu	840	46.2		43.8		48.1		42.0		50.6	
FQo	168	74.3		72.6		85.4		−		66.7	
Total	1806	58.5	.338	59.6	.375	61.6	.392	51.2	.200	61.0	.366
Prototype											
FQ−	357	75.8		85.7		73.3		69.5		79.5	
FQu	462	48.7		51.6		45.2		43.3		53.2	
FQo	168	74.3		72.6		85.4		−		66.7	
Total	987	62.9	.439	66.0	.488	63.6	.454	56.5	.277	64.2	.454
Threshold											
FQ−	441	61.8		64.0		65.5		51.0		65.9	
FQu	378	43.2		32.1		51.8		40.8		47.6	
Total	819	53.2	.156	51.2	.032	58.7	.233	45.9	.122	57.6	.217

Note. CC% = correctly classified %: refers to the % of ratings that identified the correct FQ level.

Results

Correct classifications consisted of the percentage of correct FQ classifications of all the 86 entries by the 21 raters (Table 2). The overall hit rate was 58.5% and the percentage of correct classification was low for FQu objects (46.2%), higher for FQ− entries (68.1%), and the highest for FQo entries (74.3%). Correct classifications of each card closely reflect the overall correct classification (Table 2). With regard to each card, Card VI obtained the lower overall hit rate (51.2%), whereas the highest value was obtained for Card III (61.6%). As for the highest FQ classification by card, 71.3% of FQ− entries from Card I and Card VII were recognized by the raters, 50.6% of FQu entries were correctly classified in Card VIII, and 85.4% of FQo entries were correctly classified in Card III. However, less than 50% of FQu entries from Cards I, III, and VI were correctly classified by the raters. In general, Cohen's kappa was fair ($\kappa = .338$), ranging from .200 for Card VI to .392 for Card III.

As for Prototype and Threshold entries, Table 2 shows that hit rates of Prototype entries were generally higher than of Threshold entries. The overall correct classification for Prototype entries was 62.9%, with 75.8% for FQ− entries, 48.7% for FQu entries, and 74.3% for FQo entries, whereas the correct classification for Threshold objects was 53.2%, with 61.8% of FQ− entries and 43.2% of FQu entries being correctly classified. Interestingly, considering Prototypes, 23

Table 3. Descriptive statistics of FA ratings and ICCs ($R = 1{,}806$)

	Objects (n)	FQ–		FQu		FQo		ICC
		M	DS	M	DS	M	DS	
Overall	86	1.99	0.95	2.96	1.00	4.17	1.02	.850
Prototype	47	1.81	0.94	3.18	0.92	4.17	1.02	.884
Threshold	39	2.14	0.92	2.70	1.04	–	–	.538
Card I	23	1.94	0.91	2.86	1.04	4.21	0.97	.939
Prototype	13	1.54	0.86	3.21	0.91	4.21	0.97	.943
Threshold	10	2.14	0.88	2.35	1.00	–	–	.492
Card III	19	1.97	0.92	3.04	1.01	4.41	0.71	.892
Prototype	11	1.87	0.96	3.37	0.94	4.41	0.71	.906
Threshold	8	2.10	0.84	2.63	0.96	–	–	.690
Card VI	20	2.17	1.01	3.10	1.04	–	–	.673
Prototype	10	1.98	0.96	3.13	0.99	–	–	.795
Threshold	10	2.37	1.02	3.06	1.10	–	–	.415
Card VIII	23	1.88	0.92	2.87	0.92	3.83	1.27	.828
Prototype	12	1.73	0.93	3.02	0.85	3.83	1.27	.850
Threshold	11	1.98	0.91	2.70	0.96	–	–	.656

Note. FA = Form Accuracy; FQ – = Form Quality Minus; FQu = Form Quality Unusual; FQo = Form Quality Ordinary; ICC = intraclass correlation coefficients.

FQ– entries were classified as FQo. The most misclassified FQ– entry was "Skeleton" in Card VIII (W Location), followed by "Bug" in Card VI (D1 Location), which were coded FQo by four and three raters, respectively. On the other hand, three FQo Prototype entries were classified as FQ– by the raters. The entry that was mostly misclassified was "Flower" in Card VIII (W Location), which was coded FQ– by seven raters. Cohen's kappa for Prototypes was moderate ($\kappa = .439$), ranging from .277 for Card VI to .488 for Card I, whereas Cohen's kappa for Thresholds was poor ($\kappa = .156$), ranging from .032 for Card I to .233 for Card III.

To analyze the fit (i.e., Form Accuracy) of the entries, we asked the raters to rate each object on the 5-point scale, where 1 indicated a poor fit and 5 indicated an optimum fit. According to the R-PAS manual, if one were to rely only on FA/Fit, objects with an FA rating of 2.4 or less would be classified as FQ–, objects with an FA of 3.5 or above would be classified as FQo, and objects with FA between 2.4 and 3.5 would be classified as FQu. As would be expected, mean FA ratings ($M = 1.99$, $SD = .95$) related to FQ– entries were lower than the suggested threshold of 2.4 and the mean value of FQo entries was higher than 3.5 ($M = 4.17$, $SD = 1.02$), whereas the mean FQu rating ($M = 2.96$, $SD = 1.00$) was in the intervening range (Table 3). Considering Prototypes and Thresholds, FQo Prototypes should have a mean FA above 4.15, FQu Prototypes a mean FA between 2.85 and 3.05, whereas FQ– Prototype should have a mean FA lower than 1.75. As shown in Table 3, FQ– and FQu Prototypes had a mean FA higher than the cut-off, with mean FA values of 1.81 (SD = .94) and of 3.18 (SD = .92), respectively. This pattern is consistent for Cards III and VI, whereas for Card I and VIII the mean FA ratings of FQ– Prototypes were lower than 1.75. On the other hand, FQo Prototypes showed mean FA ratings higher than 4.15, with the exception of Card VIII (M = 3.83, SD = 1.27). As for Thresholds, (Table 3) FA mean ratings were between the suggested range for both FQ– and FQu Thresholds. However, FA mean ratings for FQu Thresholds were lower than 2.55 for Card I (M = 2.35, SD = 1.00) and higher than 2.75 for Card VI (M = 3.06, SD = 1.10).

To compare the FA ratings by the raters with those used to develop the R-PAS FQ tables, we computed ICCs. Considering all the entries, the ICC value was .850, indicating an excellent reliability (Cicchetti, 1994; Shrout & Fliess, 1979). However, when looking at the different FQ codes, ICC coefficients were .403 for FQ– entries, .377 for FQu entries, and, surprisingly, .146 for FQo entries. The unexpected results for FQo entries, lead us to an in-depth analysis of the FA mean values for FQo entries. We found that one entry (i.e., "Flower [Can include leaf]" in Card VIII, Location W) had a mean FA value (M = 2.86, SD = 1.01) lower than 3.5, the cut-off used for FQo categories. Thus, excluding this entry from the analysis, the ICC value for FQo objects became .593. Thus, the results may suggest that, on aggregate ratings, raters were capable of recognizing the fit of the objects to the contour of the inkblot.

Discussion and Conclusion

The present study evaluated the extent to which Rorschach examiners agree with each other in evaluating the FQ and FA of response objects, in the absence of the FQ tables. The aim was to understand how examiners would code the FQ when objects are not listed in the FQ tables, and, thus, to investigate the examiners' judgments. We asked 21 raters to rate FA and FQ for 86 objects from Cards I, III, VI, and VIII. Considering FQ codes, the overall hit rate was 58.5% and the percentages of correct classification were 68.1% for FQ– objects, 46.2% for FQu objects, and 74.3% for FQo objects. The results indicate that examiner judgments are not reliable, and coders should not rely on their opinion in coding FQ but should use all the evidence gathered from the steps listed in the R-PAS manual in coding FQ. On the other hand, considering FA values, the ICC value was

.850, indicating an excellent reliability. Thus, examiner judgments for FQ are inaccurate, but they seem more accurate when they have to establish the degree to which an entry fits the contour of the inkblot. In other words, ICC values indicate that the raters evaluated the FA of each entry consistently with the raters who evaluated FA for the R-PAS FQ tables.

From the results of the present study, two main implications are worth noting. First, these findings may shed light on the lower inter-rater reliability values related to FQu compared with FQ– and FQo. One may speculate that when examiners are forced to make individual judgments in coding FQ because the object is not listed in the FQ tables (Step 4 of the instructions given by the R-PAS manual), they would produce inconsistent codings. In this direction, future studies should evaluate potential differences in the inter-rater reliability values for the FQ codes between FQ classifications based on the manual (Steps 1–3) and FQ classifications based on individual judgements (Step 4). Second, in terms of training, particular attention should be paid to the steps described in the manual on how to code FQ when the object is not listed in the manual. New learners who found the coding of FQ particularly difficult (Viglione et al., 2017) may find some comfort in knowing all the strategies they should adopt to deal with this challenge.

Although this study is the first to analyze the impact of examiners' judgments on the coding of FQ, some limitations are worth noting. First, we administered the survey to a small sample of graduate student collaborators. Expert researchers and clinicians may thus yield higher levels of reliability with the FQ tables, considering the experience they may have accumulated in coding objects not listed in the FQ tables. However, given that most of the studies evaluating the inter-rater reliability of Rorschach scores are based on the codings made by graduate students or young researchers and clinicians, we believe that our findings reflect the real context in which these studies were conducted. Second, we selected only single objects in W and D location, and we did not consider multiple objects or Dd locations. Given that our aim was to evaluate the extent to which raters would be able to code FQ variables correctly without using the FQ tables, we decided to maintain stable the level of difficulty of the coding. Indeed, coding one object in one location is easier than coding multiple objects in multiple or uncommon locations.

References

Acklin, M. W., McDowell, C. J., Verschell, M-S., & Chan, D. (2000). Interobserver agreement, intraobserver reliability, and the Rorschach Comprehensive System. *Journal of Personality Assessment, 74*(1), 15–47. https://doi.org/10.1207/S15327752JPA740103

Altman, D. G. (1991). *Practical statistics for medical research*. Chapman and Hall.

Cicchetti, D. V. (1994). Guidelines, criteria, and rules of thumb for evaluating normed and standardized assessment instruments in psychology. *Psychological Assessment, 6*(4), 284–290. https://doi.org/10.1037/1040-3590.6.4.284

Exner, J. E. Jr. (1974). *The Rorschach: A comprehensive system: Vol. 2. Interpretation.* Wiley.

Exner, J. E. Jr. (2003). *The Rorschach: A comprehensive system: Vol. 1. Basic foundations and principles of interpretation* (4th ed.). John Wiley & Sons.

Kivisalu, T. M., Lewey, J. H., Shaffer, T. W., & Canfield, M. L. (2016). An investigation of interrater reliability for the Rorschach Performance Assessment System (R-PAS) in a nonpatient U.S. sample. *Journal of Personality Assessment, 98*(4), 382–390. https://doi.org/10.1080/00223891.2015.1118380

Kivisalu, T. M., Lewey, J. H., Shaffer, T. W., & Canfield, M. L. (2017). Correction to: An investigation of interrater reliability for the Rorschach Performance Assessment System (R-PAS) in a nonpatient U.S. sample. *Journal of Personality Assessment, 99*(5), 558–560. https://doi.org/10.1080/00223891.2017.1325244

Landis, J. R., & Koch, G. G. (1977). The measurement of observer agreement for categorical data. *Biometrics, 33*, 159–174. https://doi.org/10.2307/2529310

Lewey, J. H., Kivisalu, T. M., & Giromini, L. (2019). Coding with R-PAS: Does prior training with the Exner Comprehensive System impact interrater reliability compared to those examiners with only R-PAS-based training? *Journal of Personality Assessment, 101*(4), 393–401. https://doi.org/10.1080/00223891.2018.1476361

Meyer, G. J., Hilsenroth, M. J., Baxter, D., Exner, J. E., Fowler, J. C., Piers, C. C., & Resnick, J. (2002). An examination of interrater reliability for scoring the Rorschach Comprehensive System in eight data sets. *Journal of Personality Assessment, 78*(2), 219–274. https://doi.org/10.1207/S15327752JPA7802_03

Meyer, G. J., Viglione, D. J., Mihura, J. L., Erard, R. E., & Erdberg, P. (2011). *Rorschach performance assessment system: Administration, coding, interpretation, and technical manual.* Rorschach Performance Assessment System.

Mihura, J. L., Meyer, G. J., Dumitrascu, N., & Bombel, G. (2013). The validity of individual Rorschach variables: Systematic reviews and meta-analyses of the Comprehensive System. *Psychological Bulletin, 139*(3), 548–605. https://doi.org/10.1037/a0029406

Pignolo, C., Giromini, L., Ando', A., Ghirardello, D., Di Girolamo, M., Ales, F., & Zennaro, A. (2017). An interrater reliability study of Rorschach Performance Assessment System (R-PAS) raw and complexity-adjusted scores. *Journal of Personality Assessment, 99*(6), 619–625. https://doi.org/10.1080/00223891.2017.1296844

Rorschach, H. (1921). *Psychodiagnostik Tafeln* [Psychodiagnostic tables]. Huber.

Shrout, P. E., & Fleiss, J. (1979). Intraclass correlations: Uses in assessing rater reliability. *Psychological Bulletin, 86*, 420–428. https://doi.org/10.1037/0033-2909.86.2.420

Su, W. S., Viglione, D. J., Green, E. E., Tam, W.C., Su, J. A., & Chang, Y. T. (2015). Cultural and linguistic adaptability of the Rorschach Performance Assessment System as a measure of psychotic characteristics and severity of mental disturbance in Taiwan. *Psychological Assessment, 27*(4), 1273–1285. https://doi.org/10.1037/pas0000144

Viglione, D. J., Meyer, G. J., Resende, A. C., & Pignolo, C. (2017). A survey of challenges experienced by new learners coding the Rorschach. *Journal of Personality Assessment, 99*(3), 315–323. https://doi.org/10.1080/00223891.2016.1233559

Viglione, D. J., Blume-Marcovici, A. C., Miller, H. L., Giromini, L., & Meyer, G. (2012). An inter-rater reliability study for the Rorschach Performancé Assessment System. *Journal of Personality Assessment, 94*(6), 607–612. https://doi.org/10.1080/00223891.2012.684118

History
Received November 6, 2020
Accepted November 12, 2020
Published online March 18, 2021

Acknowledgments
Donald J. Viglione receives royalties on the sale of the R-PAS manual and associated products.

ORCID
Claudia Pignolo
 https://orcid.org/0000-0002-6977-224X

Luciano Giromini
 https://orcid.org/0000-0002-9540-4803

Claudia Pignolo
Department of Psychology
University of Turin
Via Giuseppe Verdi 10
10124 Turin, TO
Italy
claudia.pignolo@unito.it

Summary

Form Quality (FQ) is an essential variable that has been recognized for its importance since the development of the Rorschach Inkblot test. It refers to the "goodness of fit" of visualized objects to the corresponding area of the blot used by the examinee. Moreover, FQ scores are a well-validated measure of perception accuracy, reality testing, and severity of psychological disturbance. Research studies reveal that inter-rater reliability of FQ scoring is good when visualized objects are available in FQ tables. However, many visualized objects are not found in the FQ tables so that scoring must rely on one's individual judgment. No research has directly asked the question of how reliably and accurately can individuals make these FQ judgments in the absence of the FQ tables. If the answer were to be "not very good" then such difficulty would limit the validity of FQ scoring and a remedy might be in order. To address this question about examiner judgment of fit in terms of FQ scoring accuracy and inter-rater reliability, we used the Rorschach Performance Assessment System (R-PAS) method. We asked 21 graduate students (i.e., research collaborators) from our research labs to rate Form Accuracy (FA) and FQ for 86 objects from a subset of four Rorschach card (I, III, VI, and VIII). The results clearly reveal that individual examiner making FQ judgements without using the FQ tables are not reliable. These findings shed light on the lower inter-rater reliability values related to FQu compared to FQ– and FQo. When scoring FQ, one should carefully scrutinize the empirically support of the FQ tables and base the FQ score on these rather than personal judgement. For R-PAS there are procedures to follow in the manual and online in an effort to maximize accuracy and reliability. In terms of training, new learners who found the coding of FQ particularly difficult may find some comfort in knowing all the strategies they should adopt to deal with this challenge.

Riassunto

La Qualità Formale (Form Quality; FQ) è una variabile essenziale che è stata riconosciuta per la sua importanza sin dallo sviluppo del test di Rorschach. Si riferisce alla "bontà dell'adattamento" degli oggetti visualizzati all'area della macchia utilizzata dall'esaminato. Inoltre, i punteggi FQ sono una misura validata di accuratezza della percezione, dell'esame di realtà, e della gravità del disturbo psicologico. Diversi studi hanno rivelato che l'affidabilità tra giudici delle codifiche FQ sia buona quando gli oggetti visualizzati sono elencati nella tabella FQ. Tuttavia, molti oggetti visualizzati non sono presenti nelle tabelle FQ cosicché lo scoring deve fare affidamento sul giudizio individuale del clinico. Nessuna ricerca ha indagato direttamente quanto affidabili e accurati siano i giudizi individuali sulle codifiche FQ in assenza delle tabelle FQ. Se la risposta dovesse essere "non molto" allora questa difficoltà limiterebbe la validità dello scoring di FQ. Per affrontare questo problema sul grado di accuratezza e affidabilità tra giudici dei giudizi degli esaminatori nel siglare FQ abbiamo utilizzato il metodo Rorschach Performance Assessment System (R-PAS). Abbiamo chiesto a 21 dottorandi (collaboratori di ricerca) di valutare l'Accuratezza Formale (Form Accuracy; FA) e di siglare FQ per 86 oggetti delle tavole I, III, VI e VIII. I risultati rivelano chiaramente che i singoli giudizi degli esaminatori nel valutare FQ senza l'utilizzo delle tavole FQ non sono affidabili. Questi risultati potrebbero far luce sui valori di affidabilità tra giudici più bassi relativi a FQu rispetto a FQ– e FQo. Quando si sigla FQ, si dovrebbe esaminare attentamente le tavole FQ che derivano da supporto empirico e basare la codifica FQ sulle tavole FQ piuttosto che su giudizi individuali. Nel metodo R-PAS vengono presentate le procedure da seguire sia nel manuale sia online per massimizzare l'accuratezza e l'affidabilità. In termini di training, i nuovi esaminatori che trovano particolarmente difficile codificare FQ possono trovare conforto nel conoscere tutte le strategie che dovrebbero adottare per affrontare questa sfida.

Résumé

La qualité formelle (Form Quality; FQ) est une variable essentielle qui a été reconnue pour son importance depuis le développement du test de Rorschach. Elle fait référence à la "qualité de l'ajustement" des objets visualisés aux contours de la tâche utilisée par le patient. De plus, les scores FQ constituent une mesure bien validée de la précision de la perception, du test de réalité et de la gravité du trouble psychologique. Des études ont révélé que la fiabilité inter-juges des encodages FQ est bonne lorsque les objets affichés sont répertoriés dans le tableau FQ. Cependant, de nombreux objets affichés ne sont pas présents dans les tableaux FQ, de sorte que la notation doit reposer sur le jugement individuel du clinicien. Aucune recherche n'a directement examiné la fiabilité et l'exactitude des jugements individuels sur les codages FQ en l'absence de tableaux FQ. Si la réponse était « pas beaucoup » , alors cette difficulté limiterait la validité de la notation FQ. Pour résoudre ce problème du degré d'exactitude et de fiabilité parmi les juges des jugements des examinateurs lors de la signature du FQ, nous avons utilisé la méthode du Rorschach Performance Assessment System (R-PAS). Nous avons demandé à 21 doctorants (collaborateurs de recherche) d'évaluer l'exactitude formelle (Form Accuracy; FA) et FQ pour 86 objets des planches I, III, VI et VIII. Les résultats révèlent clairement que les jugements individuels des examinateurs lors de l'évaluation de la FQ sans l'utilisation des tableaux FQ ne sont pas fiables. Ces résultats pourraient expliquer les valeurs de fiabilité des juges les plus faibles concernant FQu comparées à FQ– et FQo. Lors de l'initialisation de FQ, il faut examiner attentivement les tableaux FQ qui découlent d'un soutien empirique et baser le codage FQ sur les tableaux FQ plutôt que sur des jugements individuels. La méthode R-PAS présente les procédures à suivre à la fois dans le manuel et en ligne pour maximiser l'exactitude et la fiabilité. En termes de formation, les nouveaux examinateurs trouvant qu'il est particulièrement difficile de codifier FQ peuvent être soulagés de connaître toutes les stratégies possibles à adopter pour relever ce défi.

© 2021 Hogrefe Publishing   *Rorschachiana* (2021), 42(1), 21–34

Resumen

La calidad de la forma (FQ) es una variable esencial que ha sido reconocida por su importancia desde el desarrollo de la prueba de Rorschach. Se refiere a la "bondad de ajuste" de los objetos expuestos al área de la mancha utilizada por el examinador. Además, los puntajes FQ son una medida validada de la precisión de la percepción, las pruebas de realidad y la gravedad del trastorno psicológico. Varios estudios han revelado que la confiabilidad entre jueces de las codificaciones FQ es buena cuando los objetos mostrados se enumeran en la tabla FQ. Sin embargo, muchos de los objetos mostrados no están presentes en las tablas FQ, por lo que la puntuación debe basarse en el juicio individual del médico. Ninguna investigación ha investigado directamente qué tan confiables y precisos son los juicios individuales sobre la codificación FQ en ausencia de tablas FQ. Si la respuesta fuera "no mucho", esta dificultad limitaría la validez de la puntuación FQ. Para abordar este problema del grado de precisión y confiabilidad entre los jueces de los juicios de los examinadores al firmar FQ, usamos el método Rorschach Performance Assessment System (R-PAS). Solicitamos a 21 estudiantes de doctorado (colaboradores de investigación) que evaluaran la Exactitud de la Forma (Form Accuracy; FA) y firmaran FQ para 86 objetos en las tablas I, III, VI y VIII. Los resultados revelan claramente que los juicios individuales de los examinadores al evaluar FQ sin el uso de las tablas FQ no son confiables. Estos resultados podrían arrojar luz sobre valores más bajos de confiabilidad entre jueces para FQu en comparación con FQ– y FQo. Al inicializar FQ, se deben examinar cuidadosamente las tablas de FQ que se derivan del soporte empírico y basar la codificación de FQ en las tablas de FQ en lugar de juicios individuales. El método R-PAS presenta los procedimientos a seguir tanto en el manual como en línea para maximizar la precisión y confiabilidad. En términos de formación, los nuevos examinadores a los que les resulte particularmente difícil codificar QF pueden encontrar consuelo al conocer todas las estrategias que deben adoptar para afrontar este desafío.

要約

形態水準（FQ）は、ロールシャッハ・テストが開発されて以来、その重要性が認識されている重要な変数である。これは、被検者が使用したブロットの対応するエリアへの視覚化された対象物の「適合度」を指す。さらにQFスコアは、知覚の正確さ、現実検討力、および心理的障害の重症度を検証するに十分な尺度である。これまでの研究では、可視化された対象物が形態水準表に掲載されている場合、評価者間信頼性は良好であることが明らかにされている。しかし、可視化された対象物の多くは形態水準表にないため、スコアリングは、個人の判断に頼らざるを得ない。形態水準表にない場合、個人がこれらの形態水準の判定をどれだけ正確に行えるのか、ということについて直接問うた研究はない。もし、答えが「あまり良くない」という場合、そのような難しさは形態水準のスコアリングの妥当性を制限することとなり、救済策が必要かもしれない。FQスコアリングの正確さと評価者間信頼性の観点から、検査者の適合性の判断に関するこの疑問に答えるために、R-PASを用いた。われわれの研究室の大学院生21名（すなわち研究協力者）に、4枚のロールシャッハカード（I、III、VI、VIII）のサブセットから86個の対象物について、形態の正確さ（FA）とFQを評価してもらった。その結果、個々の検査者が形態水準表を用いずにFA判定を行うことは、信頼性が低いことが明らかになった。これらの結果は、FQ–やFQoに比べてFQuに関連した信頼性が低いことが示唆された。FQ–をスコアする時には、個人的な判断ではなく、形態水準表の経験的な裏付けを慎重に精査し、それを基にFQのスコアを行うべきである。R-PASについては、精度と信頼性を最大化するために、マニュアルやオンラインでの手順がある。トレーニングの面では、形態水準のコーディングが特に難しいと感じた初学者は、この課題に対処するために採用すべき全ての戦略を知っていることで安心感をおぼえるかもしれない。

Research Article

Color Projection in the Rorschach Test

Sanae Aoki[1] and Nobuo Kogayu[2]

[1]Division of Psychology, Faculty of Human Sciences, University of Tsukuba, Japan
[2]Correction Bureau, Ministry of Justice, Tokyo, Japan

Abstract: The purpose of this study was to examine the basic features of Color Projection (CP). This study examined how CP appeared in relation to card, position, location, development quality, form quality, determinants, contents, special scores, and projected colors. Japanese adult psychiatric patients participated in the study. A total of 68 CP responses in 37 protocols were collected from over 1,500 Rorschach protocols. The results indicated that almost 60% of CP were in response to Card I or VI, which suggests that CP may be an initial shock reaction to achromatic colors and shading. Moreover, almost all CP were shown with the card in the original position, and more than half of CP were shown with W and DQo. This suggests that coping strategies when using CP may consist of changing recognitions rather than changing behaviors. On the other hand, these results also show that almost 30% of CP responses were scored MOR, and some CP responses were changed to colors that are generally considered to be less beautiful or undesirable in Japan. Therefore, in conclusion, it is possible that the current interpretive hypothesis of denial of unpleasant feelings may not be characteristic of all CP responses.

Keywords: color projection (CP), Rorschach, affect

Color responses in the Rorschach test are regarded as variables connected to affective features (Exner, 2003; Klopfer et al., 1954; Rapaport et al., 1946; Schachtel, 1967; Shapiro, 1956, 1960). One of the most rare and unique color responses is Color Projection (CP). CP occurs when an individual projects chromatic colors into blot areas that display only varieties of black and gray (Piotrowski, 1957). Examples include "a blue bird" in response to Card I, "a bright red butterfly" in response to Card V, and "green leaves" for Card VI. The phenomenon of projecting chromatic colors onto achromatic surfaces was observed by Hermann Rorschach and many others. However, none had interpreted CP before Piotrowski, who suggested that CP could be indicative of a unique type of affective coping.

Piotrowski (1957) suggested that CP is indicative of a deliberate and conscious attempt to feel, sense, and display happiness in overt behaviors while suppressing a spontaneous and deeply felt sadness. He also explained that CP reveals a most earnest and intense attempt at self-imposed serenity to dispel the depression caused by deeply felt frustrations. Moreover, Weiner (1998) and Exner (2003) later recognized that in broader terms CP is the rejection of not only depressive feelings but also unpleasant feeling in general.

However, little research has been conducted to examine the validity of these interpretations of CP. Mihura and colleagues (2013) systematically evaluated peer-reviewed Rorschach validity literature for the 65 main variables in the Comprehensive System (CS). The result showed that CP was one of the variables with least support. However, according to Mihura et al. (2013), the lack of support for CP is not due to evidence for the absence of validity (nonsignificant findings) or low or unstable levels of validity (significant findings but with validity coefficients in the lowest quartile of the psychological assessment literature or just above this point with uncertain stability), but the absence of evidence for its validity because no studies have been conducted regarding CP, possibly due to the extremely low frequency of this response.

There are very few studies on CP, and most of them confirm its low incidence. Piotrowski (1957) stated that CP is not necessarily a psychopathologic sign, but the great majority of individuals with CP are patients who have an organic cerebral disease or incipient schizophrenia. However, Piotrowski does not specifically mention the incidence of CP in these disorders. On the other hand, some studies have reported that CP can be seen in mood disorders. Exner (2001) reported that only 3–5% of patients with schizophrenia showed CP, whereas inpatients with a depressive disorder (Lambda < 1.0) showed a higher incidence of CP at 7%. Moreover, Ishii (2003) reported on 10 cases of CP among 158 patients (6%) that he treated over 7 years.

On the other hand, depressed patients with an avoidant style showed no CP, suggesting that the incidence of the CP is not equally low in all clinical groups, and the incidence of CP differed depending on the pathological conditions and psychological mechanisms that were shown in the Rorschach. Weiner (1998) reported that individuals with CP in the protocols are at considerable risk for rapid mood swings. The co-occurrence of CP with indices of depression frequently raises the possibility of a bipolar disorder or cyclothymic tendencies. However, no quantitative evidence about this has been demonstrated.

In studies conducted with nonclinical groups, Weiner (1998) indicated that CP occurs in fewer than 2% of Rorschach records, whereas Exner (2001) suggested that it was 0.8% (N = 5/600) in the United States. In Japan, Takahashi et al. (1998) reporting on 220 nonclinical adults and Nishio et al. (2017) reporting on 400 nonclinical adults indicated that the incidence of CP was 0%. Nakamura and colleagues (2007) suggested that the incidence of CP was 3% using the Comprehensive System data of a sample of 240 adult nonpatients in Japan. Meyer et al. (2007) reported that the incidence of CP was 2% using composite adult international normative reference data from 17 countries.

Although these studies have reported more CP responses among clinical groups compared with nonclinical groups, it is obviously a rare response. However, Exner's (2001) aforementioned data are particularly noteworthy. Nakamura (2010) suggested that CP might not be surprisingly rare, and could sometimes occur. Considering this, it is probable that many clinical psychologists and counselors engaged in psychological assessment in mental health centers and mental hospitals, especially full-time and veteran psychologists, come across CP at least several times in their careers. The issue could represent the difficulty of collecting data on CP for effectively evaluating its validity by using statistical methods in short-term studies. Data on Rorschach protocols including CP responses are accumulated during spontaneous, day-to-day work in clinical settings, such as in hospitals and healthcare centers, over the long term. Therefore, when we encountered protocols that appeared to include CP in clinical practice, we began the study by asking testees to cooperate in this study, obtaining their consent, and collecting CP data. Aoki (2013) noted that those who produce CP tend to produce more than one, especially among women, and that it is relatively more common among people with posttraumatic stress disorder (PTSD) and dissociative disorders, especially survivors of abuse and bullying. Case studies (Aoki, 2009, 2011) suggested that CP was often seen in the W areas in Card I and Card VI, suggesting that it may be an initial shock to black and shading. Based on the results of the examination of 17 CPs, more than 30% of the CP responses were with MOR, contrary to the conventional interpretation hypothesis (Aoki, 2013). Ishii (2003) also pointed out from a review of 10 cases that CP may be accompanied by negative emotional expressions. Examining the characteristics of CP response may lead to future investigations of interpretive hypotheses for CP.

The purpose of this study was to examine the basic features of CP, in other words, to collect and discuss the basic findings on the characteristics with which CP appears, such as which card, position, response order, location, development quality, form quality, determinants, contents, special score, and projected colors. Although the ultimate goal of this series of studies is to examine the interpretive validity of the CP, we assume that we are at the stage of accumulating basic knowledge about the basic features of CP.

Method

Procedure

This study was performed with the cooperation and agreement of the patients and their treatment centers. The Rorschach test was administered individually for diagnosis and planning in the treatment centers. When CP appeared in Rorschach protocols, the record was placed in the set of research data after obtaining informed consent form the patient, explaining that the data were to be used only for research purposes and that personal information would be completely protected. Data from patients who signed a participation agreement were used. The research was conducted from April 1995 to July 2017. In all, 68 CP responses in 37 protocols were collected from over 1,500 Rorschach protocols. The survey was conducted with the approval of the Committee on Ethics of the Faculty for Research in Human Sciences, Tsukuba University.

Data Analysis

Certified psychologists with more than 20 years of experience in Rorschach testing, including the authors, scored protocols that were collected in the form described in the procedure independently by employing the CS (Exner, 2001). Before the scoring, the scorers agreed to use the CP principle, in which CP was coded only when the presence of chromatic coloring in the achromatic blot area was identified (Exner, 2003). In addition, prior to the score, it was confirmed among the scorers that achromatic included *white* and chromatic included both color specifications such as *red* and *blue* and noncolor specifications such as *colorful* and *multicolored*. In total, 97.0% of all scores, including CP, were in agreement. Disagreements were discussed by including another certified psychologist to determine the final scores.

Sample

The research data included 68 CP responses from adult mental health patients ($N = 37$, four men and 33 women, age range 15–47 years, $M_{age} = 28.68$ years, $SD = 9.80$). None of the patients had any visual impairments or problems with color recognition according to the attending doctor's diagnosis or medical check-ups. The diagnosis of the patients varied from PTSD, schizophrenia, depression, dissociation disorder, panic disorder, and adjustment disorder.

Results

Number of CP Responses

Among the 37 participants who produced CP, 20 participants (54.1%) produced one CP and 17 participants (45.9%) produced multiple CP responses (see Table 1).

Table 1. Number of CP per protocol

Variable	N	(%)
1	20	(54.1)
2	10	(27.0)
3	3	(8.1)
4	1	(2.7)
5	3	(8.1)
Total	37	(100.0)

Ten participants produced two CP (27.0%) and seven participants produced more than three CP (18.9%). The mean number of occurrences of CP was 1.84 (SD = 1.20), maximum being five CP (three persons). Also, four of 20 participants who produced one CP projected chromatic colors that were different from the chromatic color on the card (e.g., "yellow flowers" in red blot area on Card II, "brown monkeys" in pink blot areas on Card VIII). These different chromatic color projection responses are not CP. However, this observation leads us to assume that 57% of people who produced CP (four persons with both single CP and different color projections, and 17 persons with multiple CP) repeatedly dealt with forcibly distorting the actual colors.

Cards That Produced CP

The results indicated that Card VI produced the largest number of CP (33.8%, 23 responses) and Card I produced the second largest number (23.5%, 16 responses). Furthermore, Card V produced the third largest CP showing 11 (16.2%). Eight CP (11.8%) were shown for Card VII, and six CP (8.8%) for Card IV. CP was also shown for Cards II and III (four CP, 5.9%), which are the chromatic color cards (see Table 2).

Location

Comparing the locations of CP responses, W was the most frequent (70.6%), while D and Dd were each the second most frequent (14.7%; see Table 2).

Position of Cards

The position of the card indicated that 97.1% of CP was shown in the original position, whereas only two responses were shown in the reversed position.

Table 2. Card and location of CP

				Card				
Location	I	II	III	IV	V	VI	VII	Total
W								
N	13	0	0	5	10	14	6	48
%	19.1%	0.0%	0.0%	7.4%	14.7%	20.6%	8.8%	70.6%
D								
N	1	0	1	1	0	6	1	10
%	1.5%	0.0%	1.5%	1.5%	0.0%	8.8%	1.5%	14.7%
Dd								
N	2	1	2	0	1	3	1	10
%	2.9%	1.5%	2.9%	0.0%	1.5%	4.4%	1.5%	14.7%
Total								
N	16	1	3	6	11	23	8	68
%	23.5%	1.5%	4.4%	8.8%	16.2%	33.8%	11.8%	100.0%

Table 3. Development Quality (DQ) of CP

Variable	N	(%)
DQ+	22	(32.4)
DQo	40	(58.8)
DQv/+	3	(4.4)
DQv	3	(4.4)
Total	68	(100.0)

Developmental Quality (DQ), Form Qualities (FQ)

Comparing the DQ of CP responses indicated that DQo was the most frequent (58.8%) and DQ+ was the second most frequent (32.4%), whereas DQv/+ and DQv were the third most frequent (4.4%; see Table 3).

For FQ, 38.2% of CP was FQo, 29.4% of CP was FQu, and 32.4% of CP was FQ- (see Table 4).

Determinants

A single determinant was seen in 72.1% of CP responses and a blend determinant was seen in the remaining 27.9% of CP responses. Among the CP responses with a blend determinant, 14 responses had two determinants, and five responses had more than three determinants.

Table 4. Form Quality (FQ) of CP

Variable	N	(%)
FQo	26	(38.2)
FQu	20	(29.4)
FQ–	22	(32.4)
Total	68	(100.0)

Table 5. The percentages of determinants in CP responses

Variable	No shading			Shading		
	Form	Movement	Movement + Others	Shading	Shading + Movement	
Single	26 (38.2%)	8 (11.8%)		15 (22.1%)		49 (72.1%)
Blends			4 (5.6%)		15 (22.1%)	19 (27.9%)
Total		38 (55.9%)			30 (44.1%)	

Note. N = 68 (100%). Movement = e M, FM, and m. Shading = Y, V, and T.

Among 68 CP, shading determinants (T, V, Y) were shown in 44.1% of CP, in particular, Y was seen most often (19 of 30 CP with shading). Furthermore, form determinants were shown in 38.2% and movement determinants were shown in 39.7% of CP, of which more than half are blends with shading (Table 5).

Contents

The most popular content was Botanical (Bt) such as "red leaves," "a bouquet of pink primroses," or "a brown dead leaf," which were seen in 17 responses (25.0%). This was followed by the Whole animals (A), such as "a beautiful blue butterfly," or "tropical fishes," which were seen in 14 responses (20.6%). However, CP responses indicating wounds and damage, such as "red blood" and "a drowned body" were also present, although they occurred less frequently (Table 6).

Special Scores

Overall, 48.5% of CP responses were scored with unusual verbalizations such as DV, DR, INCOM, FABCOM, and CONTAM. Of these, 23.5% ($n = 16$) of the CP responses were scored Level 1 and 16.2% ($n = 11$) were scored Level 2. There was also one CP response with CONTAM. There were five CP responses with two

Table 6. The contents of CP

Variable	N	%	Example
A	14	(20.6)	A beautiful blue butterfly, green bats, tropical fishes
Ad	6	(8.8)	A bright red chicken crown
(A)	1	(1.5)	A skin-colored slug monster
Bt	17	(25.0)	Red leaves, brown dead leaf, a bouquet of pink primroses
Na	3	(4.4)	Blue sky and white cloud
Ls	1	(1.5)	The bluff where the green grass grew
Hh	4	(5.9)	A green lamp, a green beach parasol, a light blue bucket
Sc	4	(5.9)	The pink violin that exploded and damaged
H	1	(1.5)	A drowned body; it's bright red
Hd	1	(1.5)	Blonde child's face
(H)	3	(4.4)	Colorful life forms
(Hd)	2	(2.9)	A head of birdman with blue hair; the face of pink monster
Cg	5	(7.4)	A pink dress with ivory bows, a purple cloak with orange patterns
Fd	2	(2.9)	Brightly colored tropical fruits
Bl	1	(1.5)	Red blood
Art	1	(1.5)	Castle ornaments
H+Cg	1	(1.5)	A golden-haired yellow girl in a light blue dress.
A+Bt	1	(1.5)	Yellow loofah flowers and green bugs
Total	68	(100.0)	

special scores: one CP with two Level 1, two CP responses scoring Level 2 and Level 1, and two CP responses with two Level 2.

Among the special scores for cognitive and thinking deviations, DR was most often scored together with CP (DR = 25, 36.8%), of which 14 scored Level 1 and 11 scored Level 2 (see Table 7). On the other hand, among the special scores for content, Morbid content was the most frequently scored response (MOR = 29.4%).

Projected Colors

As shown in Table 8, 64.7% of CP had one color projection, 19.1% of CP had more than one color projection, and 16.2% of CP had a chromatic color that was not identified (e.g., a colorful chromatic color).

Next, the projected colors (hues) were compared in CP. As can be seen in Table 8, the results indicated that both red and brown were the most frequently projected colors (pure red was projected nine times, and combinations of red and other colors were projected six times; pure brown projected was 12 times,

Table 7. The special score of CP

Variable	NO		Lev1		Lev2		Total
	N	%	N	%	N	%	
DR	43	(63.2%)	14	(20.6%)	11	(16.2%)	
INCOM	60	(88.2%)	3	(4.4%)	5	(7.4%)	
FABCOM	64	(94.1%)	3	(4.4%)	1	(1.5%)	
CONTAM	67	(98.5%)					1 (1.5%)
MOR	48	(70.6%)					20 (29.4%)

Table 8. The projected color of CP

Hues	N (%)	Fre	No. of color	
			One color	More than one
Specific colors	57 (83.8%)		44 (64.7%)	13 (19.1%)
Red		15	9	6
Brown		15	12	3
Green		13	6	7
Pink		11	7	4
Violet		4	2	2
Orange		4	2	2
Yellow		4	0	4
Blue		3	2	1
Pale blue		3	2	1
Other		3	2	1
Unspecific colors	11 (16.2%)			
Total	68 (100%)			

Note. Hues = projected color phases (Hues) and specific (specific/unspecific) on CP; N = number of CP with each color specific (specific/unspecific); Fre = frequency of the hues on CP; No. of color = number of the projected color on CP.

and combinations of other colors projected three times). Green, which was projected 13 times, was the next most frequently projected color (pure green projected six times, combinations of other colors projected seven times), followed by pink, which was projected 11 times (pure pink projected 7 times, a combination of other colors projected four times).

When considering the appropriateness of the projected color to the content, an appropriate color was projected in 89.7% cases ("green leaves" or "a red blood"), and an inappropriate color was projected in 10.3% cases ("fresh green dead leaves" or "The sun. Because the color is green").

Discussion

The aim of this study was to investigate the characteristics of CP responses. Although Exner (2001) reported that both clinical and nonclinical groups produced a maximum of one CP, almost half of the participants in this study produced CP several times. This result is consistent with the results of Ishii (2003), who made similar observations with outpatients.

This suggests that some people frequently use the coping mechanism of CP for whatever purpose. To understand them, it is important to clarify whether this coping is truly a denial of unpleasant feelings and, if not, what purpose it serves.

Cards Producing CP

The results of this study indicated that Card VI produced the most CP and Card I produced the second most CP. Black is used in all of Card I, and this is the first card that people encounter black. Nishio et al. (2017) suggested that the incidence of "C" in Card I was 13.5%, which is the highest among all cards using the comprehensive system from the data of a sample of 400 adult Japanese nonpatients. In judging the impressions of Card I using the semantic differential method, the Japanese respondents~ responses were often accompanied by unpleasant emotional expressions such as "unpleasant, dark, and dirty" (Kataguchi, 1974). On the other hand, Card VI is the first soft shade of color used all over the card. More people respond to shades than colors, indicating the highest texture response (20%) of the 10 cards (Kataguchi, 1974). Nishio et al. (2017) also suggested that the incidence of T in Card VI is the highest (12.0%) and that the incidences of V and Y are the highest among all the cards. Moreover, the judgment of impressions on Card VI using the semantic differential method shows numerous responses with unpleasant feeling, including "unpleasant," "dark," and "sad," (Kataguchi, 1974). Considering that the CP generated by these two cards accounted for approximately 60% of the total, it can be speculated that CP may be one of the coping responses to the shock of first encountering an achromatic stimulus, although its features are different.

Location, DQ, FQ, and Response Position

The results for Location, DQ, and Position of the CP responses indicated several possibilities for how CP was perceived. In the present study, W was the most frequent for Location and DQo was the most frequent for DQ, accounting for approximately 70% and 60%, respectively, suggesting that CP may be caused by the overall impact of the card stimulus. The result that CP was more common in Card I and Card VI, which have a larger surface area of the figure, also supports the hypothesis.

Furthermore, the result that more than 90% of CP responses have specific forms (DQ+ and DQo) means that those who produce CPs will ignore the color but not the form of the pictorial stimulus. Nevertheless, FQ varied, with both good form quality (FQo) and poor form quality (FQ-) found about 30% of the time. These results suggest that those who exhibit CP strive to recognize the objective reality of form, but more than 30% of them deviate from the general perception.

As for the position of the card, almost all of the CP responses were also shown in the original position. These findings suggested that the coping strategy for using CP was to change perceptions rather than to change behaviors, such as rotating the cards.

Determinants

Almost half of CP responses were accompanied by shading scores. Furthermore, in particular, Y was present most, which supported Exner's findings (2001). Many studies have reported that shading responses are strongly related to unpleasant emotions, and Y in particular is related to anxiety (Klopfer et al., 1954; Rapaport et al., 1946). Taking this into account, the present results seemed to support the conventional hypothesis that when unpleasant feelings are aroused by shading stimuli, CPs cope with the unpleasant feelings by forcibly changing their perception of the stimuli, that is, denying the unpleasant feelings.

In addition, about 40% of the CP responses were accompanied by movement as a determinant. In particular, all CP responses with blended determinants were scored with movement, most of which were blends of shading and movement. In terms of creating something that does not exist on the card, Movement, which projects movement onto a nonmoving card stimulus, and CP, which projects color onto an uncolored card stimulus, are similar. However, the difference is that Movement does not deny the existence of the stimulus on the card, whereas CP is formed by denying the existence of the colorless stimulus on the card. In this way, it may be said that CP is a response that requires creativity in its production, and that creativity can sometimes be so strong that it can deviate from reality.

On the other hand, there are also more than 30% of CP responses with shape as a determinant, but it is not clear whether these CP responses are associated with anxiety and unpleasant feelings like CP responses with shading. In the future, it will be necessary to compare CPs with different determinants.

Special Scores

Concerning the special score, almost half of CP responses contained certain deviations of cognition and thinking, and half of those indicated serious deviations (Level 2). In particular, DR was the special score most often seen with CP, and the serious level of DR (DR2) accounted for 40% of DR. These results indicated that people who produce CP could easily get absorbed in inner images and deviate the focus of attention from the card, with approximately 40% of such people showing considerably serious deviations from reality. On the other hand, MOR were scored in almost 30% of the CP responses. These results suggest that the traditional CP interpretation hypothesis of denial of unpleasant feelings may not be applicable to all CP or that the denial of unpleasant feelings is actually not working properly to defend the respondent from experiencing them.

Projected Colors

When considering whether the projected colors were appropriate for the content, we found that about 90% projected appropriate colors, while the remaining 10% projected inappropriate colors. CPs that deliberately projected colors that were not appropriate for the content may have been expressed as a result of integration failures, and it is possible that CPs that projected appropriate colors may be interpreted differently than CPs that projected appropriate colors.

In projected colors (hues), both red and brown were most frequently projected. In Japan, red is the more "preferred color" while brown is less preferred. Furthermore, various surveys from 1991 to 2008 showed that few people chose brown as their favorite color (Chijiiwa, 1999; Hanari & Takahashi, 2008; Japan Color Research Institute, 2011; Takahashi & Hanari, 2005). In color impression scores using the semantic difference scale (SD) based on research in color psychology and color dynamics, red had higher SD values for positive adjectives such as "bright," "beautiful," "pleasant," and "happy," whereas brown had lower SD values regardless of the time of the survey (1991, 1993, 1995; Japan Color Research Institute, 2011; Matsuoka, 1995). On the other hand, negative adjectives such as "dark," "heavy," "blurry," and "dirty" have higher SD values in brown than in red. Thus, it seems to be necessary to consider carefully whether it is appropriate to apply the traditional interpretation of brown-projected CP as a negation of an unpleasant emotion. At this stage, although we cannot be certain, it is possible that CP may have psychological mechanisms other than the denial of unpleasant emotions, or, again, that despite trying to deny such emotions the resulting behavior falls short of achieving this scope.

Conclusion

The result that almost 60% of CPs were produced on Card I or VI suggested that CPs may be an initial shock response to achromatic or shading. Furthermore, nearly all of the CP responses were shown in the original position, and more than half of them were shown in W and DQo, suggesting that CP is a response to over-all card impact and may be a coping mechanism that changes perception rather than changing behavior. As for special scores, almost half of the CP responses included some deviation in cognition or thinking, and half of them showed a serious level (Level 2). In addition, considering the fact that approximately 30% of CP responses were FQ- and included 10% of CPs that projected colors that were not consistent with the content of the response, it was also speculated that some CP may be a failure of cognition or thought integration. Furthermore, the fact that almost 30% of the CP responses were scored on MOR and that not all CPs projected beautiful or desirable colors suggest that the traditional CP interpretation hypothesis of denial of unpleasant affect may not apply to all CP responses. However, this conclusion cannot be determined based on this study alone, and further studies are needed in the future.

Limitations

The limitations of this study are the following. First, the study relied on the incidental occurrence of CP in clinical settings to collect CP. The low frequency of occurrence of CP made it difficult to collect CP in the usual research format of recruiting study participants. Therefore, the first author asked participants to be studied when the first author encountered a response that appeared to be CP in a clinical setting, and the second author scored the data with the participant's consent. It is possible that this research setting may have acted as a bias in scoring the CPs and affected the score agreement rate. Second, because the study was conducted within the framework described above, there was no control group in the study. Third, there is a sample bias because the data were collected only in medical settings. Fourth, the data set was collected over a long period. Therefore, data from the Aoki case study (2009, 2013) were included.

It is necessary to further examine the characteristics of CP responses, such as the verbal expressions of affect in the explanation of CP responses, based on the findings of the present study, so as to accumulate the knowledge necessary to examine the validity of the interpretation of CP.

References

Aoki, S. (2009). A case report about color projection–focusing on cases with numerous CP production. *Abstracts of 13th conference of Japanese Society for the Rorschach and Projective Method, 24.*

Aoki, S. (2011). Reconsider on the color projection on the Rorschach Test. In *XX International Congress of Rorschach and Projective Methods Abstract Book* (pp. 164–165).

Aoki, S. (2013). Study of color projection in the Rorschach test. *Journal of Japanese Clinical Psychology, 31*(4), 586–596.

Chijiiwa, H. (1999). *Encyclopedia on color cognition of the world's youth – The world's first research and analysis of color cognition.* Kawade Shobo Shinsha.

Exner, J. E. (2001). *A Rorschach workbook for the comprehensive system* (5th ed.). Rorschach Workshop.

Exner, J. E. (2003). *The Rorschach: A comprehensive system, Vol. 1. Basic foundations and Principles of interpretation* (4th ed.). Wiley.

Hanari, T., & Takahashi, S. (2008). Cognitive factors in color preference (2): Generalization of previous findings by using modified procedures. *Journal of the Color Science Association of Japan, 32*(4), 282–289.

Ishii, Y. (2003). Reconsideration of color projection response. *Journal of Japanese Clinical Psychology, 21*(3), 301–306.

Japan Color Research Institute (2011). *Handbook of color science.* University of Tokyo Press.

Kataguchi, Y. (1974). *A method of psychopsy – manual and research for Rorschach psychodiagnostics.* Kaneko Shobou.

Klopfer, B., Ainsworth, M. D., & Klopfer, W. G. (1954). *Developments in the Rorschach technique, Volume 1: Technique and theory.* Harcourt, Brace & World.

Matsuoka, T. (1995). *Color and personality – the world of the image to investigate with a color.* Kaneko Shobou.

Meyer, G. J., Erdberg, P., & Shaffer, T. W. (2007). Toward international normative reference data for the comprehensive system. *Journal of Personality Assessment, 89*(Suppl. 1), S201–S216.

Mihura, J. L., Meyer, G. J., Bombel, G., & Dumitrascu, N. (2013). The validity of individual Rorschach variables: Systematic reviews and meta-analysis of the comprehensive system. *Psychological Bulletin, 139*(3), 548–605.

Nakamura, N. (2010). *Lectures on the Rorschach Test I (Basic).* Kongo Shuppan.

Nakamura, N., Fuchigami, Y., & Tsugawa, R. (2007). Rorschach Comprehensive System data for a sample of 240 adult nonpatients from Japan. *Journal of Personality Assessment, 89* (Suppl. 1), S97–S102.

Nishio, H., Takahashi, Y., & Takahashi, M. (2017). *Statistics of the Rorschach test – the variable data for numerical comparison and interpretation.* Kongo Shuppan.

Piotrowski, Z. A. (1957). *Percept analysis.* Libris.

Rapaport, D., Gill, M., & Schafer, R. (1946). *Diagnostic psychological testing* (Vol. 2). Yearbook Publisher.

Schachtel, E. G. (1967). *Experimental foundations of Rorschach's Test.* Tavistock Publications.

Shapiro, D. (1956). Color-response and perceptual passivity. *Journal of Projective Techniques, 20*(1), 52–69.

Shapiro, D. (1960). A perceptual understanding of color response. In M. Rickers-Ovsiankina (Ed.), *Rorschach psychology.* John Wiley.

Takahashi, M., Takahashi, Y., & Nishio, H. (1998). *Basic interpretation of the Rorschach by the Rorschach comprehensive system*. Kongo Shuppan.
Takahashi, S., & Hanari, T. (2005). Cognitive factors in color preference. *Japanese Journal of Color Psychology, 29*, 14–23.
Weiner, I. B. (1998). *Principles of Rorschach interpretation*. Lawrence Erlbaum Associates.

History
Received May 28, 2019
Revision received December 7, 2020
Accepted December 15, 2020
Published online March 18, 2021

Received and processed mainly under previous editorship

Acknowledgments
The data which we used in a previous publication (Aoki, 2013) are included in the data of this study. Portions of this article were originally presented at the 20th International Congress of Rorschach and Projective Methods in Tokyo, Japan, in 2011 and at the 22th International Congress of Rorschach and Projective Methods in Paris, France, in 2017.

This study is supported by the following researchers and clinicians. We would like to thank them for collecting CP dates, scoring, and helpful comments: Satoshi Ono, Yoshiyuki Takamura, Hatsue Numa, Noriko Nakamura, Munechika Ito, and Toshiki Ogawa.

ORCID
Sanae Aoki
https://orcid.org/0000-0002-4670-0876

Sanae Aoki
Division of Psychology
Faculty of Human Sciences
University of Tsukuba
1-1-1 Tennodai, Tsukuba
Ibaraki 305-8577
Japan
s-aoki@human.tsukuba.ac.jp

Summary

Color Projection (CP) is an extremely rare response in which chromatic color is projected onto an achromatic blot on the Rorschach and has been interpreted as a denial of unpleasant feelings. However, there are very few studies on CP.

The purpose of this study was to examine the basic features of CP, that is, to collect and discuss the basic findings on the characteristics with which CP appears, such as which card, position, location, development quality, form quality, determinants, contents, special score, and projected colors. Although the ultimate goal of this series of studies is to examine the interpretive validity of the CP, we assume that CP is at the stage of accumulating basic knowledge prior to the validation, since there is no basic knowledge on CP.

Japanese adult psychiatric patients (N = 37) participated in the study that was conducted between April 1995 and July 2017. A total of 68 CP responses produced in the Rorschach protocol by the participants were examined.

The result that almost 60% of CPs were produced on Card I or VI suggested that CPs may be an initial shock response to achromatic or shading. Furthermore, nearly all of the CP responses were shown in the original position, and more than half of them were shown in W and DQo, suggesting that CP is a response to overall card impact and may be a coping mechanism that changes perception rather than changing behavior. As for special scores, almost half of the CP responses included some deviation in cognition or thinking, and half of them showed a serious level (Level 2). In addition, considering the fact that approximately 30% of CP responses were FQ- and included 10% of CPs that projected colors that were not consistent with the content of the response, it was also speculated that some CP may be a failure of cognition or thought integration. Furthermore, the fact that almost 30% of the CP responses were scored on MOR and that not all CPs projected beautiful or desirable colors, as has been shown in previous studies, suggests that the traditional CP interpretation hypothesis of denial of unpleasant affect may not apply to all CP responses. However, this conclusion cannot be determined based on this study alone, and further studies are needed in the future.

要約

CPはロールシャッハ図版の無彩色領域に有彩色が投影される極めて稀な反応であり、不快な感情の否定と解釈されてきた。しかし、CPに関する研究は極めて少ない。本研究の目的は、CPの出現した図版、位置、発達水準、形態水準、決定因、反応内容、特殊スコア、そして投影された色彩についての知見を収集し、CPの基本的特徴を検討することであった。この一連の研究の最終的な目的はCPの解釈的妥当性を検討することであるが、CPの基礎知識が不足しているため、検証に先立って基礎知識を蓄積している段階が必要である。

1995年4月から2017年7月までの間に実施された研究には、日本人成人精神科患者（N=37）が参加した。参加者がロールシャッハプロトコルで作成した68のCP回答を検討した。

その結果、6割近くのCPがカードIまたはVIで産出されたことから、CPは無彩色または陰影に対する初期ショック反応である可能性が示唆された。さらに、CPの反応のほぼ全てが元の位置で示され、半数以上がWとDQoで示されていたことから、CPはカード全体の衝撃に対する反応であり、行動を変えるというよりも認知を変える対処方略である可能性が示唆された。特殊スコアについては、CP反応のほぼ半数が認知や思考の何らかの逸脱を含み、その半数が深刻なレベル（レベル2）を示していた。また、CP反応の約3割がFQ-であり、反応内容と一致しない色を投影するCPが10%も含まれていたことを考慮すると、CPの中には認知や思考の統合に失敗しているものもあると推測された。さらに、CPの約30%がMORをスコアされていることや、先行研究で示されているように、すべてのCPに美しい色や好ましいとされている色を投影しているわけではないことから、従来のCP解釈仮説である「不快な感情の否定」がすべてのCPに当てはまらない可能性が示唆された。しかし、この結論は本研究だけでは判断できず、今後のさらなる研究が必要である。

Résumé

L'objectif de cette étude était d'examiner les caractéristiques de base de la PC, en d'autres termes, de recueillir et de discuter les conclusions de base sur les caractéristiques avec lesquelles la PC apparaît, telles que la carte, la position, l'emplacement, la qualité du développement, la qualité de la forme, les déterminants, le contenu, le score spécial et les couleurs projetées. Bien que l'objectif ultime de cette série d'études soit d'examiner la validité interprétative de la PC, nous supposons que les PC en sont au stade de l'accumulation des connaissances de base avant la validation, puisqu'il n'existe aucune connaissance de base de la PC.

Des patients psychiatriques japonais adultes (N = 37) ont participé à l'étude qui a été menée entre avril 1995 et juillet 2017. 68 réponses de CP produites dans le protocole de Rorschach par les participants ont été examinées.

Le résultat, à savoir que près de 60% des CP ont été produits sur la carte I ou VI, suggère que les CP peuvent être une première réponse de choc à l'achromatique ou à l'ombrage. En outre, presque toutes les réponses de PC ont été montrées dans la position initiale, et plus de la moitié d'entre elles ont été montrées en W et DQo, ce qui suggère que les PC sont une réponse à l'impact global de la carte et peuvent être un mécanisme d'adaptation qui modifie la perception plutôt que le comportement. En ce qui concerne les scores spéciaux, près de la moitié des réponses de PC comportaient un certain écart dans la cognition ou la pensée, et la moitié d'entre elles montraient un niveau sérieux (niveau 2). En outre, compte tenu du fait qu'environ 30% des réponses CP étaient FQ- et comprenaient 10% de CP qui projetaient des couleurs qui ne correspondaient pas au contenu de la réponse, il a également été supposé que certains CP pouvaient être un échec de l'intégration de la cognition ou de la pensée. En outre, le fait que près de 30% des réponses des PC ont été notées sur MOR et que tous les PC ne projetaient pas de belles couleurs ou des couleurs désirables, comme l'ont montré des études précédentes, suggère que l'hypothèse d'interprétation traditionnelle des PC, à savoir le déni d'un effet désagréable, ne s'applique peut-être pas à toutes les réponses des PC.

Resumen

El propósito de este estudio fue examinar las características básicas de la PC, es decir, recoger y discutir los hallazgos básicos sobre las características con las que aparece la PC, como qué tarjeta, posición, ubicación, calidad de desarrollo, calidad de la forma, determinantes, contenido, puntuación especial y colores proyectados. Aunque el objetivo final de esta serie de estudios es examinar la validez interpretativa del PC, asumimos que el PC se encuentra en la etapa de acumulación de conocimientos básicos antes de la validación, ya que no existe un conocimiento básico del PC.

Los pacientes psiquiátricos adultos japoneses (N = 37) participaron en el estudio que se llevó a cabo entre abril de 1995 y julio de 2017. Se examinaron 68 respuestas de PC producidas en el protocolo de Rorschach por los participantes.

El resultado de que casi el 60% de las PC se produjeron en la tarjeta I o VI sugirió que las PC pueden ser una respuesta inicial de choque a la acromática o al sombreado. Además, casi todas las respuestas de PC se mostraron en la posición original, y más de la mitad de ellas se mostraron en W y DQo, sugiriendo que la PC es una respuesta al impacto global de la tarjeta y puede ser un mecanismo de afrontamiento que cambia la percepción más que el comportamiento. En cuanto a las puntuaciones especiales, casi la mitad de las respuestas de PC incluyeron alguna desviación en la cognición o el pensamiento, y la mitad de ellas mostraron un nivel grave (nivel 2). Además, considerando el hecho de que aproximadamente el 30% de las respuestas de PC eran FQ- e incluían un 10% de PC que proyectaban colores que no eran consistentes con el contenido de la respuesta, también se especuló que algunos PC pueden ser una falla en la cognición o en la integración del pensamiento. Además, el hecho de que casi el 30% de las respuestas de PC se puntuaran en MOR y que no todos los PC proyectaran colores bonitos o deseables, como se ha demostrado en estudios anteriores, sugiere que la hipótesis tradicional de interpretación de PC de negación del afecto desagradable puede no aplicarse a todas las respuestas de PC.

Research Article

Concurrent Validity of the Sixty-Second Drawing Test in Measuring High-Schoolers' Close Relationships and Depression

Zsuzsanna Kövi[1] , James B. Hittner[2], Zsuzsanna Mirnics[3],
Ferenc Grezsa[4], Máté Smohai[1], Nenad Jakšić[5],
Veronika Mészáros[1], Sándor Rózsa[3], András Vargha[1],
Zsuzsanna Tanyi[3], and Zoltán Vass[1]

[1]Department of General Psychology, Károli Gáspár University of the Reformed Church,
Budapest, Hungary
[2]Department of Psychology, College of Charleston, SC, USA
[3]Department of Personality Psychology, Károli Gáspár University of the Reformed Church,
Budapest, Hungary
[4]Center for Postgraduate Studies, Károli Gáspár University of the Reformed Church,
Budapest, Hungary
[5]Department of Psychiatry and Psychological Medicine, University Hospital Centre Zagreb,
Croatia

Abstract: Although clinicians have a long history of using drawings for personality and emotional assessment, the empirical validation of the drawings has been inconsistent. The goal of this study was to examine the validity of the Sixty-Second Drawing Test (SSDT) in predicting close relationships and depression. The sample consisted of 2,883 Hungarian students. The SSDT required participants to draw a series of circles, where the circles represented the self, significant others, different moods, and God. Standardized questionnaires (the Experiences in Close Relationships–Revised and the Children's Depression Inventory) were also administered. Generally speaking, small distances and relatively smaller self-circles were associated with better relationships. Depression was indicated by drawing large bad-mood circles that were close to one's self-circle, along with small happiness-circles that were distant from one's self-circle. The magnitudes of all associations were small to moderate, with explained variances ranging from 7.6% to 21.9%. The results suggest that using drawings of circles to represent important object-relations can, to some extent, predict interpersonal relations and depressive symptoms. Although we do not advocate using the SSDT as a clinical diagnostic measure, it can serve as a useful screening tool for identifying potential relational and affective difficulties.

Keywords: drawing test, validity, close relationships, depression

Validity of Projective Assessments

Psychological assessments have long been proposed to be objective if tests make direct inferences about a person based on self-report or reports from significant others in response to very clear questions, thereby producing objective scores (Lack & Thomason, 2013). Projective tests, on the other hand, are indirect measurements, in which instructions or stimuli are more ambiguous and therefore allow for more indirect inferences about a person's intelligence, personal and social qualities, and psychological state (Lack & Thomason, 2013).

Figure drawing methods are a common type of projective assessment in which individuals are asked to draw people or objects (Abell et al., 2001). The assumption is that drawings reflect the individuals' basic dispositions and attitudes toward themselves and other people (Weiner & Greene, 2008). Clinicians have long used drawings for personality assessment and the evaluation of emotional states (Bertran & Nistal, 2017; Thomas & Jolley, 1998; Veltman & Browne, 2002). Figure drawing methods are still widely used (Camara et al., 2000; Cashel, 2002; Piotrowski, 2015).

Projective measures are often linked to psychoanalytic and psychodynamic theories of personality and psychopathology (Lack & Thomason, 2013; Sartori, 2010) because these measures are supposed to reflect unconscious tendencies and implicit motives. In general, projective measures can provide valuable information not assessed by self-report techniques (Lilienfeld et al., 2000) and they are less influenced by tendencies toward social desirability responses.

On the other hand, projective techniques have been criticized for being weak and ineffective, and for lacking face validity (Sartori, 2010). According to a meta-analysis (Lilienfeld et al., 2000), the validity evidence for many of the variables calculated in projective tests is limited, although there are exceptions. One example of validity evidence comes from work by Matto and colleagues (2005), who found that a special version of the Draw-A-Person Test explained considerable variance (> .20) in emotional and behavioral measures. However, the overall empirical validation of drawing tests has been inconsistent (Piotrowski, 2015).

Quantitative Indices of Drawings

The most widely studied quantitative index of drawings has been the size of figures. Weiner and Greene (2008) noted that the size of the figure when drawing oneself may reflect either an actual self-image or an ideal image. Some researchers (Bowdin & Bruck, 1960; Gray & Pepitone, 1964; Vass, 2012) have linked the size of a self-referent figure to the subject's actual self-concept or self-esteem: Large figures are considered to reflect high self-esteem along with high energy level. Other researchers have found different results: Bennett (1966), Dalby and Vale (1977), and Prytula and colleagues (1978) did not find an association between size of the figure and self-esteem.

Lewinsohn (1964) noted that emotional states such as depression and anxiety can result in smaller drawings, and also a more recent publication (Ogdon,

2001) noted that smaller size together with placement in corners and the faintness of drawings could be indicators of depression. However, Salzman and Harway (1967) and Sandman and colleagues (1968) reported no relationship between depression and figure sizes. Gantt (2001) emphasized the ratio of empty to non-empty spaces and argued that this metric could be a more reliable indicator of depression.

Joiner et al. (1996) stated that there is no reliable relation between self-report measures of childhood depression and anxiety and drawing size, detail, and line heaviness. Their sole finding was a weak correlation between anxiety and drawing size, but in the opposite direction than expected: Higher anxiety was linked to larger drawings.

Another topic that has garnered research interest concerns the interpersonal significance and affective characteristics of the drawn person. Thomas and Gray (1992) asked participants to complete two drawings on separate papers, one of a liked person, and one of a disliked person. According to their results, the significance of a figure was reflected in its smaller distance from a self-referent figure. An assessment instrument focusing on interpersonal significance is the Inclusion of Other in the Self (IOS) Scale (Aron et al., 1992). The IOS is a semi-projective technique that uses pre-defined drawings of circles to represent different self–other relations. This single-item, pictorial measure is designed to assess interpersonal closeness. The IOS scale has good test–retest reliability; has demonstrated convergent, discriminant, and predictive validity; and is weakly correlated with measures of social desirability response bias. The IOS measures one's sense of interconnection by evaluating the overlapping of circles (larger overlapping circles indicate closer interpersonal relationships).

In addition, the relative sizes of figures/circles and their vertical positions can also reflect important aspects of relationships. For example, Thomas and Jolley (1998) pointed out that children usually draw important adults, and adults that have more power, as larger figures. Burkitt and colleagues (2003) also found that children drew positively characterized objects larger than neutrally characterized ones, and reduced the size of negatively characterized objects relative to baseline drawings.

The Sixty-Second Drawing Test

In a novel approach to studying figure size, Thomas et al. (1989) asked children to draw apples and people, and they gave them a nice, a neutral, or a nasty description of the objects. In the "nice" condition, the sizes of both the apple and men that children drew were significantly bigger than those in the neutral condition. In the "nasty" condition, the drawings of men were smaller, but the size of the apple drawings were unaffected. The authors interpreted these findings as suggesting that the significance of a topic influences the size of the drawing.

In order to simplify the complexity and ambiguity of drawings, Vass (2011, 2012) proposed a method whereby individuals draw significant others and objects not as complex drawings, but only as circles. This idea led to the Sixty-Second Drawing Test (SSDT; Vass, 2011, 2012). In this test, the participant is asked to draw a circle that represents him- or herself, and additionally, another circle that represents a significant other person or a concept. In consecutive tasks, the participant is asked to draw his/her best friend, mother, father, siblings, happiness, biggest problem, etc.

According to Vass (2012), the test evaluates personality and object relations, including conscious and not conscious aspects. Vass proposed that the size of the circles may reflect self-esteem and their shapes may indicate conformity versus opposition. Consider the case of drawing a self-referent circle and a significant other circle. The two circles could differ in size, in vertical placement on the page (thought to reflect dominance vs. submission), in degree of separation versus overlap (thought to reflect autonomy vs. symbiotic/intimacy needs), in the extent to which one circle contains another (perhaps reflecting roles in the relationship, introjection, and/or need for support), and whether the circles differ in shape/ degree of perfect circularity (thought to reflect identification, symbiosis vs. conflicts, and ambivalence; Vass, 2012). To summarize, the SSDT, like the IOS, only uses circles as the units of measurement, but has the advantage that not only the closeness of the circles is evaluated, but also relative sizes, relative positions, and multiple other characteristics as outlined above.

The overarching aim of our study was to examine how the distance and size variables of the SSDT could be linked to affective characterizations of significant others (i.e., different emotional states). Specifically, we examined the extent to which experiences in close relationships (with mother, father, and God), and depression (including low self-esteem) can be related to figure size and distance indices; thus we examined the concurrent validity of the SSDT.

We hypothesized that (1) closer attachments are linked to smaller distances (as is the case for the IOS scale; Aron et al., 1992), and (2) small size and distant placement from the center can be indicators of depression (as noted by Ogdon, 2001).

Method

Participants

Our participants were 2,883 students, 1,365 females (*M* age = 16.73 years, *SD* = 1.31) and 1,518 males (M_{age} = 16.88, *SD* = 1.39) attending secondary schools in Hungary, from Grades 9 (642 males and 578 females) and 11 (876 males and

787 females). Students were recruited from all 20 counties in Hungary, and thus are representative of the population in Hungary. Students filled out the questionnaire and completed the drawing tasks in a classroom setting.

Procedure

Ethical approval for the study was given by the ethics committee of the university of the first author. Students filled out questionnaires in their classroom settings, with help from their teacher and a research assistant. After completing the questionnaires, students were given four A4 sheets of paper that they needed to tear into four equal parts (resulting in 16 smaller pieces) and they were instructed as to which paper the various circles should be drawn on.

Measures

Sixty-Second Drawing Test (SSDT)

The SSDT was developed by Vass (Vass, 2011, 2012). It has 16 different instructions asking participants to draw 16 pairs of circles, each assessing a relation of the self to 16 different individuals, objects, or concepts.

The first instruction is: "Take this sheet and put it in landscape position. Now, draw a circle that represents yourself." Once finished: "Now, please draw a circle that represents one of your friends." In Instructions 3–16, the examiner repeats the same procedure, changing only the persons involved: (3) you and your father; (4) you and your mother; (5) you and your siblings; (6) you and your teacher; (7) you and someone you love; (8) you and a person you do not love; (9) you and the school; (10) you and a current problem that worries you seriously; (11) you and the problem in a year's time; (12) you and happiness; (13) you and bad mood; (14) you and good mood; (15) you and your mood recently; (16) you and God.

Drawings were scanned, which were then evaluated by a computer program that automatically measured:

1) Sizes of own (r_1) and other circle (r_2, length of radius);
2) Relative sizes ($r_1 - r_2$);
3) Distances (D) between center of circles; and
4) Relative distances between center of circles (distances were computed relative to the sizes of circles by this formula: $(D - (r_1 + r_2))/(r_1 + r_2)$.

Experiences in Close Relationships–Revised (ECR-RS) Questionnaire

Adult Attachment was measured by the short version of the Experiences in Close Relationships-Revised (ECR-RS) questionnaire (Fraley et al., 2011). Ten items were intended to measure one's relationship to mother and father separately.

Table 1. Confirmatory factor analyses of the ECR-RS questionnaire

	CMIN	df	CMIN/df	CFI	TLI	SRMR	RMSEA [90% CI]
Two factors (original structure) for maternal attachment	1,345.37***	34	39.57	.82	.76	.09	.12 [.12, .13]
Bifactor model for maternal attachment	532.45***	24	22.19	.93	.87	.03	.09 [.09, .10]
Bifactor model for maternal attachment (correlated e2-e3)	107.80***	23	4.87	.99	.98	.02	.04 [.03, .05]
Two factors (original structure) for paternal attachment	1,477.55***	34	26.86	.83	.77	.09	.13 [.13, .14]
Bifactor model for paternal attachment	993.37***	24	41.39	.88	.78	.07	.13 [.12, .14]
Bifactor model for paternal attachment (correlated e2-e3)	100.02***	23	4.35	.99	.98	.02	.04 [.03, .05]

Note. ECR-RS = Experiences in Close Relationships – Revised Questionnaire. ***$p < .001$.

All responses were indicated using a 5-point Likert scale. This short version along with the original version (Fraley et al., 2000) consists of two scales (avoidance and anxiety); however, it was noted by Fraley et al. (2011) that the correlations between the two subscales are relatively high (around .5) and half of the items load on both factors with at least a .25 factor weight. We tested the original two-factor model and a bifactor one, in which a global attachment factor besides the specific factors (avoidance and anxiety) is present. Table 1 lists the fit indices of the consecutive models. The bifactor model with a modification (adding correlated error terms between Items 2 and 3) yielded the best fit indices. Thus, one global and two specific factors were confirmed with two items having correlated error terms. These two items in fact measure two very similar things, namely, "talking things over" and "discussing problems."

Omega hierarchical (omegaH), which reflects the percentage of variance that can be attributed to the individual differences on the general factor, was .79 and .82, for maternal and paternal attachment, respectively. Rodriguez et al. (2016) reported that in the case of omegaH above .8, total scores can be regarded as unidimensional. Therefore, in our study we subsequently used only the global attachment scores, separately for maternal and paternal attachment measures. Reliability analyses of the global scale yielded Cronbach α values of .87 and .88 along with McDonald's ω of .86 (95% CI = [.86, .88]) and .88 (95% CI = [.88, .89]), respectively, for the mother and father relationship items.

Relationship With God

Relationship with God and religiosity were measured through several questions. First, we assessed belief in God, church attendance, and frequency of prayer ("talking to God"). Four questions asked about religious attitudes (two of them measuring fear of God's punishment, and two other questions about gratefulness to God). Lastly, three items from the Spiritual Health and Life Orientation Measurement Scale (Fisher, 2010) were used to measure the participant's opinion about how praying to or thinking about God contributes to psychological well-being.

A principal component was calculated from the 10 items to form an index of (close) relationship to God (explained variance = 62.14%, with all component scores above .6). This index is based on a formative model, which assumes that questions coming from different questionnaires can form a composite score as an index of a weighted sum of the different variables. This analysis (PCA) preserves the maximal amount of variance of observed variables while Exploratory factor analysis (EFA) accounts for common variance in the data and it assumes that all items reflect the same construct. Here we tested if different measurements and constructs (belief in God, praying to God, visiting church) could be composed as a composite score. Thus, PCA was applied, to test if one meaningful composite score could be formed with preserving as much of the original variables' variance, as possible.

Children's Depression Inventory

Depressive symptoms were measured using eight items from the Children's Depression Inventory (Kovacs, 1981, 1992), including two items on negative mood, two items on interpersonal problems, two items on anhedonia, one item on negative self-esteem and one item on ineffectiveness. The total score of the questionnaire was proved to be a reliable index over repeated administrations (Finch et al., 1987). Reliability analysis in our study yielded a Cronbach α of .76, with all item-total correlations above .3. McDonalds' ω was .76 (CI = [.74, .77]). CFA analyses confirmed a one-factor solution (χ^2 = 87.775, p < .05, df = 20; CMIN/df = 4.39; CFI = .98; TLI = .96; SRMR = .02; RMSEA = .04 [.03, .04]).

Results

Relations of Self-Circle Sizes to Self-Esteem and Emotional States

We formed an average out of the 16 drawings of self-circle sizes (the participant had to draw himself/herself 16 times). We measured whether these sizes constitute a reliable scale: Cronbach α coefficient was .95, and also McDonald's ω was .95 (CI = [.95, .96]). The average self-circle size was significantly but weakly negatively related to depression, $r(2,689)$ = −.09, p < .001. The item measuring self-esteem was weakly positively correlated with average circle size, $r(2,642)$ = .10, p < .001. These relationships were lower among boys – size and depression:

$r(1,387) = -.04$, $p = .11$, size and self-esteem: $r(1,357) = .06$, $p = .02$ - than among girls, size and depression: $r(1,288) = -.09$, $p = .001$, size and self-esteem: $r(1,270) = .10$, $p < .001$.

SSDT as a Measure of Close Relationships

Bivariate correlations were used to examine associations (1) between ECR (Experiences in Close Relationships) scores and drawing indices of "you and your mother" and "you and your father", and (2) between one's relationship to God and drawing indices calculated from the drawing "you and God" (see Table 2).

Altogether, closer relationships were indicated by significantly smaller distances between self- and other circles ($r = -.18$ to $-.25$). The relative distance measures yielded even higher correlations ($r = -.27$ to $-.33$), than the simple distance measures, for paternal attachment and relation to God, correlational coefficients were above .3 in the total sample. However, gender differences were discovered: In the case of girls, these coefficients were above .4, whereas among boys, these were below .3. For all cases, the relative distances were calculated by dividing distances by diameters of the circles.

Regarding the size of drawings, the highest correlations (.38) were found when measuring one's relationship to God. This relation was even stronger (.43) among girls. Regarding one's relationship to parents, all of the size indices yielded weak correlations (< .16).

In addition to correlations, regression analyses were performed on the total sample, in which SSDT indices served as independent variables and measures of relationships with mother, father, and God served as the dependent variables (see Table 3).

Explained variances of 8%, 13%, and 22% were achieved, respectively, for relationships with mother, $F(2, 2,599) = 106.65$, $p < .001$, father, $F(2, 2,441) = 179.60$, $p < .001$, and God, $F(3, 1,635) = 153.96$, $p < .001$. Mother attachment was negatively related to relative distance ($\beta = -.27$) and positively to relative size of mother ($\beta = .06$). Father attachment was negatively related to relative distance ($\beta = -.34$) and positively to relative size of the father ($\beta = .12$). Relationship with God was found to be positively linked to size of God ($\beta = .31$), and negatively linked to relative distance ($\beta = -.28$) and to size of self-circle ($\beta = -.20$). Regression analyses run separately for boys and girls resulted in similar significant predictors but in differences in explained variance. In the case of boys, 4%, 7%, and 21% were found, respectively, for relationships with mother (based on relative distance), father (based on relative distance and size difference), and God (based on distance, size difference and self-size). In the case of girls, 12%, 18% and 28% were found, respectively, for relationships with mother (based on relative distance and

Table 2. Correlations between SSDT indices and validity scales on total sample and separately for boys and girls

ECR-R subscales	Total sample			Boys			Girls		
	Close relationship to mother	Close relationship to father	Close relationship to God	Close relationship to mother	Close relationship to father	Close relationship to God	Close relationship to mother	Close relationship to father	Close relationship to God
Size of own circle									
r	.04	.03	−.10**	.03	.03	−.18**	.04	.04	.03
p	.06	.11	.00	.21	.33	.00	.11	.23	.38
N	2,639	2,480	1,856	1,371	1,312	933	1,258	1,158	916
Size of other circle									
r	.09**	.15**	.38**	.06*	.11**	.34**	.13**	.19**	.43**
p	.00	.00	.00	.02	.00	.00	.00	.00	.00
N	2,613	2,452	1,684	1,350	1,297	843	1,252	1,144	836
How much is the other-circle bigger than self-circle									
r	.07**	.12**	.36**	.04	.09**	.38**	.10**	.18**	.33**
p	.00	.00	.00	.16	.00	.00	.00	.00	.00
N	2,602	2,444	1,639	1,346	1,295	814	1,246	1,139	820
Distance between circle centers									
r	−.18**	−.25**	−.28**	−.15**	−.20**	−.24**	−.21**	−.33**	−.33**
p	.00	.00	.00	.00	.00	.00	.00	.00	.00
N	2,602	2,444	1,639	1,346	1,295	814	1,246	1,139	820
Relative distance (proportion of distance between circle centers and diameters of the circles)									
r	−.27**	−.32**	−.33**	−.20**	−.26**	−.26**	−.33**	−.40**	−.41**
p	.00	.00	.00	.00	.00	.00	.00	.00	.00
N	2,602	2,444	1,639	1,346	1,295	814	1,246	1,139	820

Note. SSDT = Sixty-Second Drawing Test. *Correlation is significant at the .05 level (two-tailed). **Correlation is significant at the .01 level (two-tailed).

Table 3. Results of regression analyses on predicting attachment to mother, father, and religiosity from the independent variables of the SSDT

Dependent	R^2	β	t	Sig.
Dependent: Mother attachment				
1. Relative distance	.07	−.27	−14.18	.00
2. How much bigger is mother than self	.08	.06	3.10	.00
Dependent: Father attachment				
1. Relative distance	.12	−.34	−17.75	.00
2. How much bigger is father than self	.13	.12	6.10	.00
Dependent: Religiosity				
1. Size of God circle	.14	.31	13.16	.00
2. Relative distance	.18	−.28	−11.45	.00
3. Size of self-circle	.22	−.20	−8.81	.00

Note. SSDT = Sixty-Second Drawing Test.

size difference), father (based on relative distance and size difference), and God (based on distance and size of God circle).

Predicting Depression Scores From the SSDT

In predicting depression scores, indicators of relative distance, sizes in general, and size differences were examined as independent variables in the regression model. The model was significant and accounted for 13% of the variance in depression scores, $F(6, 1,051) = 21.991$, $p < .001$ (see Table 4). As the regression coefficients indicate, depression scores were most strongly associated with a large distance between self- and happiness-circles (β = .22), a small distance between self- and bad-mood circles (β = .18), a relatively large bad-mood circle (β = .14), and a relatively small happiness-circle (β = −.10). Larger distances between one's self-circle and the circle of a rejected person (β = .10) were also associated with higher depression. Finally, big-problem circles (β = .09) and relatively small good-mood circles (β = −.08) were also associated with higher depression. We also ran regression analyses separately for girls and boys. In the case of girls, 18.5% of explained variance arose with linking depression to more distant and smaller happiness circles, less distant and bigger bad mood circles, more distant good-mood circles, bigger problem circles, and smaller school circles. Among boys, explained variance was only 9.5%. Bigger and more distant bad-mood circles, bigger problem circles, and smaller happiness circles were linked to higher depression.

Post hoc power analyses showed that all the aforementioned regressions (including ones with maternal, paternal attachment, relation with God, and depression) had an observed statistical power of 1.0.

Table 4. Regression analyses predicting depression scores from the Sixty-Second Drawing Test

	R^2	β	t	Sig.
Relative distance between self and happiness	.05	.22	7.24	.00
Relative distance between self and bad mood	.01	−.18	−5.91	.00
How much bigger is the self than bad mood	.10	−.14	−4.24	.00
How much bigger is the self than happiness	.11	.10	2.79	.01
Relative distance between self and rejected person	.12	.10	3.16	.00
How much bigger is the self than problem	.12	−.09	−2.64	.01
How much bigger is the self than good mood	.13	.08	2.17	.00

Discussion

The overarching aim of this study was to examine how size and distance indices of the SSDT are associated with quality of close relationships and depression (including low self-esteem). Average self-circle sizes were only weakly related to self-esteem and emotional state, yet the direction of these weak associations confirmed that larger sizes are linked to higher self-esteem and lower depression scores, which are findings consistent with previous research on self-esteem (Bowdin & Bruck, 1960; Gray & Pepitone, 1964; Saneei et al., 2011) and depression (Lewinsohn, 1964).

Regarding the measurement of self–other relations, our results showed that the relative distances and the size of the other-circle emerged as significant predictors. When examining the drawings of mother, father, and God, we found that closer relationships were predicted by drawing the significant other with a larger circle and closer to the self-circle. In the case of mother and father relationships, circle closeness was the most significant predictor of close relationships as measured by questionnaire data. The feeling of deep connection to God was most significantly linked to drawing God as a large circle. This result can likely be explained by the commonsense fact that religious people view God as all-powerful and almighty.

The finding that small distances were predictors of close relationships is in accordance with research by Thomas and Gray (1992) concerning the relative placement of object drawings. By contrast, the fact that we found larger relative sizes of significant others in drawings, which reflects better relationships, contradicts the findings of Thomas and Jolley (1998), who argued that larger drawings accompany perceptions of threatening adults. Regarding the sizes of correlations (and coefficients of determination, R^2 values), for the associations between circle-based and traditional scale-based indices, we found, according to Cohen's (1988) criteria, small effect sizes for self–mother close relationships and medium effect sizes for self-father and self-God relationships. However, a more recent publication on correlation effect sizes (Gignac & Szodorai, 2016) suggested treating correlation coefficients above .30 as relatively large effects. According to this suggestion, we can say that the effect sizes between circle-drawing indices and relations with both father and God were relatively large.

Our results show that although depression was not effectively predicted by the average sizes of the self-circles, there were some specific drawings (self and happiness, self and bad mood, self and good mood, self and big problem) that revealed more reliable associations with depression. The amounts of explained variance were modest, and thus the associations are not robust enough to treat the SSDT as a diagnostic tool for depression. Instead, the relative indices (relative distances and relative sizes) were more predictive of depression, and thus can be viewed as potential markers of depression-related problems. In particular, a relatively close and large bad-mood circle along with a relatively distant and small happiness-circle next to the self-circle were the strongest predictors of higher-than-average depression scores. The total explained variance of the drawing indices in relation to depression can be regarded as having a medium-sized effect according to Cohen (1988) but a relatively large-sized effect according to Gignac and Szodorai (2016).

Wright and McIntyre (1982) emphasized the need to develop standardized administration and rating techniques for drawings to assess depression levels. A general issue in the drawing test field concerns the weak-to-moderate predictive associations (Sims et al., 1983). The strongest correlation between depression, anxiety, measures of affect, and drawing test variables found by Joiner et al. (1996) was an r value of .37, which is very similar to the strongest association in the present study. Predictive associations between the IOS scale (Aron et al., 1992) and traditional self-report questionnaires typically explain around 20% of the variance, which is similar to the highest explained variance in our study (22%), received from a total sample analysis.

Finally, we have to note that there were gender differences in the amount of explained variance, with higher explained variance in the case of girls versus boys. A possible underlying factor for this difference can be a gender difference in expressing emotions through a drawing exercise. Previous research showed that women have greater emotional knowledge and are better at expressing their emotions more fluently and frequently (Brody & Hall, 2000). However, gender differences should be further studied in order to unfold the underlying determinants of these differences. Also, we have to note that lack of measurement invariances can be an underlying reason too, which should be addressed in further research. It should also be considered that traditional univariable or even multivariable statistical methods do not necessarily represent the best approach of understanding projective tests. Vass (1999, 2000, 2004, 2009, 2012) proposed a new paradigm for the interpretation of drawing tests, based on a systems analysis approach: the Seven-Step Configuration Analysis (SSCA). It is a scheme of psychological interpretation derived from studies of human expert thinking.

The SSCA was developed using artificial intelligence (Vass, 2000, 2012) to build a cognitive model of domain-specific expert thinking. Instead of the traditional psychometric approach, the model emphasizes multiple causation: It is not possible to assign certain psychological interpretations to the features of projective drawings in the manner of a dictionary. In other words, a particular feature of a picture may be the effect of several different causes. This also holds true the other way round: A single cause may be expressed in several different features of the picture.

In the SSCA, only configurations are interpreted. A configuration (Vass, 2009) is defined as an item list allocated to a psychological concept with a nonlinear certainty factor. A configuration consists of three components: (1) a psychological concept (an interpretation, e.g., a personality trait); (2) a certainty factor of the psychological concept; and (3) an item list (e.g., unusually small size, light pressure, or cautious behavior). From this systems analysis point of view, our result on the SSDT could be valuable contribution to a future expert system based on the SSCA method.

In summary, the SSDT provides researchers with a series of easily measurable and reliable drawing indices that seem to be associated with both the closeness of relationships and depression. The SSDT entails multiple drawings yet still can be administered quickly. A major strength of the SSDT is that it offers a quick and simple measurement of relationships to different individuals and objects. Because the sizes and distances of circles were the most robust indices, the test can avoid the distorting/confounding effects of drawing skill abilities and intelligence (Lilienfeld, Wood & Garb, 2000; Sims et al., 1983). Another benefit of the SSDT is that it avoids the potential bias caused by social desirability, while still allowing for the possibility of objective scoring. According to our results, the SSDT has potential for helping psychologists who work in school settings, and may be helpful as a brief screening measure of close relationships and depression. This test can be administered to small children, and even to those who cannot yet read or write.

Limitations

Our study has some limitations: The sample consisted of high school students, thus providing only nonclinical data, and we used only self-report instruments without structured interviews or reports from significant others. Further research is needed that (1) controls for demographic variables, (2) addresses the measurement invariances for gender, and (3) examines clinical samples in an effort to replicate our findings. Another limitation that arguably applies to all projective assessments is that the interpretation of scores, despite the use of quantifiable indices, remains somewhat ambiguous (see Lack & Thomason, 2013; Lilienfeld et al., 2000; Thomas & Jolley, 1998). Further psychometric evaluation of size indices should be examined.

Generally speaking, researchers should be cautious when using projective techniques to assist in assessing psychopathology. Regarding the SSDT, an important direction for future research is to elucidate those areas of psychological functioning and psychopathology that the instrument can most validly assess.

References

Abell, S. C., Wood, W., & Liebman, S. J. (2001). Children's human figure drawings as measures of intelligence: The comparative validity of three scoring systems. *Journal of Psychoeducational Assessment, 19*(3), 204–215. https://doi.org/10.1177/073428290101900301

Aron, A., Aron, E. N., & Smollan, D. (1992). Inclusion of other in the self scale and the structure of interpersonal closeness. *Journal of Personality and Social Psychology, 63*(4), 596–612. https://doi.org/10.1037/0022-3514.63.4.596

Bennett, V. (1966). Combinations of figure drawing characteristics related to drawers self-concept. *Journal of Projective Techniques, 30*(2), 192–196. https://doi.org/10.1080/0091651X.1966.10120291

Bertran, A. M. T., & Nistal, M. T. F. (2017). Cultural differences in the emotional indicators of the Two-People Drawing Test. *Rorschachiana, 38*(2), 129–142. https://doi.org/10.1027/1192-5604/a000095

Bowdin, R. F., & Bruck, M. (1960). The adaption and validation of the draw-a-person test as a measure of self concept. *Journal of Clinical Psychology, 16*(4), 427–429. https://doi.org/10.1002/1097-4679(196010)16:4<427::AID-JCLP2270160428>3.0.CO;2-H

Brody, L. R., & Hall, J. A. (2000). Gender, emotion, and expression. In M. Lewis & J. M. Haviland (Eds.), *Handbook of emotions* (pp. 338–349). . Guilford Press.

Burkitt, E., Barrett, M., & Davis, A. (2003). The effect of affective characterisations on the size of children's drawings. *British Journal of Developmental Psychology, 21*(4), 565–584. https://doi.org/10.1348/026151003322535228

Camara, W. J., Nathan, J. S., & Puente, A. E. (2000). Psychological test usage: Implications in professional psychology. *Professional Psychology: Research and Practice, 31*(2), 141–154. https://doi.org/10.1037/0735-7028.31.2.141

Cashel, M. L. (2002). Child and adolescent psychological assessment: Current clinical practices and the impact of managed care. *Professional Psychology: Research and Practice, 33*(5), 446–453. https://doi.org/10.1037/0735-7028.33.5.446

Cohen, J. (1988). *Statistical power analysis for the behavioral sciences.* Routledge.

Dalby, J. T., & Vale, H. L. (1977). Self-esteem and children's human figure drawings. *Perceptual and Motor Skills, 44*(3), 1279–1282. https://doi.org/10.2466/pms.1977.44.3c.1279

Finch, A. J., Saylor, C. F., Edwards, G. L., & McIntosh, J. A. (1987). Children's Depression Inventory: Reliability over repeated administrations. *Journal of Consulting and Clinical Psychology, 16*(4), 339–341. https://doi.org/10.1207/s15374424jccp1604_7

Fisher, J. (2010). Development and application of a spiritual well-being questionnaire called SHALOM. *Religions, 1*(1), 105–121. https://doi.org/10.3390/rel1010105

Fraley, R. C., Heffernan, M. E., Vicary, A. M., & Brumbaugh, C. C. (2011). The experiences in close Relationships – Relationship Structures Questionnaire: A method for assessing attachment orientations across relationships. *Psychological Assessment, 23*(3), 615–625. https://doi.org/10.1037/a0022898

Fraley, R. C., Waller, N. G., & Brennan, K. A. (2000). An item-response theory analysis of self-report measures of adult attachment. *Journal of Personality and Social Psychology, 78*(2), 350–365. https://doi.org/10.1037/0022-3514.78.2.350

Gantt, L. (2001). The formal element art therapy scale: A measurement system for global variables in art. *Art Therapy: Journal of the American Art Therapy Association, 18*(1), 50–55. https://doi.org/10.1080/07421656.2001.10129453

Gignac, G. E., & Szodorai, E. T. (2016). Effect size guidelines for individual differences researchers. *Personality and Individual Differences, 102*, 74–78. https://doi.org/10.1016/j.paid.2016.06.069

Gray, D. M., & Pepitone, A. (1964). Effect of self-esteem on drawings of the human figure. *Journal of Consulting Psychology, 28*(5), 452–455. https://doi.org/10.1037/h0046529

Joiner, T. E., Schmidt, K. L., & Barnett, J. (1996). Size, detail, and line heaviness in children's drawings as correlates of emotional distress: (More) negative evidence. *Journal of Personality Assessment, 67*(1), 127–141. https://doi.org/10.1207/s15327752jpa6701_10

Kovacs, M. (1981). Rating scales to assess depression in school-aged children. *Acta Paedopsychiatrica, 46*, 305–315.

Kovacs, M. (1992). *The Children's Depression Inventory (CDI) manual.* Multi-Health Systems.

Lack, C. W., & Thomason, S. P. (2013). Projective personality assessment of anxiety: A critical appraisal. In D. McKay & E. Storch (Eds.), *Handbook of assessing variants and complications in anxiety disorders* (pp. 203–216). https://doi.org/10.1007/978-1-4614-6452-5_13

Lewinsohn, P. M. (1964). Relationship between height of figure drawings and depression in psychotic patients. *Journal of Consulting Psychology, 28*(4), 380–381. https://doi.org/10.1037/h0040886

Lilienfeld, S. O., Wood, J. M., & Garb, H. N. (2000). The scientific status of projective techniques. *Psychological Science in the Public Interest, 1*(2), 27–66. https://doi.org/10.1111/1529-1006.002

Matto, H. C., Naglieri, J. A., & Clausen, C. (2005). Validity of the Draw-a-Person: screening procedure for emotional disturbance (DAP: SPED) in strengths-based assessment. *Research on Social Work Practice, 15*(1), 41–46. https://doi.org/10.1177/1049731504269553

Ogdon, D. P. (2001). *Psychodiagnostics and personality assessment: A handbook.* Western Psychological Services.

Piotrowski, C. (2015). Projective techniques usage worldwide: A review of applied settings 1995–2015. *Journal of the Indian Academy of Applied Psychology, 41*(3), 9–19.

Prytula, R. E., Phelps, M. R., Morrissey, E. F., & Davis, S. F. (1978). Figure drawing size as a reflection of self-concept or self-esteem. *Journal of Clinical Psychology, 34*(1), 207–214. https://doi.org/10.1002/1097-4679(197801)34:1<207::AID-JCLP2270340144>3.0.CO;2-F

Rodriguez, A., Reise, S. P., & Haviland, M. G. (2016). Applying bifactor statistical indices in the evaluation of psychological measures. *Journal of Personality Assessment, 98*(3), 223–237. https://doi.org/10.1080/00223891.2015.1089249

Salzman, L., & Harway, N. (1967). Size of figure drawings of psychotically depressed patients. *Journal of Abnormal Psychology, 72*(3), 205–207. https://doi.org/10.1037/h0020093

Sandman, C.A., Cauthen, N. R., Kilpatrick, D. G., & Deabler, H. L. (1968). Size of figure drawing in relation to depression. *Perceptual and Motor Skills, 27*(3), 945–946. https://doi.org/10.2466/pms.1968.27.3.945

Saneei, A., Bahrami, H., & Haghegh, S. A. (2011). Self-esteem and anxiety in human figure drawing of Iranian children with ADHD. *The Arts in Psychotherapy, 38*(4), 256–260. https://doi.org/10.1016/j.aip.2011.08.002

Sartori, R. (2010). Face validity in personality tests: psychometric instruments and projective techniques in comparison. *Quality & Quantity, 44*(4), 749–759. https://doi.org/10.1007/s11135-009-9224-0

Sims, J., Dana, R. H., & Bolton, B. (1983). The validity of the Draw-A-Person Test as an anxiety measure. *Journal of Personality Assessment, 47*(3), 250–257. https://doi.org/10.1207/s15327752jpa4703_5

Thomas, G. V., Chaigne, E., & Fox, T. J. (1989). Children's drawings of topics differing in significance: Effects on size of drawing. *British Journal of Developmental Psychology, 7*, 321–331. https://doi.org/10.1111/j.2044-835X.1989.tb00808.x

Thomas, G. V., & Gray, R. (1992). Children's drawings of topics differing in emotional significance: Effects on placement relative to a self drawing. *Journal of Child Psychology and Psychiatry, 33*(6), 1097–1104. https://doi.org/10.1111/j.1469-7610.1992.tb00899.x

Thomas, G. V., & Jolley, R. P. (1998). Drawing conclusions: A re-examination of empirical and conceptual bases for psychological evaluation of children from their drawings. *The British Journal of Clinical Psychology, 37*(2), 127–139. https://doi.org/10.1111/j.2044-8260.1998.tb01289.x

Vass, Z. (1999). La nouvelle perspective de l'examen des dessins projectifs: l'analyse psychométrique avec algorithmes [A new perspective in examining projective drawings: Psychometric analysis with algorithms]. *La Revue Française de Psychiatrie et de Psychologie Médicale, 31*, 94–97.

Vass, Z. (2000). Artificial intelligence in psychodiagnosis. In I. Jakab (Ed.), *Developmental aspects of creativity* (pp. 159–177). American Society of Psychopathology of Expression.

Vass, Z. (2004). Computergestützte Auswertung von Zeichentests [Computerized evaluation of drawing tests]. In W. Sehringer & Z. Vass (Eds.), *Dynamik psychischer Prozesse in Diagnose und Therapie beim Zeichnen und Malen, Wirken und Gestalten, Erzählen und Erfinden. Festschrift für István Hárdi* (pp. 119–143). Flaccus.

Vass, Z. (2009). A new method for configuration analysis in psychology. In *20 years: 1989–2009. The Sasakawa Young Leaders Fellowship Fund in Hungary*. Hungarian Academy of Sciences, Sasakawa Young Leaders Fellowship Fund.

Vass, Z. (2011). *A képi kifejezéspszichológia alapkérdései – szemlélet és módszer* [The basic questions in psychology of visual expression – theories and methods]. L'Harmattan.

Vass, Z. (2012). A psychological interpretation of drawings and paintings. In Z. Vass (Ed.), *The SSCA method: A systems analysis approach* (p. 928). Alexandra Publishing.

Veltman, M. W., & Browne, K. D. (2002). The assessment of drawings from children who have been maltreated: A systematic review. *Child Abuse Review, 11*(1), 19–37. https://doi.org/10.1002/car.712

Weiner, I. B., & Greene, R. L. (2008). *Handbook of personality assessment*. John Wiley & Sons.
Wright, J. H., & McIntyre, M. P. (1982). The Family Drawing Depression Scale. *Journal of Clinical Psychology, 38*(4), 853–861. https://doi.org/10.1002/1097-4679(198210) 38:4<853::AID-JCLP2270380428>3.0.CO;2-R

History

Received June 1, 2020
Revision received November 26, 2020
Accepted December 2, 2020
Published online March 18, 2021

Funding

The preparation of the present article was supported by a university grant from the Károli Gáspár University of Reformed Church (Person- and family-oriented health sciences research group, grant nu.: 20643B800). Data collection was carried out in the frame of a European Union project (TÁMOP-7.2.1-11/K-2012-0004), implemented by the National Institute of Family and Social Politics.

ORCID

Zsuzsanna Kövi
🆔 https://orcid.org/0000-0001-6970-3060

Zsuzsanna Kövi
Bécsi út 324
1037 Budapest
Hungary
kovi.zsuzsanna@kre.hu

Summary

Although clinicians have a long history of using drawings for personality assessment and the evaluation of emotional states and basic attitudes, the empirical validation of drawings has been inconsistent. The goal of this study was to examine the validity of the Sixty-Second Drawing Test (SSDT) in predicting close relationships to parents, God, and depression. The SSDT requires participants to draw a series of circles, where the circles represent the self, significant others, different moods, and God. The respondent has to draw 16 pairs of circles. The respondents can draw circles with different sizes and positions, and the parameters (diameters, vertical and horizontal positions, distances) constitute quantitative indices. In order to measure the validity of these indices, several standardized questionnaires (the Experiences in Close Relationships–Revised and the Children's Depression Inventory) were administered along with the drawing test. Also, several items were used to assess one's relationship with God, including items from the Spiritual Health and Life Orientation Measurement Scale. The sample consisted of 2,883 Hungarian students.

According to our results, drawing indices were significantly linked to scale scores measured by questionnaires. When drawing circles to represent one's self and one's parents, small distances and relatively large parent-circles marked better relationships with parents. Individuals with closer relationship to God, drew God as a larger circle that was situated closer to one's self-circle. Depression was indicated by drawing large bad-mood circles that were close to one's self-circle, along with small happiness-circles that were distant from one's self-circle. The magnitudes of all associations were small to moderate, with explained variances ranging from 7.6% to 21.9%. The results suggest that drawings of circles can be used to represent important object-relations. The sizes and positions of the drawings can, to some extent, predict interpersonal attachment, relationship to God, and depressive symptoms. Although we do not advocate using the SSDT as a clinical diagnostic measure, it can serve as a useful screening tool for identifying potential relational and affective difficulties.

Összefoglalás

Bár a klinikusok már régóta használnak rajzteszteket a személyiség, az érzelmi állapotok és az alapvető attitűdök mérésére, a tesztek validitására vonatkozó kutatási eredmények nem egybehangzóak. A tanulmányunk célja az volt, hogy megvizsgáljuk a hatvan másodperces rajzteszt (Sixty Second Drawing Test, SSDT) érvényességét a szülőkkel való szoros kapcsolat, az Istennel való kapcsolat és a depresszió előrejelzésében. Az SSDT feladatban a résztvevők köröket rajzolnak, ahol a körök képviselik az ént, a jelentős másokat, a különböző hangulatokat és Istent. A válaszadónak 16 pár kört kell rajzolnia. A válaszadók különböző méretű köröket rajzolhatnak, különböző pozíciókban, és a paraméterek (átmérők, függőleges és vízszintes pozíciók, távolságok) könnyen lemérhető kvantitatív indexeket jelentenek. Ezen indexek érvényességének mérése érdekében számos standard kérdőívet (a Gyermek depresszió kérdőív, A közvetlen kapcsolatok élményei – kapcsolati struktúrák (ECR-RS) kötődési kérdőív) a rajzteszttel együtt lettek felvéve. Emellett számos tételt használtunk az Istennel való kapcsolat mérésére, beleértve a spirituális lelki egészség és az életorientáció kérdőív egyes tételeit is. A minta 2883 magyar diákból állt.

Eredményeink szerint a rajzindexek szignifikánsan kapcsolódtak a kérdőívek által mért skálákhoz. A saját- és szülő-körök közti kis távolságok és a szülő-körök relatív nagysága jelezték előre a kérdőíven elért magas kötődési pontszámot. Az Istenhez közelebb álló egyének Istent egy nagyobb körként rajzolták, közelebb saját magukhoz. A depressziót nagy, én-körhöz közeli, „rossz hangulatot" ábrázoló körök, valamint távol eső kicsi boldogság-körök jelezték előre. A feltárt kapcsolatok erőssége kicsi vagy közepes volt, a megmagyarázott variancia 7,6% és 21,9% között mozogtak.

Az eredmények arra utalnak, hogy a körök paraméterei alkalmasak arra, hogy bizonyos mértékben előrejelezzék a hosszabb kérdőívekkel is felmérhető konstruktumokat. A rajzok méretei és pozíciói bizonyos mértékig előre jelezhetik az interperszonális kötődést, az Istennel való kapcsolatot és a depressziós tüneteket. Bár az SSDT klinikai diagnózisra nem alkalmas, hasznos szűrőeszközként szolgálhat az interperszonális kapcsolati problémák és érzelmi nehézségek veszélyének megállapításánál.

Résumé

Bien qu'il existe une longue histoire de psychologues cliniciens utilisant des dessins pour évaluer la personnalité, des états émotionnels et des attitudes de base, leur validation empirique est incohérente.

Le but de cet essai était d'examiner la validité du Test de Dessin de Soixante Secondes (the Sixty Second Drawing Test (SSDT)) pour prédire la relation étroite avec les parents, la relation avec Dieu et la dépression. Le test a requis que les participants dessinent une série de cercles, où les cercles représentent le soi, les autres significatifs, les humeurs différentes et Dieu. Les participants ont dû dessiner des cercles dessiner 16 paires de cercles. Les cercles peuvent être de tailles et de positions

                                   Rorschachiana (2021), 42(1), 52–71

différentes, les paramètres (diamètres, positions verticales et horizontales, distances) constituent des indices quantitatifs. Afin de mesurer la validité du questionnaire, plusieurs autres questionnaires standardisés (Les Expériences Dans Les Relations Étroites - révisé et L'Inventaire de Dépression de L'Enfant) ont été utilisés dans la recherche. En plus, plusieurs éléments du Questionnaire Sur La Santé Spirituelle et le Test d'Orientation de Vie ont été utilisés pour mesurer la relation de l'individu avec Dieu. L'échantillon était composé de 2883 étudiants hongrois.

Selon les résultats, les indices de dessin étaient significativement liés aux scores d'échelle mesurés par les questionnaires. En cas de dessin de cercles pour représenter soi-même et ses parents, de petites distances et des cercles de parents relativement grands marquaient de meilleures relations avec les parents. Les individus ayant une relation plus étroite avec Dieu l'ont dessiné comme un cercle plus grand qui était situé plus près de leurs propres cercles. La dépression a été indiquée en dessinant de grands cercles de mauvaise humeur proches de leurs propres cercles, ainsi que de petits cercles de bonheur qui étaient éloignés des leurs. L'ampleur de toutes les associations était petite à modérée, avec les variances expliquées de 7,6% à 21,9%.

Les résultats suggèrent que les dessins de cercles peuvent être utilisés pour représenter des relations d'objet importantes. La taille et la position des dessins peuvent, dans une certaine mesure, prédire l'attachement interpersonnel, la relation avec Dieu et les symptômes dépressifs. Bien que nous n'avons pas préconisé l'utilisation du SSDT comme mesure diagnostique clinique, le test peut servir d'outil de dépistage utile pour identifier les difficultés relationnelles et affectives potentielles.

Resumen

Aunque los psicólogos clínicos tienen una larga historia con el uso de dibujos para la evaluación de la personalidad, la evaluación de estados emocionales y actitudes básicas, su validación empírica ha sido inconsistente. El objetivo de este estudio fue examinar la validez de la Sixty Second Drawing Test (SSDT – Prueba de Dibujo de Sesenta Segundos) para predecir las correlaciones entre la relación cercana con los padres, la relación con Dios y la depresión. El SSDT requiere que los participantes dibujen una serie de círculos, donde los círculos representan a sí mismos, a los seres queridos, diferentes estados de ánimo y a Dios. La persona tiene que dibujar 16 pares de círculos. Pueden dibujar círculos con diferentes tamaños y posiciones, y durante el proceso de evaluación, estos parámetros (diámetros, posiciones verticales y horizontales, distancias) constituirán los índices cuantitativos. Para medir la validez de estos índices, se administraron varios cuestionarios estandarizados: Experiences in Close Relationships – Revised (Experiencias con Relaciones Cercanas – Versión Revisada) y Children's Depression Inventory (el Inventario de Depresión Infantil) con la prueba de dibujo. Además, se usaron varios ítems para evaluar la relación de los encuestados con Dios, incluidos los ítems de la cuestionario Spiritual Health and Life Orientation Measurement Scale (Escala de Medición de Salud Espiritual y Orientación de Vida). La muestra consistió en 2883 estudiantes húngaros.

Según nuestros resultados, los índices de dibujos se vincularon significativamente con los puntajes de cuestionarios. Al dibujar círculos para representarse a uno mismo y a sus padres, las distancias pequeñas y los círculos de padres relativamente grandes marcaban mejores relaciones con los padres. Las personas con una relación más cercana con Dios, dibujaron a Dios como un círculo más grande que estaba situado más cerca del propio círculo personal. La depresión se indicaba dibujando grandes círculos de mal humor que estaban cerca del círculo de uno mismo, y con pequeños círculos de felicidad que estaban lejos del círculo de uno mismo. Las magnitudes de todas las asociaciones fueron pequeñas a moderadas, con variaciones explicadas que van desde el 7,6% al 21,9%.

Los resultados sugieren que se puede usar los dibujos de círculos para representar importantes relaciones de objeto. Los tamaños y las posiciones de los dibujos pueden, en cierta medida, predecir el apego interpersonal, la relación con Dios y los síntomas depresivos. Aunque no recomendamos utilizar el SSDT como una medida de diagnóstico clínico, puede servir como una herramienta útil para identificar posibles dificultades relacionales y afectivas.

要約

臨床家がパーソナリティアセスメント、感情状態や基本的な態度の評価に描画を使用してきた長い歴史があるが、描画の経験的検証には、一貫性がなかった。本研究の目的は、親との親密な関係、神、及びうつ病の予測における60秒描画テスト（SSDT）の妥当性を検討することであった。SSDTでは、参加者は一連の円を書くことを要求され、円は自己、重要な他者、異なる気分、および神を表している。回答者は16個の円を描かなければならない。回答者は異なるサイズと位置の円を描くことができ、パラメータ（直径、垂直と水平の位置、距離）は定量的な指標を構成する。これらの指標の妥当性を測定するために、いくつかの標準化された質問票（親密な関係の経験―改訂版および子どもの抑うつ目録）が描画テストと一緒に実施された。また、神との関係を評価するために、スピリチュアル・ヘルスおよびライフ・オリエンテーション測定尺度の項目を含むいくつかの項目を使用した。サンプルは、ハンガリーの学生2,883人であった。

その結果、円を描く指標はアンケート調査で測定された尺度の得点と優位に関連していた。自己と親を表す円を描く場合、親との距離が小さく、親の円が比較的大きいほど、親との関係は良好であることが示された。神との関係が近い人は、自分の円に近い位置にある大きな円として神を描いていた。うつ病は、自己中心に近い大きな不機嫌な円と、自己中心から離れた小さな幸福な円を描くことで示された。すべての関連性の大きさは小さいか中程度で、説明された分散は7.6％から21.9％の範囲であった。

この結果は、円の絵が重要な対象関係を表すために使用できることを示唆している。円の絵の大きさと位置は、対人愛着、神との関係、および抑うつ症状をある程度予測することができる。われわれは、臨床診断尺度としてSSDTを使用することを提唱しているわけではないが、潜在的な関係性や感情的な困難を特定するための有用なスクリーニング・ツールとして役立てることができる。

Research Article

Motherhood Specificities With the Rorschach Method

Results of a Nonconsulting French Population in the Postnatal Phase

Rose-Angélique Belot[1] , Marie-Christine Pheulpin[2],
Pacal Roman[3], Margaux Bouteloup[1], Mathilde Pointurier[1,3],
Diane Paez[1], Nicolas Mottet[4,5], and Denis Mellier[1]

[1]Psychology Laboratory EA3188, University of Bourgogne Fanche-Comté, Besançon, France
[2]UTRPP Laboratory, University Paris XIII, Paris, France
[3]LARPSYDIS Laboratory, Institute of Psychology, University of Lausanne, Switzerland
[4]Nanomedicine Laboratory, Imagery and Therapeutics, EA4662, University of Franche-Comté, Besançon, France
[5]Department of Obstetrics and Gynecology, University Hospital Jean Minjoz Besançon, University of Franche-Comté, Besançon, France

Abstract: Motherhood, listed by the World Health Organization as a period of fragility and vulnerability, involves significant changes at the individual, family and social level. Becoming a mother entails a number of risk factors to take into account. It is therefore necessary to carry out studies on general populations not suffering from psychopathological disorders to better understand these risk factors linked to motherhood. This study was carried out in France with a nonconsulting population in the postnatal phase (N = 30) using the Rorschach test, as it presents numerous advantages to appreciate the psychic and corporeal transformations linked to birth. The quantitative results of the test were compared with recently updated norms (De Tychey et al., 2012). Eight values of the psychogram remained normative (F%, F+%, W%, Dd%, M, C, H%, P) reflecting the characteristics of a general population; conversely, eight other values of the psychogram (R, D%, S%, A%, RC%, m, E, Anguish Index%) differed significantly from general population norms. These results increase knowledge to help appreciate the complexity of the psychic processes at work during the postnatal period, and to prevent psychopathological disorders. It is thus possible to distinguish these disorders from those that are transitory and classically linked to the upheaval caused by the onset of motherhood.

Keywords: motherhood, postpartum, Rorschach

Motherhood is a particularly sensitive period, as it involves substantial changes for the individual, her family, and society as a whole, as well as numerous psychological adjustments (Gutiérrez-Zotes et al., 2016). Additionally, it is an important

Rorschachiana (2021), 42(1), 72–92
https://doi.org/10.1027/1192-5604/a000137

© 2021 Hogrefe Publishing

phase in terms of rearrangement of identity. This period can be marked by a number of disorders, which can vary significantly in severity. The "baby blues" affect 60–85% of Western women after the birth of their child (Dayan et al., 2002), postnatal depression affects 15–20% of Western women (De Tychey et al., 2005; Evans et al., 2001), and postpartum psychosis affects 0.2–0.5% of women in France (Dayan & Graignic-Philippe, 2011). Postnatal depression, in particular, is classified among the 20 most frequent and disabling illnesses according to the World Health Organization. It has been established that the risk of psychotic decompensation is much greater immediately postpartum and if the woman is primiparous (Kendell et al., 1981).

Disorders specifically linked to maternity seem to be largely underestimated according to professionals (gynecologists, obstetricians, midwives). This is also linked to the idealization of motherhood in society, in which motherhood is perceived as bringing total fulfilment. In fact, new motherhood comprises numerous readjustments: corporeal and intrapsychic, as well as environmental and contextual. For example, during pregnancy, women experience psychic life, bodily, and hormonal mutations and transformations, which bring about alterations in sleeping and eating patterns (McConnel & Daston, 1961; Fan et al., 2009). The mother's sleep is also disturbed during the first weeks, even the first few months, postpartum on account of the numerous feeds and responses to the baby's needs.

Furthermore, the birth can engender a number of obstetric incidents as well as minor complaints. It can often induce a traumatic dimension in the mother and a state of posttraumatic stress disorder (PTSD; 5% after 1 month postpartum, Denis et al., 2011). Excessive worrying and generalized anxiety have been studied in primiparous women in the postnatal phase and were found to affect 32% in a sample of 68 women (Wenzel et al., 2003). A recent study of primiparous women (Georges et al., 2013) showed that 18.8% presented with symptoms of acute anxiety before the birth, and this figure increased after the birth.

Moreover, anxiety during pregnancy impairs the complete recovery of the mother and can be a factor in the development of postnatal depression (Altshuler et al., 2008). Indeed, a study (Skouteris et al., 2009) showed that women who have a high level of stress at the end of the pregnancy are more likely to develop postnatal depression. In the postnatal period, the encounter with the baby can be the source of multiple worries linked to expected parenting ability, to the vulnerability of the baby, and to its many needs and the care it requires.

The literature review indicates a lack of recent studies of the postnatal phase using the Rorschach test among a population of women with no mental disorders. Only two very dated studies (Connell & Daston, 1961; Klatskin & Eron, 1970) demonstrate results with the Rorschach test in the postnatal period. Other studies using the Rorschach methodological tool are concerned with pregnancy (Bellion, 2001), a specific psychopathological register (depression; De Tychey et al., 1997), infertility (Setan et al., 2001), or pregnancy denial (Milden et al., 1985).

Motherhood is a unique life event that mobilizes psychological work of a particularly dense and unprecedented nature. It is therefore important to observe the postnatal psychological, corporeal, and hormonal processes outside of any psychopathological context in a general population using the Rorschach test.

Relevance of the Rorschach Test and the Mother's Psychic Life in the Postnatal Phase

During pregnancy and in the postpartum period, the interior/exterior boundaries, internal workings, and psychic life modifications of the individual are in great demand and require the mother to carry out a large amount of psychological work. The Rorschach test is an ideal tool for understanding the implications of the psychological modifications that underlie this work during the postpartum period. The Rorschach test allows us to visualize the peculiarities of the internal world and the intensity of projective movements during this period. Indeed, it promotes the updating of the internal reality of the individual, of their body image, of their representation of self and representations related to early relationships. This is all the more interesting as these elements are particularly present and at work during the postnatal phase. The cards, which are, according to Chabert (1987):

> Symmetric about one axis, make demands about the body of the participant, who projects the meaning of the images. This process gives structure to the representation of the self in its primordial essence – testing in particular the solidity of its limits and the differentiation between that which is internal and that which is external. (p. 142)

During pregnancy and in the postpartum phase, the woman's body, psychic envelope, and internal/external limits are particularly mobilized and modified, meaning that the mother carries out large-scale work on her psychic life.

The fusional relationship that unites a mother and her baby in the early period has been described by Winnicott as a very particular psychic life state sometimes approaching madness. This primary maternal preoccupation (Winnicott, 1956/1975), which is systematically accompanied by a diminished interest in social interactions, can therefore have as a corollary a decrease on the Rorschach test of the classic indicators of socialization and a simultaneous increase in human responses.

We hypothesized that in a population of women free of mental disorders and with no complications during the pregnancy and the birth, normal psychological functioning would be modified by the motherhood process. This could be assessed using the Rorschach test by comparing the quantitative results (psychogram) of nonconsulting women in the postnatal phase with adult norms (N = 310; De Tychey et al., 2012).

The norms of De Tychey et al. (2012) are representative of the general French population, divided into three age groups (25–39 years: N = 114; 40–54 years: N = 121; 55–65 years: N = 75), two sex groups (male: N = 140; female: N = 170), four groups according to marital status (single: N = 108; married: N = 172; divorced: N = 24; widower: N = 6), and three socio-professional category (CSP) groups (privileged: N = 128; intermediate: N = 62; disadvantaged: N = 120). The average age of the 310 subjects was 45.5 years (SD = 5.5).

Our exclusively female population was compared with the normative Rorschach population made up of men and women. The work of De Tychey et al. showed no statistical differences related to sex, and thus comparison with an all-female population was not necessary.

We decided to operationalize this hypothesis by estimating the effect on each quantitative Rorschach factor of the normal modification of psychic life functioning postpartum according to the description of this period in the literature and comparing this with the general population. We developed the operationalization in three ways:

1. Factors we estimated within the range of the normative data;
2. Factors we estimated to be superior to the normative data; and
3. Factors we estimated to be lower than the normative data.

Factors Estimated Within the Range of Normative Data
Considering that we had a population of women free of mental disorders, we expected to find a good adaptation to the external reality and thus to have the F+%, the Dd%, and the number of popular responses (P) within the norms.

Factors Estimated to Be Above Normative Data
Because of the mother–baby unit created by the birth and the encounter with the baby (Winnicott, 1956), we estimated that W%, S%, and F% would be increased. The creation of the mother–baby unit is linked to the construction of a whole and the necessity to strengthen the limits of the Ego. Moreover, because the postpartum phase is considered a more acutely sensitive and receptive period (Deutsch, 1933; Racamier, 1979), we hypothesized that color responses (C) and shading responses (E), and therefore also RC% (the number of responses to the pastel cards), would be significantly increased. Because of the presence of the baby

and the regressive context of the postbirth period, we expected to obtain more animal (A%) and human (H%) responses. Finally, anxiety is habitually detected in the postnatal period (Capponi & Horbacz, 2005), thus we expected to have an increased Anguish Index. The Anguish Index (AI%) is calculated as follows: (Partial human response (Hd) + Anatomic responses + Gender responses + Blood and Sex responses)/total number of protocols × 100.

Factors Estimated to Be Lower Than Normative data
Because the mother is mobilized in her dyadic adjustments (Stern, 1985), which require an additional effort of psychic life work (Belot, 2014), we hypothesized that the psychic life functioning would be saturated and inhibited. We therefore expected to have a lower number of responses (R) and movement responses (M and m), which are three indicators of capacity to deal with internal and external excitations according to the Parisian School (Chabert, 1983). We also expected that the focus on the baby will lead to less frequent detailed location responses (D%), linked to the increase in other locations of the answers.

Method

This study was approved by the local clinical ethics committee (number: P/2019/434). It obtained all legal authorizations and was registered (research not under the jurisdiction of the French "Jardé law": hospital certification number ISO900:v2015).

Inclusion Criteria

The participants were recruited out according to the following inclusion criteria.
1. Women living in a couple with the child's father. The child was desired by the couple.
2. Absence of complications during the pregnancy and the birth.
3. Women without psychopathological disorders at the clinical interview. (The research interviews carried out by a clinical psychologist confirm the absence of proven psychopathological disorders.) Absence of psychotropic medication.
4. Full-term baby without acute fetal suffering, without any intrauterine growth restriction, and whose state of health at birth required no particular medical assistance.
5. Women having experienced pregnancy and labor without obstetrical complications or somatic illness.

Recruitment of women took place through gynecologists and midwives. The postnatal follow-up gynecologist or midwife proposed the study to the participant after verification of the strict inclusion criteria on specialized medical software. Midwives have access to a database that allows them to find out if there is a history of mental health issues. If the participant fulfilled the inclusion criteria, the gynecologist or midwife proposed the study. If agreed, the research psychologist telephoned the participant to arrange a home appointment.

A clinical research interview was always carried out before the presentation of the Rorschach test to verify the absence of psychopathological disorders. Data collection took place exclusively at the participant's home. This allowed the participant to stay with her baby and to not travel unnecessarily, which reduced her anxiety and prioritized her organization of daily living activities, while encouraging participation in the study. A debrief interview was systematically offered to the participant after the end of the research data collection. Out of the 32 women who requested to participate, two were not accepted in the study (due to separation of the couple and social difficulties). For this study, it was important for all participants to be emotionally, socially, and relationally stable, and to be involved in a stable relationship with their husband or partner. Sociodemographic data were obtained for all patients including age, educational level, and professional status (see Table 1).

No refusal to participate in this study was recorded. All participants gave their written informed consent. The assessment was conducted from 3 to 16 weeks after the birth. As such, all the women remained very close to what is habitually called the "post-natal period" and belonged to a "general population". In addition, follow-up of these women by midwives and the physician after the study confirmed that no participant presented with any psychopathological disorder during the year following the birth of their child.

The sample was composed of 30 French women including 18 primiparous women. All participants were between 24 and 37 years old (average age: 31). All were living as a couple with the father of the child (average age: 33) and the pregnancy was desired. All the socio-professional categories were evenly represented in our population (French CSP classification from 2 to 6) according to the current INSEE criteria (National Institute for Statistics & Economic Studies in France). All personal details were anonymized.

Each response to the Rorschach cards was scored according to the criteria and technical standards of the Parisian School (Azoulay, et al., 2012; Chabert, 1983). This approach has positive psychometric indicators in France (Azoulay et al., 2007). Initially, scoring was done by the administrator.

The most difficult responses were checked with the other projective method specialist colleagues who coauthored this article and teach the projective methods at Université Paris René Descartes. They are graduates of the Parisian School with

Table 1. Demographic characteristics of the group

Demographic characteristics	Women ($N = 30$)
Number of children before this pregnancy	
Primiparous (0 child)	60%
1 Child	26.6%
2 Children	13.3%
Age: *Mean* (years)	33
Educational level	
GNVQ Intermediate or under	23.3%
High-school diploma	23.3%
Bachelor's degree	33.3%
Degree higher than bachelor's	20%
Family status	
Single	0%
Common-law couple	20%
Married	46.6%
PACS	33.3%

Note. PACS = civil union in France.

a "Diplôme Universitaire de Psychologie Projective" (DUPP; this university diploma is a 2-year complementary training on projective methods). They are also experienced Rorschach users who have been using the test for research purposes for many years. The psychogram results of our population were compared with the current norms of the Rorschach test (De Tychey et al., 2012).

Data Analysis

SPPS version 20.0 was used in all quantitative analyses. We performed a two-tailed one-sample Student test (*t*) to compare our averages with the standards of De Tychey et al. (2012). We also report the Cohen's *d* statistic as a measure of effect size.

Results

General Comments

A comparison between the clinical group and the adult norms ($N = 30$) is provided in Table 2. Of the 16 indications of the Rorschach psychogram, eight indications did not diverge from the current standards of the French population (De Tychey et al., 2012) and were not significant: These indications appear not to be modified by the context of motherhood. The other half of the indications diverge from the norms with a high threshold of significance ($p < .05$ for one indication and $p < .01$ for seven indications), showing that in spite of our relatively small group size, there is a statistical validity in our results. Some results validated what we expected with the operationalization we proposed for the examination of the psychic life functioning of nonconsulting women in the postnatal phase. Other results were surprising because they did not match our expectations.

Results That Were Expected According to Our Operationalization

Factors Within the Range of the Normative Data

We observed a number of popular responses within the norms: P = 4.47 on average in our sample for a norm of 4.83, $t(29) = -1.41$, $p = .168$, $d = -0.258$; a nonsignificant F+%, 65.27 on average versus a norm of 60.86, $t(29) = 1.19$, $p = .244$, $d = 0.217$; and a normative Dd%, 3.25 on average versus a norm of 3.13, $t(29) = 0.14$, $p = .892$, $d = 0.025$. These results reflect the norms of the classic nonconsulting population and confirm that our population is suitable, with a well-adjusted relationship to exterior reality.

Factors Significantly Different From the Normative Data

As expected, we noticed that some factors were significantly weaker than in the general population: D%, mean 49.61% instead of the expected 57.24, $t(29) = -3.71$, $p < .001$, $d = -0.677$; small movements, Sum m = 1.87 on average versus a norm of 3.82, $t(29) = -8.36$, $p < .001$, $d = -1.527$; and R, mean 23.47, instead of the expected 28.16, $t(29) = -2.91$, $p = .007$, $d = -0.531$. The quantity of representations mobilized within this group is therefore reduced. The RC% was significantly higher in our group, 39.7 on average versus a norm of 35.94, $t(29) = 2.23$, $p = .03$, $d = 0.407$, as was the S%, 3.98 on average versus a norm of 1.99, $t(29) = 3.41$, $p = .002$, $d = 0.622$. Finally, the index of anxiety (Anguish Index%) was very clearly higher in our population: 25.77 on average versus a norm of 13.3, $t(29) = 4.65$, $p < .001$, $d = 0.849$.

Results That Were Not Expected According to Our Operationalization

Factors Within the Range of the Normative Data That Were Expected to Be Significantly Different

Contrary to what we expected, the number of human movement responses was not lower than but was close to the norm, Sum M = 2.33 on average versus a norm of 2.42, $t(29) = -0.28$, $p = .781$, $d = -0.051$. The W% score, 41.54 on average

Table 2. Comparison of Rorschach variable means with adult norms

Rorschach variable	M (SD)	Standards	t(19)	p	Cohen's d
R	23.47 (8.83)	28.16	−2.91	.007	−0.531
W%	41.54 (15.87)	36.83	1.63	.115	0.297
D%	49.61 (11.27)	57.24	−3.71	.000	−0.677
Dd%	3.25 (4.97)	3.13	0.14	.892	0.025
S%	3.98 (3.20)	1.99	3.41	.002	0.622
F%	60.81 (16.32)	57.81	1.01	.322	0.184
F+%	65.27 (20.33)	60.86	1.19	.244	0.217
A%	36.29 (12.29)	42.55	−2.79	.009	−0.509
H%	15.42 (10.26)	15.85	−0.23	.822	−0.041
Anguish Index %	25.77 (14.68)	13.30	4.65	.000	0.849
Sum M	2.33 (1.69)	2.42	−0.28	.781	−0.051
Sum m	1.87 (1.28)	3.82	−8.36	.000	−1.527
Sum C	2.92 (2.16)	3.36	−1.12	.271	−0.205
Sum E	0.28 (0.63)	1.04	−6.63	.000	−1.210
RC%	39.70 (9.24)	35.94	2.23	.034	0.407
P	4.47 (1.41)	4.83	−1.41	.168	−0.258

versus a norm of 36.83, $t(29) = 1.63$, $p = .115$, $d = 0.297$, was likewise normative, as were the H%, 15.42 on average versus a norm of 15.85, $t(29) = −0.23$, $p = .822$, $d = −0.041$, and the F%, 60.81 on average versus a norm of 57.81, $t(29) = 1.01$, $p = .322$, $d = 0.184$, while we had hypothesized that these factors would be increased. We also noted a normative number of color responses, Sum C = 2.92 on average where the norm is 3.36, $t(29) = −1.12$, $p = .271$, $d = −0.205$. This result is surprising because we hypothesized that the hypersensitivity of the subjects in our group of postpartum mothers would increase this index.

*Factors Significantly Different From the Normative Data
and Contrary to What We Expected*
Finally, two indications differed from the norms but were in contrast to our expectations. We thought that the shading responses and A% would be increased. The significantly lower number of (E) shading responses is a surprising result given the mother's state of sensitivity in this postnatal period, 0.28 on average in our sample for a norm at 1.04, $t(29) = −6.63$, $p < .001$, $d = −1.210$). Another unexpected result was the diminished value of A%, 36.29 on average compared with a norm of 42.55, $t(29) = −2.79$, $p = .009$, $d = −0.509$, while we had hypothesized that the postnatal period would be conducive to psychic life regression regarding animal content.

Qualitative Results: Response Contents Without Normative Data

Even though we did not specifically operationalize the response contents because there are no normative data with which to compare them, we were surprised to find specific contents in numerous protocols. Anatomic responses appeared clearly and in large numbers. We counted 21 responses with "uterus" and "cervix," 16 "pelvis" responses, two "sonography" responses, and 10 "birth-giving" responses. They are of a "sexual" or "visceral" type, but "object" responses related to sonography were also given.

The non-symbolized nature of the anatomic responses concerned 14 of the 30 protocols. The responses ranged from "less symbolized" in the majority of the protocols (visceral and sexual responses) to "highly symbolized" in four protocols, with responses such as "the passage," "a cavity open at the top and closed at the bottom," "a cavern with an entrance," "symbolic opening and closing," example, "a zip." The non-symbolized responses observed for the Rorschach test mostly concerned primiparous women. Indeed, 11 out of the 18 primiparous participants gave more of this type of response than other types of response. Some of the response contents were specific and were directly related to the conception phase and to female anatomy (22 responses concerned the "female sexual organ" and 17 responses included "ovaries," "fallopian tubes," or "vagina"). Blood responses were quasi-nonexistent, while the sexual responses, "vagina, uterus, cervix, ovaries, labia, period," were predominant. We likewise noted a strong prevalence of visceral responses in the protocols "inside of a belly, heart, lungs, inside the body, organs, etc."

The theme of birth (animal or human) concerned 18 of the 30 protocols. Conception and implantation were also evoked: "a baby in its mother's belly" (eight responses). The real presence of the baby was evoked (17 "baby" responses, eight protocols).

Finally, even if the number of shading responses (E) was low, we noted that when this type of response was present, it concerned texture shading. We only noted one diffusion response on Card III: "smoke rising from the pot there." All other shading responses were texture shading, for example: Card I, "a hairy black butterfly"; Card III, "two birds with their feathers"; Card IV, "a kind of hairy beast"; Card V, "a beast with lots of hair"; Card VI, "a rug-shaped animal skin." Texture responses characterize tactile sensitivity and indicate the reactivation of very early experiences in relationships, particularly the quality of the infant environment. Also, the presence of this type of response shows that new motherhood is indeed a context linked to early childhood reactivation.

Discussion

A Psychic Life Functioning That Remains Adapted

Despite the recognized habitual phase of primary maternal preoccupation, our participants presented an adequate relationship with external reality (normative F+%) and maintained normal perceptual control (normative F%). The adequate number of popular responses (P) shows that we are studying a population where the socialization is no different from that of a classic general population.

The nonsignificantly reduced number of human movement responses (M) demonstrates the preservation of thinking capacities among the women. Psychological work and reflexivity remain proficient, but nevertheless more difficult for certain criteria. In effect, a high kinesthesis score clearly reflects the presence of a transitional space and the participants' capacities for development of their psychic life via the Rorschach (Chabert, 1983). The normative human responses (H%) show the participants' capacities for creation and mentalization. These results confirm the fact that we are indeed dealing with a general population.

With regard to F%, we believe the presence of formal control demonstrates efforts to master the reality linked to the desire to control instinctual impulses. It also shows how much these women put up internal boundaries to guarantee the integrity of the Self.

We also note the relatively high number of human movement responses, normative (M), whereas the small movements (m) were seemingly absent in our group. This is interesting because it shows that in these women in the postnatal phase, the intensity of the underlying and identifying investments is turned more toward the human, rather than toward the animal or objects. Finally, all of these indications remain normative and confirm that we are dealing with a nonconsulting population that does not suffer from any proven psychopathological disorder. This population does, however, show aspects of fragility of the psyche that should be taken into account.

Specificities That Should Be Taken Into Account in the Postpartum Period

General Indications

We draw attention first and foremost to the reduced number of responses (R) of our group, which was significantly lower than the norm. The work of putting ideas into words that is required by the presentation of the Rorschach cards was more difficult for this group of participants in the postpartum phase. We hypothesize that confrontation with the Rorschach test mobilizes archaic elements not yet formulated in words and shareable representations. Primary maternal preoccupation (Winnicott, 1956) hinders the mother's psychological work (her available psychological representations are weaker). The R translates the quantity of the representations available. In the postpartum period, in fact, the number of responses to the Rorschach is significantly lower. The archaic elements are more present during the postpartum period. This is visualized in the Rorschach by the significantly lower "Sum m and Sum E" indications and by a significantly higher RC% index. We observe dominant regression processes with the significantly higher index S% (Dbl) as well as the RC%. The regression phenomenon is also proven with the significant weakness of the Sum m and E indications. These indications also show the weakness of psychological work.

Our clinical experiments among women who had given birth recently showed us that the psychological work is more laborious during this period. The representations are therefore more difficult to express, which explains the significantly reduced number of R responses. The intensity of the transformations that occur in this phase of life (Belot, 2014) confirms a context of saturation in terms of the mother's psychic life, a weaker investment in external reality, and a centering on the internal world.

Although we observed a lesser investment in the activity of representations (significantly low R), the number of responses to the pastel cards (RC%) increased significantly. In effect, the average of the RC% of our group highlights an increased permeability compared with the norm and the hypersensitivity of the participants in our group of postpartum mothers. However, the number of color responses (C) remained within the norms. Women in the postnatal phase are very sensitive to situations that encourage regressive tendencies without leading to psychic disorganization, as shown by F% and F+%, which are normative.

The earliest and most archaic material brought to the surface by the Rorschach is expressed by the *shading* responses named "E." For this operation, the flexibility of the psychological apparatus is brought into play. The texture shading we described in the qualitative results clearly indicates the mother's sensitivity and investment in corporeal experiences, such as skin-to-skin contact with her baby. We assume that this result is related to the difficulty of psychological work and the reduced availability of mothers during this period – they are very concerned with the concrete and constant care for their babies. The shading E responses appear later because the archaic materials later manage to make their way through the psyche.

Modes of Approach

Although the W% is within the norms we observe a sensitivity to emptiness and to absence, shown in the significantly higher number of S% responses. The increase in this type of response can be connected to the increased feeling of emptiness after the birth of the baby. The aspects of fullness and completeness in the final stages of pregnancy end brutally with the birth of the baby and loss of the fetus. Moreover, encountering and adjusting to the baby can also present the mother with new difficulties, which can relate to the unknown.

The significant increase in S% responses can also be connected to mourning for the imaginary child and the reactivation of the infantile in the mother, or the necessity of regression to adjust to the needs of her baby and the newness of the relational experience.

Certain defense mechanisms, such as isolation, are reduced (number of D responses in our protocols was smaller than in a classic population). These aspects can be linked to a defense against reactivation of undesirable instinctual movements but can also be related to the specific nature of the primary maternal preoccupation and the mother–baby unit in the postnatal period.

In addition, we know that the increased internal and external excitation during the postnatal phase can engender difficulties to think in mothers. The mother's internal psychic life reality is subjected to great pressure on account of the internal and external modifications she faces. The mother accepts the birth event from multiple angles. Several studies (Belot, 2014; Belot et al., 2016) show the weakness of the maternal excitation barrier system because the mother must adapt to a new lifestyle and simultaneously manage the emotional regulation of her baby.

Not only does the new mother encounter her baby but, prior to this, she lived through a pregnancy, the modifications of her body image, and the testing experience of childbirth, which can be classified as *ordinary trauma*. This succession of events can produce the effect of psychological paralysis.

The reduced presence of small movements can demonstrate both difficulties in the psychological work and a lack of ability to let go with regard to certain cards, and the difficulty for mothers to deal with solicitations encouraging regressive tendencies in psychological terms. (Regression as we consider it here concerns a *topical regression* linked to different states of the psychological apparatus – unconscious, preconscious, conscious – a *temporal regression*, as it concerns the recovery of anterior psychological formations, and finally *a formal-type regression*, as the modes of expression and figuration in this context are more primitive.) The divergences here are the greatest in our study and we believe they are linked to the intensity of underlying instinctive reactivations, which the participant seeks to control.

Anxiety Indication

Concerning the anxiety indication (AI%), which was significantly higher in our population, we observed a majority of non-symbolized responses, sexual representations, and notably responses related to female sexual anatomy ("vagina," "labia," "uterus," "ovaries"), which were present in 16 protocols out of the 30 studied.

Response Contents

We observed a significant decrease in A% responses (36.29 while the norm is 42.55). This result can be explained by the increase in attention to the human and a parallel deficiency in the contents of animal responses. Furthermore, the state of primary maternal preoccupation can weaken the indications of socialization. The mother is indeed completely dedicated to her baby and its care.

The number of human responses was slightly lower (15.42 for a norm of 15.85) without being statistically significant. However, the human responses were interesting, as the majority centered on "baby" representations and the experiences of mothering, as if motherhood was directly reflected in the Rorschach responses. It is therefore relevant to inquire as to the other contents of responses.

The anatomic responses reflect the impact of the corporeal event of childbirth, and may even reflect earlier preoccupations linked to the state of pregnancy. Preoccupations linked to the body are central at this time of life and appear more or less directly. The intensity of psychological and corporeal readjustments can interfere with the activities of symbolization and secondarization and reveal more numerous emergences of primary processes without, however, modifying these participants' connection to reality (normative F%).

Among the findings resulting from the research with Rorschach tests, it appears that the psychic life functioning processes that are the most flexible and accessible to regression are those that offer the easiest access to motherhood.

Conclusion

This preliminary research demonstrates the nature and amplitude of psychic life modifications inherent in the postnatal period, which are clearly demonstrated by the Rorschach test. These periods of profound adjustment and of psychological vulnerability in mothers, habitually described in the literature, are given here a pertinent as well as unexpected and complex reading.

Even if the sample may seem small ($N = 30$), the results of this study show that among a sample of women coming from the general population and not suffering from any psychopathological disorders, there exist psychological resonances and particularities specific to the postnatal phase. Of the 16 usual psychogram indications in the Rorschach test, although eight remained normative (adaptation to the outside world, quality of mentalization, human representations, indication of socialization, and relationship with reality), eight other indications diverged significantly from the norms of the general French population. Thus, the psychological upheaval in the postnatal phase operates subtly and with regard to certain values only. Improved knowledge of the different phases of motherhood can aid professionals in the prevention of disorders specific to pre- and postpartum (baby blues, post-natal depression, and postpartum psychosis) periods.

The psychological factors involved at the time of pregnancy, birth, and the arrival of the infant necessitate further in-depth investigation to enable the provision of care that is both appropriate and preventive, in order to reduce disorders. These disorders can be linked to the postpartum phase, but may also emerge prepartum. Effectively, the great vulnerability existing during this period requires improved knowledge about the psychological impact involved in the experience of new motherhood.

Indeed, it appears necessary to increase the size of our sample in a subsequent study. We are currently conducting a longitudinal study to better understand the impact of psychic life and bodily transformations before the birth, in particular for primiparous women. This research is being duplicated internationally to compare intercultural differences with the experience of motherhood.

Limitations

The absence of psychological disorders among the women encountered was evaluated according to three essential criteria: strict adherence to the inclusion criteria, absence of proven depressive disorders (confirmed during the clinical interview), and the absence of use of psychotropic medications (confirmed during the clinical interview). We envision subsequently consolidating these criteria with the use of a self-assessment questionnaire (to evaluate depression and anxiety as well as levels of stress) within the framework of a new study.

The anxiety present in certain women in our sample population corresponds to the norms in a general population of women in the post-natal phase. However, a detailed evaluation of anxiety, including its intensity and frequency, would have allowed us to create different and more relevant subgroups. In the same way, although the birth took place with no apparent difficulties in the case of all the women in our population, a more careful examination of the circumstances surrounding the birth should be taken into account in our subsequent study.

An additional Rorschach protocol in the antenatal period is necessary for a subsequent study. This will enable us to observe changes longitudinally and more closely. Furthermore, studies of longitudinal cases from the beginning of the pregnancy to just after birth and the postnatal period would allow us to measure the extent of the changes throughout the pregnancy, the birth, and motherhood.

References

Altshuler, L. L., Cohen, L. S., Vitonis, A. F., Faraone, S. V., Harlow, B. L., Suri, R., Frieder, R., & Stowe, Z. N. (2008). The Pregnancy Depression Scale (PDS): A screening tool for depression in pregnancy. *Archives of Women's Mental Health, 11*, 277–285. https://doi.org/10.1007/s00737-008-0020-y

Azoulay, C., Corroyer, D., & Emmanuelli, M. (2012). *Nouveau manuel de cotation des formes au Rorschach* [New Rorschach form dimensioning manual]. Dunod.

Azoulay, C., Emmanuelli, M., Rausch de Traubenberg, N., Corroyer, D., Rozencwajg, P., & Savina, Y. (2007). Les données normatives françaises du Rorschach à l'adolescence et chez le jeune adulte [The French normative data of Rorschach in adolescents and young adults]. *Psychologie Clinique et Projective, 13*(1), 371–409. https://doi.org/10.3917/pcp.013.0371

Bellion, E. (2001). Agressivité et grossesse. Pour un cheminement nécessaire vers la naissance de la relation mère/bébé: Le fonctionnement psychique chez la femme enceinte à la lumière du Rorschach et du TAT [Aggression and pregnancy. For a necessary journey towards birth of the mother/baby relationship: Psychic functioning in women with Rorschach and TAT]. *Devenir, 1*(1), 67–83. https://doi.org/10.3917/dev.011.0067

Belot, R. A. (2014). Changes in maternal protective shield system pre- and postpartum and somatic expression of baby. From an observation, Elise (1 month 19 days). *Neuropsychiatrie de l'enfance et de l'adolescence, 62*(4), 218–225. https://doi.org/10.1016/j.neurenf.2014.02.002

Belot, R. A., Maïdi, H., Givron, S., & Arcangelli, E. (2016). Dépression maternelle et processus de co-identification mère-bébé. L'archaïque en soi dans la rencontre primordiale [Maternal depression and mother-baby co-identification process. The archaic in itself in the primordial encounter]. *Annales Médico-Psychologiques, 174*(9), 748–756. https://doi.org/10.1016/j.amp.2016.04.011

Capponi, I., & Horbacz, C. (2005). Evolution et déterminants éventuels de l'anxiété périnatale de primipares: du huitième mois de grossesse au troisième mois post-partum [Evolution and possible determinants of perinatal anxiety in first-time mothers: From the eighth month of pregnancy to the third month postpartum]. *Devenir, 17*(3), 211–231. https://doi.org/10.3917/dev.053.0211

Chabert, C. (1983). *Le Rorschach en clinique adulte. Interprétation psychanalytique* [The Rorschach in adult clinic: Psychoanalytic interpretation] (3rd ed.). Dunod 2002

Chabert, C. (1987). *La psychopathologie à l'épreuve du Rorschach* [Rorschach-tested psychopathology]. Bordas.

Connell, M. C., & Daston, P. G. (1961). Body image in pregnancy. *Journal of Projective Techniques, 25*(4), 451–456. https://doi.org/10.1080/08853126.1961.10381065

Dayan, J., Andro, G., & Dugnat, M. (2002). *Psychopathologie de la périnatalité* [Psychopathology of the perinatal period]. Masson.

Dayan, J., & Graignic-Philippe, R. (2011). Prescrire des antipsychotiques en postpartum [Prescribing postpartum antipsychotics]. *Devenir, 23*, 69–85. https://doi.org/10.3917/dev.111.0069

De Tychey, C., Bei, M., Tenenbaum-Partouche, M., & Touvenot, V. (1997). Dépression postnatale et imago maternelle: Approche comparative à travers le test de Rorschach [Postnatal depression and maternal imago: Comparative approach through the Rorschach test]. *Psychologie Clinique et Projective, 3*, 61–73.

Rorschachiana (2021), 42(1), 72–92

De Tychey, C., Huckel, C., Rivat, C., & Claudon, P. (2012). Nouvelles normes adultes du test de Rorschach et évolution sociétale: quelques réflexions [New adult standards of the Rorschach test and societal evolution: Some thoughts]. *Bulletin de Psychologie, 5*(521), 453–466. https://doi.org/10.3917/bupsy.521.0453

De Tychey, C., Spitz, E., Briancon, S., Lighezzolo, J., Girvan, F., Rosati, A., Thockler, A., & Vincent, S. (2005). Pre- and postnatal depression and coping: A comparative approach. *Journal Affective Disorders, 85*(3), 323–326. https://doi.org/10.1016/j.jad.2004.11.004

Denis, A., Parant, O., & Callahan, S. (2011). Post-traumatic stress disorder related to birth: A prospective longitudinal study in a French population. *Journal of Reproductive and Infant Psychology, 29*(2), 125–135. https://doi.org/10.1080/02646838.2010.513048

Deutsch, H. (1933). *Maternité et sexualité in La Psychanalyse des névroses* [Maternity and sexuality in The Psychoanalysis of Neuroses]. Payot.

Evans, J., Heron, J., Francomb, H., Oken, S., & Golding, J. (2001). Cohort study of depressed mood during pregnancy and after childbirth. *BMJ, 323*, 257–260. https://doi.org/10.1136/bmj.323.7307.257

Fan, F., Zou, Y., Ma, A., Yue, Y., Mao, W., & Ma, X. (2009). Hormonal changes and somatopsychologic manifestations in the first trimester of pregnancy and post partum. *International Journal of Gynecology & Obstetrics, 105*(1), 46–49. https://doi.org/10.1016/j.ijgo.2008.12.001

Georges, A., Luz, R. F., De Tychey, C., Thilly, N., & Spitz, E. (2013). Anxiety symptoms and coping strategies in the perinatal period. *BMC Pregnancy and Childbirth, 13*, 233. https://doi.org/10.1186/1471-2393-13-233

Gutiérrez-Zotes, A., Labad, J., Martin-Santos, R., Garcia-Estève, L., Gelabert, E., Jover, M., Guillamat, R., Mayroral, F., Gornemann, I., Canellas, F., Gratacos, M., Guitart, M., Roca, M., Costas, J., Ivorra, J.-L., Navinés, R., De Diego-Otero, Y., Vilella, E., & Sanjuan, J. (2016). Coping strategies for postpartum depression: A multi-centric study of 1626 women. *Archives of Women's Mental Health, 19*, 455–461. https://doi.org/10.1007/s00737-015-0581-5

Kendell, R. E., Rennie, D., Clarke, J. A., & Dean, C. (1981). The social and obstetric correlates of psychiatric admission in the puerperium. *Psychological Medicine, 11*(2), 341–350. https://doi.org/10.1017/S0033291700052156

Klatskin, E. H., & Eron, L. D. (1970). Projective test content during pregnancy and postpartum adjustment. *Psychosomatic Medicine, 32*(5), 487–493. https://doi.org/10.1097/00006842-197009000-00006

McConnel, O. L., & Daston, P. G. (1961). Body image changes in Pregnancy. *Journal of Projectives Techniques, 25*(4), 451–456. https://doi.org/10.1080/08853126.1961.10381065

Milden, R., Rosenthal, M., Winegardner, J., & Smith, D. (1985). Denial of pregnancy: An exploratory investigation. *Journal of Psychosomatic Obstetrics & Gynecology, 4*(4), 255–261. https://doi.org/10.3109/01674828509016727

Racamier, P.-C. (1979). *La maternalité psychotique in De psychanalyse en psychiatrie-Etudes psychopathologiques* [Psychotic motherhood in from Psychoanalysis to Psychiatry – Psychopathological Studies]. Payot.

Setan, A. K., Theis, A., & De Tychey, C. (2001). Réflexions sur l'approche psychodynamique des stérilités féminines [Reflections on the psychodynamic approach to female sterility]. *L'Évolution Psychiatrique, 66*(1), 61–74. https://doi.org/10.1016/S0014-3855(01)90005-2

Skouteris, H., Wertheim, E. H., Rallis, S., Milgrom, J., & Paxton, S. J. (2009). Depression and anxiety through pregnancy and the early postpartum: An examination of prospective relationships. *Journal of Affective Disorders, 113*(3), 303–308. https://doi.org/10.1016/j.jad.2008.06.002

Stern, D. (1985). *The interpersonal world of the infant.* Basic Books.
Wenzel, A., Haugen, E. N., Jackson, L. C., & Robinson, K. (2003). Prevalence of generalized anxiety at eight weeks postpartum. *Archives of Women's Mental Health, 6,* 43–49. https://doi.org/10.1007/s00737-002-0154-2
Winnicott, D. W. (1975). *The primary maternal preoccupation. Paediatrics to psychoanalysis* (pp. 168–174). Payot (Original work published 1956).

History
Received September 4, 2019
Revision received December 9, 2020
Accepted December 15, 2020
Published online March 18, 2021

Received and processed mainly under previous editorship

Acknowledgments
We would like to express our very great appreciation to Claire Giboudeaux-Baumes, translator–revisor, University of Franche-Comté, and Jennifer Dobson, translator and clinical research administrator, Besançon University Hospital, for the proofreading of our manuscript.

Conflict of Interest
The authors have none to declare.

ORCID
Rose-Angélique Belot
https://orcid.org/0000-0001-9348-3707

Rose-Angélique Belot
Psychology Laboratory EA3188
University of Bourgogne Fanche-Comté
32 rue Mégevand
25030 Besançon Cedex
France
rose-angelique.belot@univ-fcomte.fr

Summary

Motherhood, listed by the World Health Organization as a period of fragility and vulnerability, involves significant changes at the individual, family, and societal level.

Becoming a mother entails a number of risk factors to be taken into account. Although the extremely widespread psychopathological disorders ("baby blues," pre- and postnatal depression, puerperal psychosis, denial of pregnancy) are well known, they remain largely underdiagnosed.

It is therefore necessary to conduct studies on general populations without psychopathological and obstetric disorders to better understand all the risk factors associated with motherhood. The literature review indicates a lack of research on motherhood and the Rorschach in a general population at low risk.

This study was carried out in France with a nonconsulting population in the postnatal phase ($N =$ 30) using the Rorschach test, because this tool has many advantages for assessing the mental and bodily transformations linked to becoming a mother.

We compared the quantitative results of the test with the recently updated standards (De Tychey et al., 2012). We made specific operational assumptions for all of the psychogram indices based on our knowledge of the postpartum period. Some assumptions were validated, others were not. Eight values of the psychogram remained normative (F%, F+%, G%, Dd%, K, C, H%, Ban) and reflected the characteristics of a general population, whereas the eight other values of the psychogram (R, D%, Dbl%, A%, CR%, k, E, Anxiety index%) differed considerably from the norms of the general population. These periods of deep adjustment and psychic vulnerability in mothers, which have been generally described in the literature, are revealed by a relevant, unexpected reading with the Rorschach.

These results increase our understanding of the complex psychic processes that occur during the postnatal period, and make it possible to identify the areas of weakness associated with access to maternity more precisely. They also make it possible to distinguish proven disorders from transient and classic disorders linked to the upheavals caused by becoming a mother. They can help prevent psychopathological disorders, which are too frequent in the perinatal period.

Résumé

La maternité, répertoriée par l'OMS (Organisation Mondiale de la Santé) comme une période de fragilité et de vulnérabilité, implique des changements conséquents au niveau individuel, familial et sociétal. Devenir mère comporte un certain nombre de facteurs de risques à repérer et prendre en compte.

Si les troubles psychopathologiques extrêmement répandus (baby-blues, dépression anté et post-natale, psychose puerpérale, déni de grossesse) sont bien répertoriés, ils restent encore largement sous-diagnostiqués.

Il est donc nécessaire de mener des études sur des populations générales qui ne souffrent pas de troubles psychopathologiques et obstétriques pour mieux appréhender tous les facteurs de risque liés à la maternité. La revue de la littérature indique en effet l'absence de travaux de recherche sur « maternité et Rorschach » auprès d'une population « tout venant » à bas risque.

La recherche est menée en France sur une population non consultante en phase postnatale ($N =$ 30) à l'aide du test de Rorschach, car cet outil présente de nombreux avantages pour apprécier les transformations psychiques et corporelles liées au « devenir mère ».

Les résultats quantitatifs du test ont été soumis à une comparaison avec les normes récemment mises à jour (De Tychey & al., 2012). Nous avons émis pour tous les indices du psychogramme des hypothèses opérationnelles spécifiques en fonction de nos connaissances sur la période post-partum. Certaines sont validées, d'autres non. Huit valeurs du psychogramme restent normatives (F% - F+% - G% - Dd% - K - C - H% - Ban) et reflètent les caractéristiques d'une population générale, à l'inverse, huit autres valeurs du psychogramme (R - D% - Dbl% - A% - RC% - k - E - Indice d'angoisse%) diffèrent considérablement des normes de la population générale. Ces périodes d'ajustements profonds et de vulnérabilités psychiques chez les mères, habituellement décrites dans la littérature, sont révélées par une lecture pertinente et inattendue au Rorschach.

Ces résultats augmentent les connaissances pour apprécier la complexité des processus psychiques durant la période postnatale et permettent de discriminer plus finement les zones de fragilités liées à l'accès à la maternité. Ils permettent également de distinguer les troubles avérés de ceux transitoires et classiques liés aux bouleversements provoqués par l'accès à la maternité. Ils peuvent favoriser la prévention des troubles psychopathologiques, trop répandus en périnatalité.

Resumen

La maternidad, catalogada por la OMS (Organización Mundial de la Salud) como un período de fragilidad y vulnerabilidad, implica cambios significativos a nivel individual, familiar y social. Ser madre implica varios factores de riesgo. Si los trastornos psicopatológicos extremadamente generalizados (melancolía, depresión prenatal y postnatal, psicosis puerperal, negación del embarazo) también están bien documentados, todavía están en gran medida sin diagnosticar.

Por lo tanto, es necesario realizar estudios en poblaciones generales que no padecen trastornos psicopatológicos y obstétricos para comprender mejor todos los factores de riesgo asociados con la maternidad. La revisión de la literatura indica la ausencia de trabajo de investigación sobre "maternidad y Rorschach" en una población de "todos los que vienen" con bajo riesgo.

Esta investigación se lleva a cabo en Francia con una población que no consulta en la fase postnatal (N = 30) utilizando la prueba de Rorschach, porque esta herramienta tiene muchas ventajas para evaluar las transformaciones psíquicas y corporales vinculadas a "convertirse en madre".

Los resultados cuantitativos de la prueba se sometieron a una comparación con los estándares recientemente actualizados (De Tychey y otros, 2012). Hemos emitido hipótesis operativas específicas para todos los índices del psicograma basados en nuestro conocimiento del período posparto. Algunos están validados, otros no. Ocho valores del psicograma siguen siendo normativos (F% - F+% - G% - Dd% - K - C - H% - Ban) y reflejan las características de una población general, por el contrario, otros ocho valores del psicograma (R - D% - Dbl% - A% - CR% - k - E - Índice de ansiedad%) difieren considerablemente de las normas de la población general. Estos períodos de ajustes profundos y vulnerabilidades psíquicas en las madres, generalmente descritos en la literatura, se revelan mediante una lectura relevante, inesperada con el Rorschach.

Estos resultados aumentan el conocimiento para apreciar la complejidad de los procesos psíquicos durante el período posnatal y permiten discriminar más finamente las áreas de debilidad vinculadas al acceso a la maternidad. También permiten distinguir trastornos probados de trastornos transitorios y clásicos relacionados con los trastornos causados por el acceso a la maternidad. Pueden ayudar a prevenir los trastornos psicopatológicos, que son demasiado comunes en el período perinatal.

要約

WHOは、母性を脆弱性の時期として挙げている。そしてそれは、個人、家族、社会レベルで大きな変化を伴う。母親になることは、考慮すべきおおくの危険因子を伴う。極めて広範な精神病理的障害（"マタニティブルー"、出生前及び出生後のうつ病、産褥期精神病、妊娠の否定）はよく知られているが、それらは、ほとんど診断されないままである。

したがって、母性に関するすべての危険因子をよりよく理解するために、精神病理的障害や産科的障害のない一般集団を対象とした研究が必要である。文献を精査してみると、リスクの低い一般集団における母性とロールシャッハに関する研究が不足していることを示している。

この研究は、ロールシャッハ・テストを使用して、このツールが母親になることに関連した精神的・身体的変化を評価するために多くの利点があると考え、産後期の非相談集団（N=30）を対象にフランスで実施された。

テストの定量的な結果と、最近更新された基準（De Tychey ら, 2012）と比較した。われわれは、産後期間に関する知識に基づいて、全てのサイコグラム指標について特定の運用上の仮説を設定した。いくつかの仮説は支持されたが、他の仮説は検証されなかった。サイコグラムの8つの値（F%, F+%, G%, Dd%, K, C, H%, Ban）は、標準値と変わらず、サイコグラムの他の8つの値（R, D%, Dbl%, A%, CR%, k, E, Anxiety index%）は、一般集団の基準とはかなり異なっていた。一般的に文献に記載され

ている母親の中にある深い適応と精神的脆弱性のこれらの期間は、ロールシャッハを使った意外な読み方に関連させることによって明らかにされた。

　これらの結果は、産後期に起こる複雑な精神的プロセスの理解を深め、より正確に母性に立ち入る際の弱点領域をあぶり出すことが可能になる。それらはまた、明らかとなった障害を、母親になることによって引き起こされる激変に関連する一過性および古典的な障害と区別することを可能にする。それらは、周産期に頻繁に起こる精神病理学的障害の予防に役立つ。

Original Article

The Development of the Rorschach Test in China

Jiang Yanhua[1,2] and Fonny Dameaty Hutagalung[2]

[1]College of Education Science, Hengyang Normal University, China
[2]Faculty of Education, University of Malaya, Kuala Lumpur, Malaysia

Abstract: This article summarizes the development and research status of the Rorschach Test in China as comprehensively as possible. The development of the Rorschach Test in China can be divided into two stages: the initial stage and the developing stage. At the initial stage the research mainly includes: introduction and localization of the Rorschach Test, studies on schizophrenia, and the measurement of intelligence and personality. In the developing stage the research mainly includes: spreading and localization of the Rorschach Test, the variables, indices, and derivative scales, clinical psychology, talent assessment, combination with eye movement techniques, the Group Rorschach Inkblot Test, and reviews. Based on the domestic development and research status of the Rorschach Test, the article also summarizes the achievements and issues present in existing studies and puts forward the prospect of researching the Rorschach Test in China.

Keywords: China, research status, Rorschach Test

This study reviews the studies conducted in China using the Rorschach Test since its introduction in the country, summarizes the research achievements and the issues existing in the studies, and puts forward the future work of researching the Rorschach Test in China. On the basis of Zhang Yu's viewpoint (2016), we divided the development of the Rorschach Test in China into the initial stage and the developing stage. At the initial stage, the Rorschach Test was introduced to China, and researchers began to make a systematic study. In the developing stage, the introduction of the Rorschach Test gradually increased, and the research on the Rorschach Test began to diversify.

The Initial Stage of the Rorschach Test (1940s to 2000)

Introduction and Localization of the Rorschach Test

The introduction of the Rorschach Test to China goes back to Ling Minyou, Gong, and Luo Chuanfang in the 1940s and 1950s. Tentative research was conducted (e.g., a study on the Beck System and a trial to establish a national norm, etc.), but in the following 20 years, the Rorschach Test was not further developed (Exner, 2001/2013b). Gong et al. began the establishment of a norm again in 1985, the Comprehensive System (CS) was selected, and a preliminary norm was established by 1987 (Exner, 2001/2013b). Then Gong et al. published the *Rorschach Test Manual* in 1991. In addition, Ling Wenquan and Bing (1988) made a comprehensive introduction of the Klopfer System in their book *Method of Psychology Test* and J. Yuan translated and published *Psychodiagnostik* in 1997 (Rorschach, 1921/1997).

M. Chen et al. (1997) collected the CS data of 666 healthy Chinese adults and compared these with the data of 1990 in the United States. The results indicated the scores of variables (Zf, Blends, W, S, M, m, FC, CF, WsumC, T + V + Y + C', H, (H), (Hd), Ad, INCOM, AG, and MOR) were higher in the American sample than the Chinese sample, while F, A, An, and PSV were lower. The differences were all statistically significant ($p < .01$).

Studies on Schizophrenia

L. Li (1987) reported the Rorschach features of patients diagnosed with chronic schizophrenia. S.-G. Li and Gong (1988) compared differences between the schizophrenia group and the control group. The analyses indicated the schizophrenia group displayed many responses related to mental disorders and their perceptual accuracy was lower than that of the control group. Q.-X. Li (1986) concluded that perception and thinking disorders of schizophrenia were associated with perception or mediation distortion according to the Rorschach Test perception theory. Furthermore, she and her colleagues reported that the values for F+%, M, Ma, FM, and FC of the schizophrenia group were lower than the control group, and the differences were significant (Li et al., 1989). L.-Y. Li et al. (1993) indicated that the neurosis group had more emotional instability and personality introversion than the control group. A study conducted by B. Wang et al. (1993) described the Rorschach characteristics of patients with schizophrenia, with depression, and with mania and found significant differences between these three groups on a number of variables (R, P, W, M, H, Sx, F+%, X+%, X−%, Afr, Zf, Zd, D score, S-CON, DEPI, SCZI; $p < .01$). T.-N. Chen (1999) compared the Rorschach results of children diagnosed with schizophrenia with a control group in a sample of 13–15-year-olds. Mean comparisons showed that the children with schizophrenia scored significantly lower than the control children in the total test time and in Fx% (all age groups), S, M, Fc, Clob, and F% (13-year-old group), D, F, Hd, and Ad (14-year-old group) and in FM, Ad (15-year-old group). Frequency analyses showed that the children with schizophrenia scored significantly lower than the control group in M, H (13-year-old group), EC, Ad (14-year-old group), and FM,

Ad (15-year-old group). Mean comparisons and frequency analyses both showed that the children with schizophrenia scored significantly higher than the control children in Dd (15-year-old group). H.-B. Jiang et al. (2000) analyzed the Rorschach features of patients diagnosed with schizophrenia and found they had abundant association ability, weak integration ability, the perception of the part was enhanced, more M, fewer color responses, the type of experience was introverted, poor form quality, and impaired ability to identify reality. Moreover, they could not respond well when emotionally stimulated.

The Measurement of Intelligence and Personality

Hu and Gong (1989) used the Rorschach Test and Eysenck Personality Questionnaire (EPQ; Gong, 1983) to measure personality differences between writers and math teachers and the results showed the values for R, H/R, Isolate/R, AG/R, number of content categories, Id/R, Zsum/Zf, M/R, FM/R, m/R, C', CF', and Blends/R of the writers were higher than those of the math teachers, while the average time to the first reaction, Hd/H, Zf/R, FC/R, and F/R were lower. The differences were all statistically significant ($p < .01$). X.-F. Zhu and Gong (1995) conducted a correlational study between the Rorschach Test and the Wechsler Adult Intelligence Scale-Chinese Revision (Gong, 1982) and the results indicated that the variables R, W, DQ+, DQv/+, DQo, M, Zf, Zsum, EA, Blend, CS, X+%, and F+% had positive correlations with intelligence ($r = .32$–$.62$), while X−% had a negative correlation with intelligence ($r = -.35$). Y.-H. Wu et al. (1998) used the Rorschach Test and the EPQ with college students and found that there were significant differences in the Rorschach Test between the extroverted group and the introverted group, suggesting that the Rorschach Test can distinguish different personalities. Guo (1999) conducted a comparative study between the CS and 16PF (Zhu B-L. & Dai, 1988) and the results indicated there were significant correlations between a number of Rorschach variables and 16PF ($r = -.4$–$.4$).

The Developing Stage of the Rorschach Test (2000 to Present)

Spreading and Localization of the Rorschach Test

Xu has taught the Rorschach Test in postgraduate classes since 2000 (Ma, 2016). Moreover, he introduced the Rorschach Test and reported some Rorschach cases in his books: *Study Abroad Life of Intercultural Adaptation – Mental Health and*

Assistance for Chinese Students (2000) and *Clinical Psychology – Knowledge of Mental Health and Aid* (2001).

X.-Z. Meng introduced the Lerner Defense Scale (LDS; Lerner & Lerner, 1980) in *Practical Psychological Measurement* (Jie & Dai, 2006) and the CS in *Psychological Assessment* (Yao, 2007). At the same time, he published two translated books: *A Rorschach Workbook for the Comprehensive System* (Exner, 2001/2013b) and *A Primer for Rorschach Interpretation* (Exner, 2000/2013a). Ren (2007) studied the localization of AgC and established a Chinese AgC list including 60 contents with excellent reliability. T.-Y. Li (2016) collected data from 326 healthy adults in Guangdong Province according to the CS and established a Guangdong adult norm for the Rorschach Test. The results showed that this norm had good-to-excellent reliability (i.e., the intraclass correlation coefficients of test–retest reliability and inter-rater reliability were .44 to .98 [except DQv and Hx] and .51 to 1.00, respectively), and it also had good content validity and criterion validity. Xiong (2014) compared Chinese, Israeli, and American samples, and He (2015) compared Chinese, American, and Japanese samples of the Rorschach Test. The results showed differences between the Chinese, Israeli, and American samples on the variables D, Dd, X+%, Xu%, X−%, FQxo, FQxu, FQx−, P, Afr, EB, EA, FC: CF + C, FC, CF, FD, p, FM + m, SumV, SumT, PHR, COP, HVI, DEPI, CDI; significant differences between the Chinese and American samples on the variables Dd, DQo, FQx+, FQxo, FQxu, FQx−, MQ−, CF, WSumC, FD, F, Lambda, EA, D score, AdjD, A (active), Ma, Afr, P, XA+%, WDA%, X+%, X−%, Xu%, A, Idio, ALOG, PSV; finally, there were significant differences between the Chinese and Japanese samples on the variables CF, EA, AdjD, Ad, Idio, SumT, A, and S−. These two studies both indicated that the Rorschach Test had significant cultural differences, and therefore a norm corresponding to the local culture was required.

Additional publications include Yang and Ji Yuanhong's (2008) *Practical Rorschach Ink Test* and Kong and Y.-Q. Li's (2013) *Rorschach Ink Test: A Clinical Application Study on Comprehensive System*. Meanwhile, Tsinghua University has held several international Rorschach Test advanced training courses by Bruce Smith, board member of the International Society of the Rorschach and Projective Methods, since 2010 (Ma, 2016).

The Variables, Indices, and Derivative Scales

G.-H. Liu and Meng (2003) summarized studies on the aggression variables and identified some problems in the research. Furthermore, they modified and established a new framework including 12 aggression variables: AG, MOR, AgC, AgPot, AgPast, Active Aggression (AAg), Passive Aggression (PAg), Overt Aggression

(OAg), Covert Aggression (CAg), Aggressive emotion (AgE), Mental Harm (Mh), Physical Harm (Ph; Liu & Meng, 2007b). In samples of criminals and college students, they examined the new framework's reliability and validity and explored the correlations between the EPQ and the new aggression variables. Analyses revealed good inter-rater agreement but the validity and the correlations required further study (Liu & Meng, 2007a, 2007b). Yan and Meng (2007) examined this new framework again and the results indicated that AgC, AgPot, AgE, Mh, and total aggression scores were significantly correlated with the hostility factor of the Brief Psychiatric Rating Scale (BPRS), and AgC and the total aggression score showed significant differences between high and low scores on the BPRS hostility factor. X.-J. Liu (2006) studied MOR, AgPast, and impaired object relations and found that MOR and AgPast were associated with depression and suicide. Ying (2006) examined five aggression variables (AgPast, MOR, Ag, AgC, and AgPot) and the Type A Behavior Pattern Questionnaire. This study indicated that the Type A group had significantly less Ag than the non-Type A group ($p < .01$). Factor analysis showed that aggressive variables could be divided into three factors: aggression on the object (AgPast, MOR), the object of aggression (Ag, AgC), and potential aggression (AgPot).

D.-D. Li (2007) conducted a study of Ag and AgC in a sample of criminals. The results indicated that AgC had good empirical validity, Ag was negatively associated with scores on the Pd scale (MMPI), and AgC was positively associated with scores on the Pd scale. Y.-H. Jiang (2006) studied children's aggressive behaviors using the Rorschach Test and concluded that the aggression variables proposed by foreign researchers also had some value in measuring children's aggressive behaviors in China. C.-F. Wang (2006) examined the validity of AgC and reported that the reliability was excellent (Cohen's $k = .87$). AgC could distinguish between high and low aggressive groups and college boys' AgC scores were significantly higher than those of college girls.

Yu's research on the Depression Index (DEPI; 2008) indicated that its reliability was acceptable (Cohen's $k > .70$), and it could effectively distinguish patients diagnosed with depression from healthy people. Hong (2008) compared the DEPI of patients diagnosed with depression before treatment with that of those after treatment and found that the DEPI scores after treatment were significantly lower than before, providing support that the DEPI had some empirical validity. Y.-H. Jiang et al. (2015) also used the DEPI to measure college students' depression and found that it could measure depression. Sun (2011) studied the DEPI and the Coping Defect Index (CDI) and the results indicated the κ coefficients of DEPI and CDI were acceptable. The study also indicated that using the CDI could bring incremental validity to the DEPI and increase its diagnostic accuracy. X.-L. Li (2007) conducted a study on the Suicide Constellation (S-CON), and the results indicated that all variables of S-CON had sufficient inter-rater agreement. The study also showed that S-CON was valuable in identifying patients diagnosed with depression and suicide ideation and behaviors.

H.-X. Liu (2009) conducted a study on the Egocentricity Index (Ego) to investigate the relationship between Ego, MOR, and the Self-Esteem Scale (SES) and an Implicit Association Test (IAT) in samples of normal, depressive, and manic patients. The results did not support Exner's view about Ego (i.e., high Ego is associated with high self-esteem) but indicated MOR could reflect explicit self-esteem (i.e., low MOR is associated with high self-esteem). Y.-C. Tang (2011) examined the reliability and validity of the Ego Impairment Index (EII-2) and indicated the inter-rater reliability of the EII-2 was acceptable. Moreover, the EII-2 could distinguish patients with mental disorders from the controls, and could differentiate between various severities and types of mental disorders. X.-L. Wu (2013) examined the reliability and validity of the EII-2 and Rorschach Alexithymia Scale (RAS). The results were as follows: (1) The EII-2 had excellent inter-rater reliability and certain discriminant validity; (2) the RAS had excellent inter-rater reliability but validity needed further study and verification. Meng and T.-Y. Li (2015) studied the differences of the EII between patients diagnosed with schizophrenia and controls and the results indicated the ego functions of these patients had severe damage compared with the controls. The EII could discriminate these patients with schizophrenia from the controls.

Y.-X. Chen (2007) examined the reliability and validity of the LDS and the results indicated good reliability and validity in a small-scale study with a small sample. Different populations had different defense mechanisms and the LDS can be used as an auxiliary tool in clinical diagnosis. In addition, Peng et al. (2008) indicated that the reliability and validity of the Mutuality of Autonomy Scale (MOA) were acceptable. The study by J. Tang (2004) also showed that the MOA could distinguish healthy people from patients, especially the low-level object relationship.

Cai and Shen (2007) studied the Rorschach self-concept variables in college students. The results indicated that the reliability of the self-concept variables was acceptable and that they could measure the self-concept well. The variables were divided into four factors by factor analysis: introspection [(2), FD, Hd + (H) + (Hd)], positive regard (Fr + rF, Ego), feeling of reality [H: Hd + (H) + (Hd), H, SumV, An + Xy], and negative regard (MOR).

Qin et al. (2015) explored gender differences in the Rorschach variables related to pressure in patients diagnosed with schizophrenia. The results indicated there were significant gender differences in some variables (CDI, D, es, Adjes, m, SumY, FM + m, SumC' + SumT + SumV + SumY, L).

X.-X. Chen and Zhou (2007) discussed the construct validity of the Rorschach Test and introduced the Rorschach Rating Scale (RRS) and its application by reviewing the literature. Guo et al. (2007) correlated RRS with some Rorschach variables about self-concept and the results indicated that the variables (Pure H, H%, An + Xy, and Sx) could measure healthy people's self-concept. Y.-H. Wang et al. (2009) found that there was a significant correlation between the interpersonal relationship variables in the Rorschach Test and the interpersonal relationship indices in the RRS.

Clinical Psychology

J. Liu (2001) introduced two Chinese cases scored and interpreted by the CS and explored its application in clinical psychology. X.-Q. Wang (2009) reported a case of a heroin addict assessed with the Rorschach Test. Qi (2010) combined SCL-90 and an emotional experiment with a clinical case study to explore the psychological diagnosis validity of the Rorschach Test. The results indicated that the Rorschach Test in clinical psychological diagnosis and assessment was valid. Tu and Yuan (2010) used a case-study method combined with a semi-structured interview method and suggested that the Rorschach Test had distinct advantages over other diagnostic methods and was a unique and efficient tool for the diagnosis of college students' emotional disorders.

Zhong et al. (2007) explored the characteristics and possible projection mechanism of children with attention deficit hyperactivity disorder (ADHD) using the Rorschach Test. The results indicated that the values for Zf, COP, $3r + 2/R$, Zd, X+%, and Sum6 of children with ADHD were lower than those of the controls, while AG, Lambda, Sum Shading, X−%, SCZI, DEPI, and CDI were higher ($p <$ .05) and the Rorschach Test could project some characteristics of the inner world of children with ADHD. In addition, N. Zhang (2008) found the Rorschach data of children had significant differences in some variables depending on their psychological adjustment (i.e., lower R, shorter average reaction time; more human An and the ratio of human An in the control group).

X.-X. Chen (2008) examined the validity of the Rorschach Test in psychological health assessment. The results supported the validity of the Rorschach Test in a clinical psychology health context. Nan Zhang (2013) used the Rorschach Test as a measure of adult attachment. The results indicated that males had a lower level of anxiety than females. Furthermore, she established a structural equation model of adult attachment. The variables representing the anxiety dimension in the model are CF, Color-shading Blends, Y, m, Food, and T > 1. The variables representing avoidance dimensions are FM, Mp, Hum con, p, MOR, Cg, (Hd) + (Ad) + (H) + (A), (Hd) + (Ad) + Hd + Ad, and T = 0. The model had good reliability, construct validity, and criterion validity. Cai et al. (2014) explored the Rorschach Test's activating complex characteristic and its application to clinical practice. It was found that the Rorschach images could stimulate more negative feelings and the homogeneous complex manifestations associated with them had the evident characteristics of activating complex.

Talent Assessment

W.-L. Wang (2008) confirmed the validity of the Rorschach Test in personnel assessment and its potential in selecting talents by a comparative study of the Rorschach Test, interview, and 16PF. Guo et al. (2009) conducted a study on the effectiveness of the Rorschach Test in personnel quality assessment. The results indicated that the Rorschach Test could measure the abilities of information processing, emotion management, self-perception, and interpersonal communication. Qu (2010) also used the Rorschach intelligence variables (F+, Fo, Fu, F−, Ab, Art, Ay, F) to evaluate the intelligence of enterprise employees and the results indicated that the Rorschach Test could make up for the defects of traditional intelligence tests and was a useful tool for enterprise managers to evaluate employees' intelligence. X. Li (2010) synthesized the relevant research on the Rorschach Test, reviewed the controversy, and discussed the problems and practical value of the Rorschach Test in talent assessment.

Combination With Eye Movement Techniques

D. Zhang et al. (2009) examined the objectivity of the Rorschach Test with the eye movement technique. The results indicated that there were significant differences in the first reaction time, the fixation count, and the average fixation time of 10 images. X.-B. Zhang (2011) confirmed that there were significant differences in eye movement between individuals with depressions and those without depression; at the same time, there were significant differences in the average fixation time, track map, and hot spot map of eye movement between two types of cards (Black\white and color). J. Li and Jia (2014) compared the eye movement characteristics between patients with depression and controls during the response phase. The results indicated that the fixation count, total fixation duration, and saccade count of patients with depression were significantly lower than those of the normal controls ($p < .05$). The average saccade amplitude of the group with depression was significantly larger than that of the control group ($p < .05$). Zou and Jia

(2014) studied eye movement characteristics of participants with different cognitive styles when they viewed the Rorschach images. The results also indicated there were distinct differences between field-independent and field-dependent participants.

The Group Rorschach Inkblot Test

Japanese researcher Ben Ming Kuan developed the Group Rorschach Test (GRIT) based on the classic Rorschach Test and established its standardized norm (Li M., 2001). In China, there are mainly two relative pieces of research about the GRIT. M. Li (2001) studied the diagnostic criteria and reliability of the GRIT in a Chinese sample. The results indicated there were no significant cultural differences between Chinese and Japanese samples, and on this basis, the researcher put forward the Chinese diagnostic criteria. Qu (2007) revised and developed the GRIT and examined her new GRIT in an adolescent sample. The results showed the new GRIT had test–retest reliability, inter-rater agreement, convergent validity, and empirical validity.

Reviews

There are also some relevant literature reviews and meta-analyses. For example, Guo and Q.-M. Meng (2003) summarized the development history and research status of the Rorschach Test in the Western world, affirming its value and putting forward some questions based on previous research. Cong (2009) promoted a more fair and objective understanding of the Rorschach Test and its use in personality testing, psychological counseling, and other areas of clinical psychology through understanding the development history, implementation process, and analyzing the existing problems. Kong et al. (2015) summarized the research of "Faking Good" and Malingering Reaction in the Rorschach Test based on foreign research, and pointed out that the research was still at a preliminary stage, and it was necessary to conduct further research and to establish specific Faking Good and Malingering scales.

Y.-Q. Li et al. (2014) used a meta-analysis method to compare the results of 18 studies on the Rorschach CS from normal adult samples with Exner's norm (2005) from 16 countries. The results indicated that 23 of the 113 variables in the CS revealed significant differences between the joint sample of 16 countries and Exner's norm. They concluded that Exner's norm had a certain deviation and a tendency of preference.

Summary and Future Perspectives

This article comprehensively summarizes studies on the Rorschach Test in China. The aforementioned research results indicate that some achievements have been made: (1) Researchers in China have done much work regarding the popularization and localization of the Rorschach Test. Some books were published and translated and some universities teach this test in their courses (including some training). There is some exploratory work to establish Chinese norms for the Rorschach Test, which indeed have made certain achievements, such as the establishment of the initial Guangdong Province norm. (2) Researchers in China have also carried out much research on the theory and application of the Rorschach Test, including reliability and validity, various indices (variables, indices, and derivative scales), and the applications to clinical and management settings, etc. (3) Researchers in China have applied new technologies in researching the Rorschach Test, such as eye movement technologies and the GRIT. This shows that the Rorschach Test in China is in continuous development.

However, the following specific issues have arisen: (1) There are some attempts to localize the Rorschach Test, but this is in the initial stages, some of which is regional work, and national norms have a long way to go. (2) Research and experience in clinical applications are not enough to support persuasive conclusions. Clinical research has mainly focused on schizophrenia. The data are not sufficient enough to support conclusions about the reliability and validity of the test itself and all indices in the test. Studies have been exploratory research and involve only a few fields. (3) Research has not been in line with Western countries, and mostly is involved with the CS. However, Western countries have already developed a new Rorschach Test system. (4) There is not a specialized organization to study and apply the Rorschach Test. There is no authoritative institution to buy the original Rorschach images and reference books in China.

Future work should include: (1) A wider dissemination of the Rorschach Test. In line with international standards, regular Rorschach training courses should be held in high-level universities, inviting authoritative overseas experts to train and update the Rorschach Test latest approaches (such as R-PAS). A Chinese Rorschach Association should be established to discuss and explore the Rorschach Test regularly and introduce the original images and reference books. A Chinese version of the software should be developed based on the introduction of foreign computer-assisted Rorschach software and efforts to establish the Chinese norm of the Rorschach Test should begin. (2) The whole test and all kinds of Rorschach indices should be further studied to improve the Rorschach Test reliability and validity. There should be more clinical application research. The Rorschach Test is a valuable tool for clinical measurement, psychological consultation, diagnosis, and treatment of mental disorders and personnel management, etc. Therefore, domestic researchers and clinical workers should pay more attention to the application of the Rorschach Test and help it become a really useful and valuable tool. At the same time, we can continue to explore the application of the Rorschach Test in new fields. (3) With the development of new technologies, Rorschach research combined with these technologies will be emphasized, such as EEG technology, eye movement technologies, and meta-analyses.

References

Cai, C.-H., & Shen, H.-Y. (2007). Self-concept reflected by Rorschach Test in private and public college students. *Chinese Mental Health Journal, 21*(8), 539–543. https://doi.org/10.3321/j.issn:1000-6729.2007.08.009e

Cai, C.-H., Li, Q., Yu, M., Shen, H.-Y., & Fang, J. (2014). Rorschach inkblot method's activation effect on complex. *Chinese Mental Health Journal, 28*(11), 853–858. https://doi.org/10.3969/j.issn.1000-6729.2014.11.010

Chen, M., Gong, Y.-X., Li, S.-G., & Xie, Y.-N. (1997). The cross cultural comparison of result of Rorschach Test between American and Chinese adults. *Chinese Mental Health Journal, 11*(4), 209–212. http://www.cnki.com.cn/Article/CJFDTOTAL-ZXWS704.004.htm

Chen, T.-N. (1999). A control study on Rorschach responses of children with schizophrenia and normal. *Chinese Journal of Clinical Psychology, 7*(2), 86–88+104. http://www.cnki.com.cn/Article/CJFDTOTAL-ZLCY902.005.htm

Chen, X.-X. (2008). *The validity of the Rorschach Inkblot Test in the psychology health assessment* [Master's thesis]. China Master's Theses Full-text Database. http://cdmd.cnki.com.cn/Article/CDMD-10165-2009122600.htm

Chen, X.-X., & Zhou, Q. (2007). Construct validity of the Rorschach ink technique. *Business Culture (Academic Edition), 11*, 259+242.

Chen, Y.-X. (2007). *A study in reliability and validity for Lerner Defense Scale LDS in Rorschach Test* [Master's thesis]. China Master's Theses Full-text Database. http://cdmd.cnki.com.cn/Article/CDMD-10559-2007192586.htm

Cong, J.-W. (2009). On the cognition and practical application of the Rorschach Inkblot Test. *Theory Research, 4*, 24–25. https://doi.org/10.3969/j.issn.1002-2589.2009.04.009

Exner, J. E. (2013a). *A primer for Rorschach interpretation.* (X.-Z. Meng, B.-H. Ren, & H.-H. Liu, Trans.). Jinan University Press. (Original work published 2000)

Exner, J. E. (2013b). *A Rorschach workbook for the Comprehensive System.* (X.-Z. Meng & Y.-C. Tang, Trans.). Jinan University Press. (Original work published 2001)

Gong, Y.-X. (1982). *Wechsler Adult Intelligence Scale – Chinese revision.* Hunan Map Press.

Gong, Y.-X. (1983). *Revised Eysenck Personality Questionnaire manual.* Hunan Medical College.

Gong, Y.-X. (1991). *Rorschach Test manual.* Hunan University Press.

Guo, Q.-K. (1999). A comparative study of the Rorschach Test and 16PF in personality measurement. *Psychological Science, 6*, 565–566. https://doi.org/10.16719/j.cnki.1671-6981.1999.06.026

Guo, Q.-K., Chen, X.-X., & Shan, Z.-Y. (2009). The effectiveness of the Rorschach ink technology in the assessment of personnel quality. In The 12th National Academic Conference of Psychology (Eds.), *Collection of abstracts: The 12th National Academic Conference of Psychology, Jinan, China* (pp. 397–398). https://cpfd.cnki.com.cn/Article/CPFDTOTAL-ZGXG200911001A29.htm

Guo, Q.-K., Chen, X.-X., & Wang, W.-L. (2007). Validity of self-perception score in Rorschach Rating Scale. *Journal of Clinical Rehabilitative Tissue Engineering Research, 11*(48), 9768–9770. https://doi.org/10.3321/j.issn:1673-8225.2007.48.041

Guo, Q.-K., & Meng, Q.-M. (2003). History and present study of the Rorschach Inkblot Method in the western world. *Advances in Psychological Science, 11*(3), 334–338. https://doi.org/10.3969/j.issn.1671-3710.2003.03.016

He, L.-Y. (2015). *The cross-cultural research on the Rorschach – The comparison sample among China, Exner's normative, and Japans* [Master's thesis]. China Master's Theses Full-text Database. http://cdmd.cnki.com.cn/Article/CDMD-10559-1015977598.htm

Hong, H.-J. (2008). *The variation of the Rorschach Depression Index before and after the treatment of depression* [Master's thesis]. China Master's Theses Full-text Database. http://cdmd.cnki.com.cn/Article/CDMD-10559-2009010737.htm

Hu, C.-Y., & Gong, Y.-X. (1989). Personality difference between writers and mathematics teachers. *Chinese Mental Health Journal 3*(3), 119–123. http://www.cnki.com.cn/Article/CJFDTOTAL-ZXWS198903008.htm

Jiang, H.-B., Yan, S.-M., Chen, D.-Y., Yu, J.-H., Qi, S.-G., Sun, J.-H., Xia, Y.-C., Tian, Z.-H., & Zhang, Z. (2000). Analysis of Rorschach Test in patients with "positive" schizophrenic symptoms. *Health Psychology Journal, 8*(1), 16–17. https://doi.org/10.3969/j.issn.1005-1252.2000.01.011

Jiang, Y.-H. (2006). *Validity of Rorschach aggression variables: A school age children sample* [Master's thesis]. China Master's Theses Full-text Database. http://cdmd.cnki.com.cn/Article/CDMD-10559-2007045068.htm

Jiang, Y.-H., Xia, L.-N., Deng, J., & Wang, Z.-Y. (2015). On Rorschach measurement of college students' depression. *Journal of Hengyang Normal University, 36*(5), 142–s144. https://doi.org/10.13914/j.cnki.cn43-1453/z.2015.05.031

Jie, Y.-N. & Dai, X.-Y. (Eds.). (2006). *Practical psychological measurement*. China Medical Science Press.

Kong, D.-S., & Li, Y.-Q. (2013). *Rorschach ink test: A clinical application study on the Comprehensive System*. National Defense Industry Press.

Kong, D.-S., Li, Z.-N., & Li, Y.-Q. (2015). Research on "faking good" and malingering reaction and development in Rorschach inkblot test. *Journal of Psychological Science, 38*(5), 1207–1212. https://doi.org/10.16719/j.cnki.1671-6981.2015.05.023

Lerner, P., & Lerner, H. (1980). Rorschach assessment of primitive defenses in borderline personality structure. In J. Kwawer, H. Lerner, P. Lerner, & A. Sugarman (Eds.), *Borderline phenomena and the Rorschach Test*. International Universities Press.

Li, D.-D. (2007). *A study on the correlation between Rorschach aggression variables AG, AgC and sociopathic tendencies* [Master's thesis]. China Master's Theses Full-text Database. http://cdmd.cnki.com.cn/Article/CDMD-10559-2007192239.htm

Li, L. (1987, September). *Characteristics of the Rorschach Test in patients with chronic schizophrenia* Paper presented at the 6th National Psychology Academic Conference, Hangzhou, China. https://cpfd.cnki.com.cn/Article/CPFDTOTAL-ZGXG198709001247.htm

Li, L.-Y., Hu, X.-X., & Yang, L.-C. (1993). A comparative study of the Rorschach Test between neurosis and normal subjects. *Chinese Journal of Nervous and Mental Diseases, 2*, 101–103. https://www.cnki.com.cn/Article/CJFDTOTAL-ZSJJ199302019.htm

Li, J., & Jia, D.-M. (2014). Eye movement characteristics of depression patients during the Rorschach inkblot test. *Medical Innovation of China, 11*(9), 29–31. https://doi.org/10.3969/j.issn.1674-4985.2014.09.011

Li, M. (2001). *The study on Group Rorschach Inkblot Test* [Master's thesis]. China Master's Theses Full-text Database. http://cdmd.cnki.com.cn/Article/CDMD-10269-2004033171.htm

Li, Q.-X. (1986). Rorschach Test. *Foreign Medical Sciences (Section of Psychiatry), 2*, 69–73.

Li, Q.-X., Zuo, C.-Y., Li, S.-T., & Yang, L.-L. (1989). Rorschach Test in schizophrenic patients. *Chinese Journal of Neurology, 22*(5), 269–273. http://www.cqvip.com/qk/90113x/198905/5095023.html

Li, S.-G., & Gong, Y.-X. (1988). A comparative study of the Rorschach Test between schizophrenic patients and normal people. *Psychological Science, 6*, 19–24. https://doi.org/10.16719/j.cnki.1671-6981.1988.06.005

Li, T.-Y. (2016). *The construction for the Guangdong adult norm of Rorschach Comprehensive System* [Master's thesis]. China Master's Theses Full-text Database. http://cdmd.cnki.com.cn/Article/CDMD-10559-1016733575.htm

Li, X. (2010). On the effectiveness of the Rorschach inkblot method in personnel assessment. *Technology & Management, 11*, 48–49. https://www.cnki.com.cn/Article/CJFDTOTAL-KXZC201011035.htm

Li, X.-L. (2007). *Researches on reliability and validity of Rorschach Suicide Constellation (S-CON)* [Master's thesis]. China Master's Theses Full-text Database. http://cdmd.cnki.com.cn/Article/CDMD-10559-2007192705.htm

Li, Y.-Q., Ding, X., Jin, L.-L., An, M.-L., Kong, D.-S., & Li, Z.-N. (2014). A meta-analysis of Rorschach Comprehensive System. *Studies of Psychology and Behavior, 12*(2), 199–206. https://www.cnki.com.cn/Article/CJFDTOTAL-CLXW201402010.htm

Ling, W.-Q., & Bing, S.-Z. (1988). *Method of psychology test*. Science Press.

Liu, G.-H., & Meng, X.-Z. (2003). A review of Rorschach aggression variables over the past decade. *Chinese Journal of Applied Psychology, 9*(3), 62–64. https://doi.org/10.3969/j.issn.1006-6020.2003.03.012

Liu, G.-H., & Meng, X.-Z. (2007). Correlation between personality and Rorschach aggression variables. *China Journal of Health Psychology, 15*(2), 177–178. https://doi.org/10.3969/j.issn.1005-1252.2007.02.035

Liu, G.-H., & Meng, X.-Z. (2007). Rorschach aggression variables: A study of reliability and validity. *Chinese Journal of Clinical Psychology, 15*(1), 13–14. https://doi.org/10.3969/j.issn.1005-3611.2007.01.005

Liu, H.-X. (2009). *The study on the Egocentricity Index in Rorschach Test* [Master's thesis]. China Master's Theses Full-text Database. http://cdmd.cnki.com.cn/Article/CDMD-10559-2009111359.htm

Liu, J. (2001). *Application and practical exploration of the Rorschach Comprehensive System in Chinese clinical psychology* [Master's thesis]. China Master's Theses Full-text Database. http://cdmd.cnki.com.cn/Article/CDMD-10269-2004033090.htm

Liu, X.-J. (2006). *Researches on Rorschach aggression variables MOR, AgPast and impaired object relations* [Master's thesis]. China Master's Theses Full-text Database. http://cdmd.cnki.com.cn/Article/CDMD-10559-2007045335.htm

Ma, C.-L. (2016). Development of Rorschach Test in China. *Journal of Harbin University, 37*(5), 133–135. https://www.cnki.com.cn/Article/CJFDTOTAL-HEBS201605032.htm

Meng, X.-Z., & Li, T.-Y. (2015). Differences of Ego Impairment Index of Rorschach Test between patients with schizophrenia and normal individuals. *Chinese Mental Health Journal, 29*(7), 522–527. https://doi.org/10.3969/j.issn.1000-6729.2015.07.008

Peng, H.-J., Meng, X.-Z., Long, Y., & Yang, C.-J. (2008). A study of reliability and validity for Mutuality of Autonomy Scale (MOA) in Rorschach Test. *Chinese Journal of Clinical Psychology, 16*(2), 141–143. https://doi.org/10.3969/j.issn.1005-3611.2008.02.010

Qi, F. (2010). *The effectivity of Rorschach Ink-blot Method (RIM) in psychological diagnosis* [Master's thesis]. China Master's Theses Full-text Database. http://cdmd.cnki.com.cn/Article/CDMD-10165-1011012941.htm

Qin, J.-M., Li, C.-H., & Li, Jun. (2015). Gender characteristics about stress related indexes of Rorschach ink-blot test in schizophrenia patients. *China Journal of Health Psychology, 23*(5), 666–670. https://doi.org/10.13342/j.cnki.cjhp.2015.05.008.

Qu, X.-L. (2007). *The reliability and validity researches of group Rorschach inkblot test for teens* [Master's thesis]. China Master's Theses Full-text Database. http://cdmd.cnki.com.cn/Article/CDMD-10285-2007202920.htm

Qu, X.-L. (2010). The case study of the application of the RT intellectual variables in the enterprise's personnel assessment. *Business Research, 18*, 47–49. http://www.cnki.com.cn/Article/CJFDTOTAL-QYYJ201018025.htm

Ren, B.-H. (2007). *The localization of the AgC variable in Rorschach* [Master's thesis]. China Master's Theses Full-text Database. http://cdmd.cnki.com.cn/Article/CDMD-10559-2007192206.htm

Rorschach, H. (1997). *Psychodiagnostik*. (J. Yuan, Trans.). Zhejiang Education Press. (Original work published 1921)

Sun, M. (2011). *The study of the Depression Index (DEPI) and Coping Deficit Index (CDI) in Rorschach Test* [Master's thesis]. China Master's Theses Full-text Database. http://cdmd.cnki.com.cn/Article/CDMD-10559-1011127654.htm

Tang, J. (2004). *Study of the Mutuality of Autonomy Scale (MOA) in Rorschach ink test* [Master's thesis]. China Master's Theses Full-text Database. http://cdmd.cnki.com.cn/Article/CDMD-10559-2004119289.htm

Tang, Y.-C. (2011). *A review on the Ego Impairment Index of Rorschach's reliability and validity* [Master's thesis]. China Master's Theses Full-text Database. http://cdmd.cnki.com.cn/Article/CDMD-10559-1011127421.htm

Tu, R.-S., & Yuan, R.-X. (2010). An empirical study of Rorschach inkblot method in psychodiagnosis on college students with emotional disturbance. *Journal of Shihezi University (Natural Science), 28*(4), 474–477. https://doi.org/10.3969/j.issn.1007-7383.2010.04.017

Wang, B., Li, C.-M., & Li, Ling. (1993). A comparative study of RT, MMPI between schizophrenic patients and emotional disorder patients. *Chinese Journal of Nervous and Mental Diseases, 19*(5), 296–297. http://www.cnki.com.cn/Article/CJFDTOTAL-ZSJJ199305020.htm

Wang, C.-F. (2006). *Rorschach Aggressive Content (AgC) Variable: A study of validity – From the undergraduate sample* [Master's thesis]. China Master's Theses Full-text Database. http://cdmd.cnki.com.cn/Article/CDMD-10559-2007045067.htm

Wang, W.-L. (2008). *The effectiveness of Rorschach ink-blot method (RIM) in personnel assessment* [Master's thesis]. China Master's Theses Full-text Database. http://cdmd.cnki.com.cn/Article/CDMD-10165-2009122602.htm

Wang, X.-Q. (2009). A case report of heroin addicts using Rorschach Test. *Chinese Journal of Drug Abuse Prevention and Treatment, 15*(1), 47–48. https://doi.org/10.3969/j.issn.1006-902X.2009.01.016

Wang, Y.-H., Guo, Q.-K., Chen, X.-X., & Wang, W.-L. (2009). Rorschach ink technology on inter-personal relationship construct validity of measurement and diagnostic research.

Clinical Journal of Medical Officers, 37(6), 1090–1092. http://www.cnki.com.cn/Article/
CJFDTOTAL-JYGZ200906090.htm

Wu, X.-L. (2013). Rorschach Ego Impairment Index: The analysis of validity and its influencing factors [Master's thesis]. China Master's Theses Full-text Database. http://cdmd.
cnki.com.cn/Article/CDMD-10559-1013027905.htm

Wu, Y.-H., Zhu, X.-F., & Zhou, S.-H. (1998). Personality characteristics of typical introverted and extroverted college students in Rorschach Test. Chinese Mental Health Journal, 12(3), 171–172. http://www.cnki.com.cn/Article/CJFDTOTAL-ZXWS803.019.htm

Xiong, B. (2014). The cross-cultural research on the Rorschach–the comparison sample among China, Israel and Exner's normative [Master's thesis]. China Master's Theses Full-text Database. http://cdmd.cnki.com.cn/Article/CDMD-10559-1015002423.htm

Xu, G.-X. (2000). Study abroad life of intercultural adaptation – Mental health and assistance for Chinese students. Shanghai Lexicographic Publishing House.

Xu, G.-X. (2001). Clinical psychology – Knowledge of mental health and aid. Shanghai Education Press.

Yan, Y.-Y., & Meng, X.-Z. (2007). Relationship between Rorschach aggression variables and explicit hostility. Chinese Journal of Clinical Psychology, 15(6), 569–571. https://doi.org/
10.3969/j.issn.1005-3611.2007.06.004

Yang, D., & Ji Yuanhong. (2008). Practical Rorschach ink test. Chongqing Press.

Yao S.-Q. (Ed.). (2007). Psychological assessment. People's Medical Publishing House.

Ying, D.-N. (2006). The correlation between Rorschach aggression variables and Type A Behavior Pattern Questionnaire [Master's thesis]. China Master's Theses Full-text Database. http://cdmd.cnki.com.cn/Article/CDMD-10559-2007045766.htm

Yu, X. (2008). Study of the Depression Index (DEPI) in Rorschach Test [Master's thesis]. China Master's Theses Full-text Database. http://cdmd.cnki.com.cn/Article/CDMD-10559-2009010671.htm

Zhang, D., Kong, K.-Q., & Wang, X.-F. (2009). Exploring the objectivity of the Rorschach Inkblot Test – a research from an eye movement experiment. Psychological Science, 32(4), 820–823. http://www.cnki.com.cn/Article/CJFDTOTAL-XLKX200904012.htm

Zhang, N. (2008). The exploratory research on Rorschach Test used in children (4–6 years old) from China [Master's thesis]. China Master's Theses Full-text Database. http://
cdmd.cnki.com.cn/Article/CDMD-10269-2008148068.htm

Zhang, Nan. (2013). The research about using Rorschach as a measure of adult attachment [Master's thesis]. China Master's Theses Full-text Database. http://cdmd.cnki.com.cn/
Article/CDMD-10217-1014133221.htm

Zhang, X.-B. (2011). Experimental study on eye movement in depressed individuals with the Rorschach inkblot test [Master's thesis]. China Master's Theses Full-text Database. http://cdmd.cnki.com.cn/Article/CDMD-10418-1011302061.htm

Zhang, Y. (2016). Research status of Rorschach ink test in China. Chinese Journal of Critical Care Medicine (Electronic Edition), 9(4), 279–282. http://www.cnki.com.cn/Article/
CJFDTOTAL-ZWZD201604017.htm

Zhong, S.-B., Jing, J., Wang, L.-H., & Yin, Q.-Y. (2007). Analysis on Rorschach inkblot test in Children with attention deficit hyperactivity disorder. Chinese Journal of Clinical Psychology, 15(5), 545–547. https://doi.org/10.3969/j.issn.1005-3611.2007.05.033

Zhu, B.-L., & Dai, Z.-H. (1988). The revision of the Chinese norm of the 16 PF. Psychological Science, 6, 14–18. https://doi.org/10.16719/j.cnki.1671-6981.1988.06.004

Zhu, X.-F., & Gong, Y.-X. (1995). The correlative study between some variables of Rorschach Test and intelligence. Chinese Journal of Clinical Psychology, 3(3), 140–143. http://www.
cnki.com.cn/Article/CJFDTOTAL-ZLCY503.003.htm

Zou, J., & Jia, D.-M. (2014). The study on eye movements in Rorschach inkblot test with field cognitive style of college students. *Studies of Psychology and Behavior, 12*(1), 26–29. http://www.cnki.com.cn/Article/CJFDTOTAL-CLXW201401005.htm

History
Received August 9, 2020
Revision received December 8, 2020
Accepted December 15, 2020
Published online March 18, 2021

Funding
This research was supported by grants from Hunan Province "the 13th Five-Year Program of Education Science" in China.

Fonny Dameaty Hutagalung
Faculty of Education
University of Malaya
Kuala Lumpur 50603
Malaysia
fonny@um.edu.my

Summary

This article provides a comprehensive summary of the development and research status of the Rorschach Test in China. The authors reviewed the literature on the Rorschach Test in China and wrote the article by reading and analyzing the literature. The introduction of the Rorschach Test to China goes back to Ling Minyou, Gong Yaoxian, and Luo Chuanfang in the 1940s and 1950s. The development of the Rorschach Test in China can be divided into two stages: the initial stage and the developing stage. During the initial stage (1940s to 2000), the Rorschach Test was introduced to China and researchers began a systematic study. The article mainly introduces these fields: introduction and localization of the Rorschach Test, studies of schizophrenia, and the measurement of intelligence and personality. In the developing stage (2000 to present), the introduction of the Rorschach Test gradually increased, and research on the Rorschach Test began to diversify. The article presents these aspects: spreading and localization of the Rorschach Test, the variables, indices, and derivative scales, clinical psychology, talent assessment, combination with eye movement techniques, the Group Rorschach Inkblot Test, and reviews. Finally, the authors also summarize the achievements and issues present in existing studies and put forward the prospect of researching the Rorschach Test in China. The issues existing in the present studies are mainly: (1) There are some attempts to localize the Rorschach Test, but this is in the initial stages, some of which is regional work, and national norms have a long way to go. (2) research and experience in clinical applications are not enough to support persuasive conclusions. Clinical research has mainly focused on schizophrenia. The data are not sufficient to support conclusions about the reliability and validity of the test itself and all indices in the test. Studies have been exploratory and involve only a few fields. (3) Research has not been in line with Western countries, and is mostly involved with the CS; however, Western countries have already developed a new Rorschach Test system. (4) There is not a specialized organization to study and apply the Rorschach Test. There is no authoritative institution to buy the original Rorschach images and reference books in China.

总结

本文尽可能全面地综述了罗夏测验在中国的发展和研究现状。作者收集了中国有关罗夏测验的文献，并通过阅读和分析文献撰写了这篇文章。将罗夏测验引入中国的历史可以追溯到上个世纪40年代和50年代的凌敏猷、龚耀先以及罗传方三位学者。罗夏测验在中国的发展可以分为两个阶段：初始阶段和发展阶段。在初始阶段（从1940年代到2000年），罗夏测验被引入中国，研究人员开始进行系统的研究。本文主要介绍以下领域：罗夏测验的引入和本地化；精神分裂症人群的研究；智力和人格的测量。在罗夏测验的发展阶段（从2000年到现在），罗夏测验的引入逐渐增多，对罗夏测验的研究也开始多元化。作者从这些方面进行了介绍：罗夏测验的普及和本地化；罗夏测验的变量、指数和导出量表；临床心理学的研究；人才评估；结合眼动技术的研究；团体罗夏墨迹测验；综述研究。最后，文章总结了中国关于罗夏研究的成果和存在的问题，并提出了将来研究罗夏测验的前景。当前研究中存在的问题主要有：**(1)** 对罗夏测验的本地化和建立常模的工作还处于起步阶段，有的只是些区域性工作。**(2)** 临床应用的研究不足以支持有说服力的结论，也没有足够的材料来支持有关测验信度和效度的结论。**(3)** 还未与国际接轨，大部分研究是综合系统的研究。但是，西方国家已经发展了新的罗夏测验系统。**(4)** 没有专门的机构来研究和应用罗夏测验。甚至在中国都购买不到正版的罗夏测验图片和参考书。

Résumé

Cet article résume le développement et l'état de la recherche du test de Rorschach en Chine de manière aussi complète que possible. L'auteur a ramassé les articles et les documents sur le test de Rorschach en Chine et a rédigé cet article tout en les lisant et en les analysant. L'introduction du test de Rorschach en Chine est due aux trois savants : LING Minyou, GONG Yaoxian et LUO Chuanfang, remonte dans les années 1940 et 1950. Le développement du test de Rorschach en Chine est divisé en deux phases : la phase initiale et celle de développement. Dans la phase initiale (depuis des années 1940 jusqu'en 2000), le test de Rorschach a été introduit en Chine et les chercheurs ont commencé à faire une étude systématique. Pour cet article, on va présenter principalement les domaines suivants : l'introduction et la localisation du test de Rorschach; les études sur le groupe des gens de schizophrénie; la mesure de l'intelligence et de la personnalité. Dans la phase de développement (de l'année 2000 à aujourd'hui), l'introduction du test de Rorschach devient de plus en plus nombreuse et la recherche sur ce test commence à se diversifier. L'auteur effectuera sa présentation à partir de ces aspects : la vulgarisation et la localisation du test de Rorschach; les variables, les indices et les échelles dérivées du test; la recherche sur la psychologie clinique; l'évaluation des talents; la recherche sur la combinaison avec les techniques de mouvement oculaire; le test de tache d'encre du groupe Rorschach et le sommaire. Finalement, l'article résume les réalisations et quelques problèmes qui se posent au cours de ses études en Chine, tout en prévoyant la perspective de recherche sur le test de Rorschach. Les problèmes qui existent dans les études actuelles sont principalement suivants : (1) Il y a quelques tentatives pour localiser le test de Rorschach, mais il n'en est qu'à ses débuts, dont certains sont des travaux régionaux; (2) La recherche et l'expérience dans les applications cliniques ne suffisent pas à étayer des conclusions convaincantes. La recherche clinique s'est principalement concentrée sur la schizophrénie mais n'est pas encore entrée en profondeur. Les données ne sont pas suffisantes pour étayer des conclusions sur la fiabilité et la validité du test lui-même et de tous les indices du test; (3) La recherche n'a pas rendu conforme à la pratique internationale, la plupart des recherches sont synthétiques et systématiques. Cependant, les pays occidentaux ont déjà développé un nouveau système de test Rorschach; (4) Il n'existe pas une organisation spécialisée pour étudier et appliquer le test de

Rorschach. En Chine, on ne peut pas acheter les images originales de Rorschach et les livres de référence en version originale.

Resumen

En este documento se ofrece un panorama lo más amplio posible del desarrollo de la prueba de Rorschach en China y del estado actual de la investigación. El autor recopiló literatura sobre el test de Rorschach en China y escribió este artículo leyendo y analizando las tesis.

La introducción de la prueba de Rorschach en China se remonta a los tres eruditos, LING Minyou, GONG Yaoxian y LUO Chuanfang en las décadas de 1940 y 1950. El desarrollo de la prueba de Rorschach en China puede dividirse en dos fases: la fase inicial y la fase de desarrollo. Durante la fase inicial (del decenio de 1940 al 2000), la prueba de Rorschach se introdujo en China y los investigadores comenzaron a realizar estudios sistemáticos. Este artículo se centra en las siguientes áreas: la introducción y localización de la prueba de Rorschach, la investigación sobre poblaciones esquizofrénicas y la medición de la inteligencia y la personalidad. Durante la fase de desarrollo de la prueba de Rorschach (desde 2000 hasta la actualidad), la introducción de la prueba de Rorschach ha aumentado gradualmente y la investigación sobre la prueba de Rorschach se ha diversificado. Los autores presentan estos aspectos: la popularización y localización de la prueba de Rorschach; variables, índices y escalas derivadas de la prueba de Rorschach; investigación en psicología clínica; evaluación de talentos; investigación que incorpora técnicas de rastreo ocular; pruebas de manchas de tinta de Rorschach en grupo; y estudios de revisión. Por último, el artículo resume los resultados y problemas de la investigación sobre el Rorschach en China, y sugiere perspectivas para futuras investigaciones sobre las pruebas de Rorschach. Los principales problemas del presente estudio son: (1) la localización de la prueba de Rorschach y el establecimiento de un modelo normativo están todavía en sus comienzos, y algunos de los trabajos son de carácter regional. (2) Las investigaciones sobre las aplicaciones clínicas son insuficientes para apoyar conclusiones persuasivas y no hay suficiente material para apoyar las conclusiones sobre la fiabilidad y la validez de las pruebas. (3) No está todavía en consonancia con las normas internacionales y la mayor parte de las investigaciones son integradas y sistemáticas. Sin embargo, en Occidente se han desarrollado nuevos sistemas de prueba de Rorschach. (4) No hay un cuerpo especial para estudiar y aplicar el test de Rorschach. Ni siquiera se pueden comprar fotos de pruebas de Rorschach auténticas y libros de referencia en China.

要約

本論文では、中国におけるロールシャッハテストの発展と研究状況をまとめている。著者らは、中国におけるロールシャッハテストに関する文献を精査し、それらを分析して論文化した。中国でのロールシャッハテストの導入は、1940年代から1950年代にかけてのLing Minyou、Gong Yaoxian、Luo Chuanfang にまで遡る。中国におけるロールシャッハテストの8点は、初期段階と発展段階の2つの段階に分けることができる。初期段階（1940年代から2000年まで）では、ロールシャッハテストが中国に導入され、研究者たちは提携的な研究を始めた。本稿では、主にロールシャッハテストの導入と地方で独特の発展をした、統合失調症の研究、知能や性格の測定などの分野を紹介している。発展期（2000年〜現在）では、ロールシャッハテストの導入が徐々に増え、ロールシャッハテストの研究が多様化し始めた。本稿では、ロールシャッハテストの普及と局在化、変数・指標・派生尺度・臨床心理学・才能評価・眼球運動法との組み合わせ、集団ロールシャッハ・インクブロットテスト、レビューなどの側面を提示している。最後に、既存の研究の成果と課題をまとめ、中国におけるロールシャッハテストの展望を述べている。既存の研究に存在する問題点は、主に以下の通りである。(1) ロールシャッハテストの地域化の試みはあるが、これば初期段階のも

のであり、その一部は地域的なものであり、国の規範はまだ長い道のりを辿っている。(2) 臨床応用における研究や経験は、説得力のある結論を支持するには十分ではない。臨床研究は、統合失調症を中心に行われてきた。試験自体や試験中のすべての指標の信頼性や妥当性についての結論を支持するにはデータが十分ではない。研究は探索的なものであり、いくつかの分野にしか関与していない。(3) 欧米諸国の研究が追随しておらず、ほとんどがCSに関わるものであるが、欧米諸国ではすでに新しいロールシャッハテストのシステムが開発されている。(4) ロールシャッハテストを研究・応用する専門機関がない。中国には、ロールシャッハのオリジナル図版や参考書を購入できる権威ある機関がない。

Editorial

Celebrating 100 Years

Kari Carstairs

Private Practice, London, UK

This special edition of *Rorschachiana* is a celebration of the centenary of the publication in 1921 of Hermann Rorschach's book *Psychodiagnostics*. Authors were invited to submit review articles that summarize the research in particular areas of study. The aim is to offer an update on the White Paper from the Society of Personality Assessment that was published in 2005 in response to criticisms of the Rorschach that called for a moratorium on the use of the test in clinical practice. Based on a review of the scientific literature, the White Paper concluded "the Rorschach possesses documented reliability and validity similar to other generally accepted test instruments used in the assessment of personality and psychopathology and that its responsible use in personality assessment is appropriate and justified" (Society for Personality Assessment, 2005, p. 221).

The question to authors was, "What does the scientific literature from 2005 to the present tell us now about the reliability and validity of the Rorschach as a tool for the assessment of personality?" Then, in order to broaden the discussion and reach out to the wider psychological community, each article was sent to another psychologist with specialist knowledge on the topic. The discussants were invited to comment on how the Rorschach literature informed their area of practice.

Nancy Kaser-Boyd gives us an update on the research into how the patient's experience of trauma is manifested on the Rorschach (Kaser-Boyd, 2021). She discusses the two main symptom clusters of avoidance and intrusions and links these to "constricted" and "flooded" protocols. There are sections on torture, interpersonal abuse, and combat trauma. She also considers the research on malingering. The discussant for this article is Steven Gold and he writes convincingly about the value of the patient's experience being given full rein in the test (Gold, 2021).

In a very different vein, Koji Jimura, Tomoki Asari, and Noriko Nakamura plunge into neurophysiological studies of brain functioning during the administration of the Rorschach and provide fascinating links between individual differences in particular Rorschach scores and patterns of brain activity, looking at the human movement response, achromatic determinants, form quality, chromatic responses, oral dependent responses, and complexity (Jimura et al., 2021).

© 2021 Hogrefe Publishing

Rorschachiana (2021), *42*(2), 113–117
https://doi.org/10.1027/1192-5604/a000150

L. Andre van Graan, a neuropsychologist with additional training in neuroscience and neuroimaging, is the discussant. He shares his thoughts on how the Rorschach has potential to bring ecological validity to such studies (van Graan, 2021).

Corine de Ruiter takes us into the courtroom with a case study of a 20-year-old man accused of attempted manslaughter (de Ruiter, 2021). She introduces her case by reviewing the research on violent crime and the Rorschach, noting that it provides "a mixed picture." Anita Boss is the discussant and she picks up on the point that the Rorschach cannot be used to predict violent acts; it comes into its own as a clinical tool when the psychologist needs to advise on treatment. She also discusses some current concerns about forces in the USA that have led American forensic psychologists away from considering performance-based tests, including the Rorschach, whereas in other jurisdictions, there is more scope for a wider remit when carrying out assessments for the courts (Boss, 2021).

Silvia Monica Guinzbourg de Braude, Sarah Vibert, Tommaso Righetti, and Arianna Antonelli took on the challenging task of integrating the findings from studies with patients with eating disorders across two different approaches with the Rorschach, the Comprehensive System and the French School (Guinzbourg de Braude et al., 2021). Katarina Meskanen and Massiliano Pucci discuss the research with an eye to spelling out methodological issues and how to account for confounding variables (Meskanen & Pucci, 2021). Once again, we find the theme of how an assessment with the Rorschach is helpful in treatment planning.

It is therefore very fitting to have a discussion of the use of the Rorschach in the assessment of treatment outcome from Filippo Aschieri and Giulia Pascarella (Aschieri & Pascarella, 2021). They take as their starting point a meta-analysis by Grønnerød (2004) and provide us with an update. Their discussants, Christopher Hopwood, Mathew Yalch and Xiaochen Luo, respond with a tightly reasoned critique of methodology and recommendations for future research (Hopwood et al., 2021).

Last but certainly not least, we have the contribution from James Kleiger and Joni Mihura in the US on the Rorschach and thought disorder. They set out some conceptual issues, give an overview of recent research findings and provide recommendations (Kleiger & Mihura, 2021). Their discussants are two psychologists from The Netherlands (Boyette & Noordhof, 2021).

In my experience, upon first coming across the Rorschach, many psychologists balk at it and find it unlikely that it really tells us anything reliable about the examinee. As Rorschach himself said in *Psychodiagnostics:*

> It is always daring to draw conclusions about the way a person experiences life from the results of an experiment. To try it on the basis of the findings of so simple an experiment as this may, at first glance, appear absurd. (p. 87)

This common response of assuming that it is absurd to draw conclusions about a person's psychological functioning from the results of the test is expressed by the discussants who begin their commentary on Kleiger and Mihura's article with this question, "Why on earth would one use the Rorschach to assess disordering thinking?" (Boyette & Noordhof, 2021, p. 281). As they delve into the research, they are persuaded that the Rorschach is a reliable and valid tool for this purpose. This is my hope for this special edition – that we can widen our audience to reach psychologists who previously would have dismissed the test as no better than tea leaf reading.

The apparent simplicity of presenting the examinee with an inkblot and asking, "What might this be?" means that the examinee "settles himself for a harmless test of the imagination and what he is subjected to is far more than that" (Rorschach, 1921, p. 121). The contributions to this special issue give a window onto the different ways in which the test is indeed "far more than that" and describe some of the different applications of Rorschach's original work. Many important topics are missing, such as the assessment of suicide risk, work with children, normative studies, and forensic assessment in the civil and family courts, but I hope that the selection of topics provides something of interest for all our readers.

In his letter to Roemer on June 18, 1921, Hermann Rorschach described how the test was based on two kinds of thinking about the data:

> analytical and psychological. The result is that psychologists perceive it to be too analytical and often do not understand it, while analysts want to stick to the content of the meaning and do not care about the origins. And it will only become worse. (Rorschach, 1921, p. 12)

We can see that this divide remains true today in the range of articles in this special issue. There is a wide spectrum of different approaches to the Rorschach, from those that emphasize psychometric rigor as the central organizing principle to those that consider that the key strength of the method is its ability to capture the particular subjectivity of each individual who takes the test.

Much of the work for this special issue took place during a pandemic that has had a profound impact on all of our lives. As I write this editorial, a huge international effort is on-going to roll out a vaccination program for the whole world. In this same spirit of international collaboration, it is a pleasure to see that the authors who have contributed to this special issue come from eight different countries: Argentina, Finland, France, Italy, Japan, The Netherlands, UK, and the USA; the article on eating disorders wins the prize in this category, with four different countries represented between the authors and the discussants!

In that same letter to Roemer on June 18, 1921, Hermann Rorschach expressed his sense of how more work was needed if we are going to realize the full promise of the test. He wrote:

There is a lot more still in the experiment not to mention the question of a more or less acceptable theoretical underpinning and factors are certainly still buried in the findings that also have their own strict value. One just has to find these. (Rorschach, 1921, p. 11)

One hundred years later, this is most certainly still true. I am sure that we have not unearthed all that the test offers and several of the discussants have outlined their recommendations for future research. We look to the next generation of psychologists to carry this work forward.

References

Aschieri, F., & Pascarella, G. (2021). A systematic narrative review of evaluating change in psychotherapy with the Rorschach Test. *Rorschachiana, 42*(2), 232–257. https://doi.org/10.1027/1192-5604/a000142

Boss, A. L. (2021). A commentary on "The Rorschach and violent crime" (de Ruiter, 2021). *Rorschachiana, 42*(2), 196–201. https://doi.org/10.1027/1192-5604/a000144

Boyette, L.-L., & Noordhof, A. (2021). A commentary on "Developments in the Rorschach assessment of disordered thinking and communication" (Kleiger & Mihura, 2021). *Rorschachiana, 42*(2), 281–288. https://doi.org/10.1027/1192-5604/a000145

de Ruiter, C. (2021). The Rorschach and violent crime: A literature review and case illustration. *Rorschachiana, 42*(2), 175–195. https://doi.org/10.1027/1192-5604/a000134

Gold, S. N. (2021). A commentary on "The Rorschach and trauma" (Kaser-Boyd, 2021). *Rorschachiana, 42*(2), 139–142. https://doi.org/10.1027/1192-5604/a000143

Grønnerød, C. (2004). Rorschach assessment of changes following psychotherapy: A meta-analytic review. *Journal of Personality Assessment, 83*(3), 256–276. https://doi.org/10.1207/s15327752jpa8303_09

Guinzbourg de Braude, S. M., Vibert, S., Righetti, T., & Antonelli, A. (2021). Eating disorders and the Rorschach: A research review from the French School and the Comprehensive System. *Rorschachiana, 42*(2), 202–224. https://doi.org/10.1027/1192-5604/a000136

Hopwood, C. J., Yalch, M. M., & Luo, X. (2021). A commentary on "A systematic narrative review of evaluating change in psychotherapy" (Aschieri & Pascarella, 2021): More rigor is needed in research on the Rorschach and treatment change. *Rorschachiana, 42*(2), 258–264. https://doi.org/10.1027/1192-5604/a000146

Jimura, K., Asari, T., & Nakamura, N. (2021). Can neuroscience provide a new foundation for the Rorschach variables? *Rorschachiana, 42*(2), 143–165. https://doi.org/10.1027/1192-5604/a000147

Kaser-Boyd, N. (2021). The Rorschach and trauma – an update. *Rorschachiana, 42*(2), 118–138. https://doi.org/10.1027/1192-5604/a000133

Kleiger, J. H., & Mihura, J. L. (2021). Developments in the Rorschach assessment of disordered thinking and communication. *Rorschachiana, 42*(2), 265–280. https://doi.org/10.1027/1192-5604/a000132

Meskanen, K., & Pucci, M. (2021). A commentary on "Eating disorders and the Rorschach" (Guinzbourg de Braude et al., 2021). *Rorschachiana, 42*(2), 225–231. https://doi.org/10.1027/1192-5604/a000148

Rorschach, H. (1921, June 18). Letter to Georg A. Roemer (Dictate2Us, Trans.). The Rorschach Archives (HR 2:1:29), University of Berne, Switzerland.

Rorschach, H. (1921/1951). Lemkau P., & Kronenberg B. (1921/1951). *Psychodiagnostics: A diagnostic test based on perception* (5th ed.). Verlag Hans Huber.

Society for Personality Assessment (2005). The status of the Rorschach in clinical and forensic practice: An official statement by the Board of Trustees of the Society for Personality Assessment. *Journal of Personality Assessment, 85*(2), 219–237. https://doi.org/10.1207/s15327752jpa8502_16

van Graan, L. A. (2021). A commentary on "Can neuroscience provide a new foundation for the Rorschach variables?" (Jimura et al., 2021). *Rorschachiana, 42*(2), 166–174. https://doi.org/10.1027/1192-5604/a000149

Published online September 15, 2021

Acknowledgements

I floated a proposal for a special issue of *Rorschachiana* in July 2018 in Montreux at the executive board meeting of the International Society for the Rorschach. Sadegh Nashat, who was then the Editor-in-Chief, suggested that I might be the guest editor. I had very little idea then about how much work would be involved and perhaps this is just as well because if I had realized, I might not have volunteered! However, I am grateful to him for encouraging me to take on this project. Thank you also to Lionel Chudzik and Filippo Aschieri who helped me along the way. It has been rewarding to see it come together. Thank you, Hermann Rorschach, for giving us this unique and special test!

Kari Carstairs
Private Practice
London
UK
kari@carstairspsych.co.uk

Special Issue: The Rorschach Test Today: An Update on the Research
Original Article

The Rorschach and Trauma – An Update

Nancy Kaser-Boyd

Geffen School of Medicine, University of California Los Angeles, CA, USA

Abstract: Early research on trauma employing the Rorschach found it to be an ideal instrument, with its red, black, gray, and vibrant colors, to elicit trauma content. Two patterns of Rorschach responses emerged: the constricted pattern, where the evaluee kept to a form-based, avoidant approach to the blot, as if defending against the memories of the trauma, and a flooded pattern, where morbid and aggressive images paralleled that of psychosis. The Rorschach as an instrument continues to demonstrate high sensitivity to the experience of trauma, and research since 2005 has added complexity and additional validation for the use of the Rorschach in the evaluation of the effects of trauma.

Keywords: constriction, flooding, malingering, Rorschach, trauma

The Rorschach has a history of sensitivity to trauma, calling out or triggering images from experienced trauma with its dark, red, colorful, shaded, and ambiguous stimuli. The Rorschach as an instrument continues to demonstrate high sensitivity to the ˙experience of trauma, and research since 2005 has added complexity and additional validation for the use of the Rorschach in the evaluation of the effects of trauma. Trauma disorders take varied but well-described forms. The Rorschach accesses psychological processes not tapped by self-report measures, allowing the patient to communicate trauma images in the ambiguous and unstructured Rorschach that were avoided in the direct examination by the evaluator and not called out by more structured psychological tests. There is now a robust literature on the Rorschach and trauma, and presenting this is the focus of this paper. Few psychological assessment instruments have as broad an international usage as the Rorschach (Viglione & Meyer, 2008; Evans & Hass, 2018). The Rorschach has a large body of international norms, which include international norms for the Exner Comprehensive System (CS; Meyer et al., 2007) and for the Rorschach Performance Assessment System (R-PAS; Meyer et al., 2011, 2017).

Posttraumatic stress disorder (PTSD) as a diagnostic entity has been modified by both *The Diagnostic and Statistical Manual of Mental Disorders (DSM-5;* American Psychiatric Association, 2013) and by the *International Classification of Diseases (ICD-11;* World Health Organization, 2019). In addition to the historical enumeration of symptoms of (a) re-experiencing, (b) avoidance, and (c) hyperarousal,

DSM-5 has added the following: "Negative alterations in cognitions and mood associated with the traumatic event(s)." The ICD-11 has added a stand-alone diagnosis of complex posttraumatic stress disorder, which outlines symptoms when the trauma has been longstanding, as in repetitive child abuse or domestic violence, or torture. Complex PTSD is widely discussed in the United States in domains such as children's courts and veterans' treatments, but it is acknowledged in DSM-5 only as PTSD "with associated features supporting diagnosis." PTSD and complex PTSD are only two of many possible trauma outcomes and there are often comorbid disorders such as major depressive episode, anxiety disorder, and, commonly, substance abuse disorders. Trauma symptoms can also be misunderstood and diagnosed as borderline personality disorder, bipolar disorder, or even schizophrenia.

Sadly, there is no shortage of sufferers of trauma, either in the United States or worldwide, with ongoing wars, gang violence, political repression, and cataclysmic weather events. Psychological assessment documents symptoms of trauma for asylum-seekers, personal injury for litigation, symptoms pertinent to mental state in criminal court, and targeting treatment approaches. Careful assessment includes a battery of psychological tests, among which the Rorschach is a valuable tool, often described as a "screen" for traumatic memories. The Rorschach can also offer important information on whether the patient has the psychological resources to tolerate the stress of treatments like exposure therapy (Foa et al., 2000).

Brief History

The earliest studies of Rorschach and trauma involved service people in wartime. Shalit (Shalit, 1965) administered the Rorschach to 20 servicemen in the Israeli navy while they were in the midst of a severe storm at sea. He found a rise in inanimate movement (m) that has been replicated in subsequent studies of trauma of multiple origins. Van der Kolk and Ducey (1989) and Salley and Teiling (1984) studied Vietnam combat veterans and became the first researchers to document traumatic intrusions on the Rorschach. Tori (1989) studied Mexican homosexuals, both those illegally in the United States and those in Mexico. He concluded that the Rorschach elucidated dysphoric mood, distorted perceptions, and difficulties coping with a perceived dangerous social environment. Franchi and Andronikof-Sanglade (1999) studied a group of West African immigrant women in Paris who had genital circumcision (clitoridectomies). Although none of these women complained of being sexually mutilated, images of intact and clitoridectomized organs, along with scores associated with emotional distress, emerged as a dominant theme in 40% of their protocols.

The Rorschach was used early on to evaluate traumatized children. Zivney and colleagues (1988), using the CS (Exner, 1974), examined the Rorschach records of 80 girls with histories of sexual abuse, aged 9–16. Dividing them into two groups according to their age at the beginning of molestation, these researchers found that the most disturbed girls were those who experienced early abuse. Over half of these girls manifested disturbed cognition (M-, low X+% and more DVs and FABCOMs.) They also found scores associated with anxiety and helplessness (m and Y), a damaged self (Morbids), and a "preoccupation with themes of primitive supply and transitional relatedness" (food and clothes, X-rays, and abstracts). Leifer et al. (1991) administered the Rorschach to 38 sexually abused girls aged 5–16 and 32 age-matched controls. Scored with the CS (Exner, 1974), the sexually abused girls had more disturbed thinking and impaired reality testing (X-% and high WSum6). Leifer found higher levels of distress with a preponderance of negative affect (higher DEPI, higher SumShading) more primitive, disturbed human relationships, and more sexual responses. Holaday and Whittenberg (1994) used the Rorschach to study children with burn injuries. Scored with the CS (Exner, 1993), one fourth of these children met the diagnostic criteria for schizophrenia, mostly on the cognitive variables, yet they did not exhibit psychosis. They had significantly lower Egocentricity Indices, reflecting their impaired sense of self, and significantly less Texture, which is associated with comfort with intimacy.

Van der Kolk and Ducey (1989) and Levin and Reis (1996) were the first to describe two patterns in Rorschach responses, one that revealed traumatic flooding, with contents of danger and injury, and, by contrast, a second involving emotional constriction, with a record that was largely form-based and brief; also described were records where responses alternated between flooding and constriction. This came to be known as the biphasic response to trauma. Kaser-Boyd (1993) administered the Rorschach to battered woman waiting trial for murder. Scored with the CS (Exner, 1974), she found that they typically delivered brief, constricted records with the occasional emergence of trauma images. However, some of the women delivered Rorschach records that seemed almost psychotic.

Other early researchers made similar findings; for example, Cerney (1990) reported finding two distinct response modes among her study participants: either constriction with no color determinants, or flooding with unmodulated color. Swanson and colleagues (1990), Hartman et al. (1990), Armstrong (1991), and Brand et al. (2006) all noted a biphasic trauma pattern within their study participants' protocols. The biphasic pattern was seen in children as well (Holaday & Whittenberg, 1994).

Over time, the constricted protocol came to be identified by: High Lambda, low R, low Affective Ratio and few Blends, low EB, focus on Populars, and a bland, form-based protocol. This is a cognitive strategy that appeared to reflect avoidance and numbing. The extreme end of constriction or avoidance is dissociation. Labott and colleagues (1992) developed a dissociative index. Scored apart from the Exner CS, it included objects in the distance and objects shifting or rapidly changing. Leavitt and Labott (1997) found that the presence of these responses in their Rorschach sample correlated with scores on the Dissociative Experiences Scale (Carlson & Putnam, 1992).

The "flooded" protocol was identified by: traumatic content, responsivity to color in CF + C responses, scores reflecting painful affect (Y and V), poor reality testing (high X-%, low Xo% and X+%), inanimate movement and a high HVI, negative D, and Adjusted D. Individuals with flooded protocols can be mistaken as psychotic. The trauma content in flooded protocols was described as a window into the trauma experience. For example, Ephraim (2002) presents a torture victim's response to Card II: "If I take the card this way, I see a mask. A bad person behind the mask. Can I talk about the most repulsive face I ever saw in my life? Because this reminds me exactly of that face." He was recalling the circumstances of a friend's execution. Armstrong and Kaser-Boyd (2003) present responses from a 14-year-old male victim of molestation by a violent father: (Card I) "A crippled guy with some kind of writing on his chest." (Card III) "A dead frog with blood all over. A person looking at a reflection and there is blood on the wall." (Card IV) "A dead animal, his skull has been crushed and there are parts everywhere. It's shattered." (Card V) "A lady putting her hands up to a mirror and her leg has been cut off." (Card VII) "A pig that's been blown up and the parts of him are all separated, and two elephants that got shot and got all blown up."

Content reflecting the trauma experience was found to be so pervasive that Armstrong and Loewenstein (1990) developed the Trauma Content Index (TCI). The TCI is based on the Exner CS scores of Sex, Blood, Anatomy, Morbid, and Aggressive Movement, divided by the total number of responses (TC/R). A TC/R of 0.3 and above was hypothesized to suggest traumatic intrusion. A number of studies have shown support for the TCI. For example, Kamphuis and colleagues (2000) documented the ability of the TCI to distinguish between patients with confirmed sexual abuse and those without abuse. A mean of 0.25 has shown specificity and sensitivity for trauma, which means scores greater than 0.30 have been suggested to indicate traumatic intrusions and can differentiate traumatized and nontraumatized patients (Armstrong, 2002). This has been replicated in studies after 2005 (Arnon et al., 2011; Kamphuis et al., 2008).

Sloan et al. (1995) developed a Combat Content Score (CC), which included perceptions of weapons and personalized responses referring to experience that occurred during the course of military operations. They found a positive correlation between their CC scale and the MMPI-PK Scale.

Rorschach researchers, overall, have worked to map the effects of trauma on cognitive processing, reality testing, problem-solving, and coping with stress, emotional control, world view, and self and object relations. Researchers of trauma of various types have found a high incidence of impaired reality testing and thought disorder on the Rorschach. This includes atypical views of reality (low X+%, high Xu%), illogical combinations of ideas (INCOMs and FABCOMs), and loss of task focus (DR). Armstrong (2002) hypothesized that these scores reflect a "traumatic thought disorder." The Rorschach has been proposed as the best instrument to assess cognitive disturbances associated with traumatic intrusion, defense patterns, issues of identity and relatedness, and problems with self-regulation and dissociation (Opaas & Hartmann, 2013).

Although not directly related to the Rorschach, the neurobiology of trauma received focused attention in the work of van der Kolk (1987) and was amplified by others: Schachter (1996), LeDoux (1996, 1998), Yehuda et al. (1992), van der Kolk and Greenberg (1987), Bremner (1999), and DeBellis et al. (1994).

Malingering Trauma

There was little research before 2005 on whether trauma could be malingered on the Rorschach. Perry and Kinder (1992) and Frueh and Kinder (1994) explored the malingering of combat-generated PTSD, and created the Dramatic Content Score, which consisted of responses with sex, aggression, blood, fire, explosions, and morbidity. These contents, however, are similar to those on Armstrong's Trauma Content Index. Also, the authors noted that their PTSD sample was many years postcombat and the authors did not appear to be aware of the tendency for the defensive process of constriction to set in as combat veterans tried to cope and go back to a "normal" life.

2005 to the Present

By 2005, when *Rorschachiana* published a whole volume on the Rorschach and trauma, much was known about the value of the Rorschach in evaluating trauma. That volume presented Rorschach research on torture (Ephraim, 2002), traumatic dissociation (Armstrong, 2002), trauma in sexually abused children (Gravenhorst, 2002), and combat veterans (Sloan et al., 2002). Ephraim summarized the articles noting that the Rorschach elucidated cognitive disturbances associated with intrusive recollections, illustrated avoidant and numbing defense patterns, and demonstrated deviations in identity and relatedness and complications with self-regulation. Researchers pointed out that there was no standard set of data that was seen in trauma, as the data were often dependent on the variability in processing Rorschach data, the type of trauma, and other variables. Studies since 2005 have confirmed earlier findings and expanded knowledge about Rorschach indicators of trauma; the past 10 years have seen the emergence of the Rorschach Performance Assessment System (R-PAS; Meyer et al., 2011) with the publication of R-PAS national norms (Meyer et al., 2011; Meyer et al., 2015; Viglione & Giromini, 2016). Research published in the past 15 years has employed the Exner CS (Exner, 1974), or the R-PAS (Meyer et al., 2011), or sometimes scores from both systems. For the convenience of the reader, this will be organized according to type of trauma, with a summary to follow.

Torture

The past 15 years have seen a great influx of refugees fleeing war, gang violence, and political oppression. The torture victim may appear for treatment, may apply for government benefits, or may apply for asylum. Evans (2008) suggests the Rorschach is valuable as a vehicle that evokes trauma memories and is useful when it is unclear whether the individual is malingering symptoms of trauma or being deceptive about a torture experience. He recommends that the Rorschach be used with careful consideration of the state of the examinee as its black, gray, red, and bold colors may elicit memories of terror and anguish. From his experience of assessing over 100 torture victims, Evans noted that the horrific and relentless intrusive experiences of the torture in many evaluees overwhelmed attempts at avoidance and numbing. He cited the concept of "terrible knowledge" (Jay, 1991) that torture victims experience through witnessing the terrible acts of other human beings. He suggests caution in using the Rorschach if there has been recent torture, as it has the potential for overpowering brittle defenses.

Evans (2008) and Opaas and Hartmann (2013) present nuanced differences about the merits of the Rorschach with this population. Opaas and Hartman reported a Rorschach study of 51 traumatized refugees from 15 different countries where the Rorschach seemed easier to complete than more formal questionnaires. The Opaas and Hartmann study is unique in choosing variables from both the CS and R-PAS and relating them to external measures of adaptation and functioning. The participants were all in Norway, where their mean stay was 11 years. The majority of the participants came from the Middle East and a few came from East Africa. Overall, 53% confirmed having been tortured and 22% having been raped. Almost all had experienced military attacks, being forced to evacuate, and the violent death or murder of a family member or friend. About 75% had witnessed others being killed or dying due to violence, and 75% had been close to being killed themselves. As far as diagnosis, 78% qualified for a diagnosis of PTSD. Keeping Evans's (2008) cautions in mind, the authors altered the standard administration when clinical and ethical considerations made it necessary. The variables they chose were: m, M, CF+C, Blends, D, and R, from Exner, the TCI, and R-PAS variables SevCog, FQo%, and FQ-%. In total, 33% of the protocols were short, which others have found to be common in survivors of torture (Arnon et al., 2011). TCI, SevCog, and FQ-% were found to be especially high, pointing to a relationship among trauma content, thought disturbances, and perceptual distortions. The TCI was especially high (0.44). Their analysis also supported the biphasic response to trauma. The authors note that the Rorschach results of the group as a whole indicated limited productivity, limited fantasy and creativity, perceptual and emotional restrictedness, anxiety, and fluctuation between rigidity and deficits of emotional control. When the authors examined correlations between the Rorschach and measures of adaptability (such as the ability to work), they found the participants who were emotionally constricted to be more impaired, and constriction did not seem to protect these participants against the pain of past trauma. Evans makes this point as well (Evans & Hass, 2018).

Trauma From Interpersonal Abuse

Brand and colleagues (2006) studied traumatized inpatients with dissociative disorder (DD), comparing their Rorschach scores with those of non-DD with PTSD, inpatients with depression, and nonpatient adults. They note that severely traumatized individuals with dissociative identity disorder (DID) tend to be flooded by traumatic material, while paradoxically having defenses that permit distancing and detachment from their experience. They comment that the Rorschach is generally the most challenging but most informative test because it opens up intense emotions and conflicts that patients who have DD habitually "turn off." They note that, as with other severely traumatized individuals, it is common for patients who have DD to give fewer responses than other patients, likely in order to limit and escape from painful associations. Their study included 100 inpatients, 78 with DID and 22 with dissociative disorder not otherwise specified (NOS). No significant differences between the DID and DDNOS groups were found on 17 Rorschach variables, and thus the groups were collapsed. All participants met DSM criteria for PTSD. The DD group was compared with several other diagnostic groups: Non-DD patients with PTSD, inpatients with depression, and nonpatient adults. While the DD records were often short, the responses themselves tended to be lengthy because of a high number of blends and special scores, and the DD group was low on Lambda. The group showed a highly ideational, obsessive style of managing stress (highly introversive), which contrasts with the extratensive style of individuals with borderline or hysterical personality disorders. They had more M responses, which was hypothesized as a heightened ability to fantasize. However, they had more M- responses, suggesting distorted views of others. The DD patients had FD scores higher than the other groups, which suggested a greater capacity for emotional distance and insight, which was hypothesized to be a positive predictor for engagement in therapy. They showed as much interest in others as the non-patients (COP, H) and less alienation than the other patient groups. They had a low Afr, indicating an attempt to avoid emotion. The DD group was not high on m, contradicting the consistent finding of high m among other trauma groups. The average score on the Trauma Content Index was 0.50. They were preoccupied by a sense of their bodies being damaged and the world being filled with aggression.

The patients with DD blatantly misperceived reality less than the other patient groups, but showed the most distorted perceptions and illogical thought on trauma-related percepts. The authors conclude that traumatized individuals whose defense is dissociation retain some resilience by protecting some intellectual and emotional abilities.

In a follow-up study, Brand and colleagues (2006) compared Rorschach scores of patients with DID ($N = 67$), borderline personality disorder ($N = 40$), and generally psychotic inpatients ($N = 43$). As in the study by Brand et al. in 2006, a number of the DID patients gave records with fewer than 14 responses, but in consultation with Greg Meyer, the researchers removed cases with fewer than 14 responses only if Lambda was greater than 0.50. Brand et al. (2009) note that the Rorschach was difficult for DID patients, whom they described as showing their distress by rocking, showing fear, experiencing flashbacks, and sometimes switching personality states. Findings were similar to those reported in the previous study by Brand et al. (2006). In terms of cognitive variables, the DID patients showed significantly more complex thinking (Blends/R). Patients with DID had lower WSum6 scores than both BPD patients and those with psychotic disorders. The level of M- was similar across the groups. In terms of unmodulated emotion, DID patients had lower CF+C:FC scores. Patients with DID provided more FD and COP responses than did patients with BPD or psychotic disorders. The DID patients had a TCI score that was similar to the other two groups but appeared to be able to remain more reality focused, based on the WSum6 Score comparison. The authors concluded that patients with DID, compared with patients with BPD and psychotic disorders, showed a greater interest in collaborative engagement and a much greater capacity to be self-reflective (FD), which suggested a greater capacity for participation in therapy.

Kaser-Boyd (2008) re-analyzed the records of battered women who killed their partner (Kaser-Boyd, 1993), separating the women by high Lambda and low Lambda scores, and opined that the high Lambda scores reflected emotional constriction or the avoidance symptoms of PTSD, and the low Lambda scores reflected the re-experiencing phase of PTSD. Like earlier research, the low-Lambda or flooded protocols graphically illustrated the experience of trauma. For example, Kaser-Boyd (2008) presents a battered woman's response to Card II:

A broken chest, somebody busted 'em in the chest, broken, bleeding. *Inquiry*: It's like your chest here, and they hit you here in the heart, the heart exploded from the top because they hit you there, and then part of your lungs or kidneys or whatever would be down here. It would be like an x-ray of the chest here somebody just punched it and there's blood spots just where it's bruised. (*Bruised?*) The color. (*Exploded?*) The burst of the fingers. The splatter effect there, you know how when you hit a water balloon, how it just splatters?

Smith et al. (2020) employed the Rorschach Trauma Content Index (Armstrong & Loewenstein, 1990) in a sample of women prisoners, where the experience of child sexual trauma was high; 44.4% met criteria for PTSD and 55% had a trauma-related disorder. They explored the relationship between the Rorschach Trauma Content Index (Armstrong & Loewenstein, 1990) and a number of other personality test measures such as the Personality Assessment Inventory (Morey, 1991) and the Trauma Symptom Inventory-2 (Briere, 2011). The mean TCI in the inmates diagnosed with PTSD was 0.26 (*SD* = 0.19). The TCI was significantly correlated with the total number of reported traumatic events and the total reported sexual abuse events. In this population the authors note that the TCI components consisted of aggression, a damaged sense of self, sexual preoccupations, blood, and anatomy responses. To illustrate, one victim of rape saw:

A ballet dancer. These are her feet. She's on her toes and this is her torso. I don't know why the body would be open in the middle. Maybe it's some sort of emblem hanging on a chair. Maybe her body is not present, just the pieces she wears, almost as if on a hanger. I see it both ways, as a costume with a medallion and as a woman ripped apart with her heart torn out, and blood all over her clothes. I see it both ways but it scares me this other way, so I said clothing on a hanger.

This woman's response process illustrates, by itself, the process of constriction and distancing from the traumatic imagery.

In an interesting study of PTSD in first responders, Mrevlje (2018) examined Rorschach scores of a group of crime scene investigators (CSIs) in Slovenia. Distinguishing CSIs with higher levels of trauma from those with lower levels using the Detailed Assessment of Posttraumatic Stress (DAPS; Briere, 2001), the authors found that the group with higher scores (17.2%) had Rorschach protocols marked by lower XA% scores (proportion of responses with a good form fit) and significantly higher X-% scores (answers that disregard reality). The CSIs as a group tended toward an avoidant cognitive style, ignoring, denying, or simplifying complexity, which may enable them to distance themselves from becoming overwhelmed. The authors note that a similar finding was made by Brewster and colleagues (2010) with police officer candidates, suggesting there is already an inclination toward an avoidant cognitive style. The Trauma Content Index in the CSI sample did not reach significance, likely as a result of the avoidant style.

Ephraim (2020), presents clinical findings of youths with complex PTSD. He notes that severely and repetitively traumatized youths commonly give constricted or defensive protocols, those that are form-based, with high Lambdas. He cautions that the traditional interpretation of such protocols as defensive underestimates the strong ongoing efforts of these youths to avoid feeling overwhelmed by memories, thoughts, or emotions associated with their painful experiences. Ephraim notes that even in such protocols, trauma content may be elicited and significant windows into the trauma experience can be given. He notes that the Rorschach protocols of these youths with complex PTSD often included danger-related themes that were directly or indirectly associated with specific trauma memories and/or reflected their strong negative expectations about the world. Ephraim revisits the Preoccupation with Danger Index (Ephraim & Kaser-Boyd, 2003), which was culled from response categories of two trauma groups: victims of torture/state violence, and severely battered women. A thematic content index, the DI contains four categories: Fear, Threat, Harm, and Violent Confrontation. Both trauma groups obtained significantly higher DI scores than a group of normal volunteers (5.55 for battered women, 6.33 for torture victims, compared with 1.25 for the normal).

Combat Trauma

There were fewer studies of combat trauma with the Rorschach after 2005, perhaps due to the end of the Vietnam war in the United States, perhaps with fewer combat veterans to study, or with Iraq and Afghanistan, more interest in the impact of physical injury such as brain trauma from improvised explosive devices. Arnon and colleagues (2011) examined the records of military, prison, and police personnel diagnosed with PTSD, employing the CS (1974), and subjected the data to linear regression to attempt to determine which Rorschach variables were sensitive to PTSD. They attempted to find an index, a cluster of Rorschach indicators, for diagnosing PTSD. The lapse in time from the date of injury averaged 4 years. About one third of the subjects produced Rorschach records with fewer than 14 responses. This has come to be known as a common pattern of emotional constriction in trauma survivors. They were, nevertheless, included in the analysis. Anatomy was the first component selected by the analysis, which the authors believe resulted from subjects who had been injured. INC1 was the second component, and the authors suggest this was the result of the experience of the implausible, unsuspected occurrence of a horrific event. Bt was the third component, hypothesized to reflect avoidance, and Fi was the last component, which, like anatomy, was often part of traumatic military events. The stepwise linear regression analyzed 220 RIAP5 variables. A 13-item model was proposed by the computed analysis. This was the PTSD Predictive Score (PPS). The PPS was calculated for the PTSD group (N = 116) and a comparison non-PTSD group (N = 71). The two groups were found to differ significantly on the PPS. However, the sensitivity and specificity of the PPS were below acceptable levels.

Illustrating the pervasive experience of combat trauma, Kaser-Boyd and Evans (2008) present the response of a combat veteran on Card VII:

> Two dead wolves and something is stuck to their neck, an apparatus, and I guess it looks like they are sucking something out and waste is coming out of this end. Actually, this kind of looks like a rifle here. It's got two scopes here, and this looks like blood or do-do. It's like a rifle but it's connected to their neck and it looks like it is sucking something out of the wolves. It's got the scopes, the grips, the barrel. You see the colors? It's red but it's got a little bit of yellow and it looks like guts and waste. It looks really dirty and messy, stuff you wouldn't touch. These are animals and they really look dead, and these two really look like rifles, just the kind of scope I had. This is the flash suppressor. This has the grip, the magazine, and it's pointing right at their neck.

The Rorschach Performance Assessment System

The Rorschach Performance Assessment System (R-PAS) was introduced in 2011 (Meyer et al., 2011), and research employing R-PAS variables to evaluate trauma is slowly emerging.

Viglione et al. (2012) combine findings from the Exner CS R-PAS to suggest five interpretive areas for evaluating trauma with the Rorschach: (1) cognitive constriction; (2) trauma-related imagery; (3) trauma-related cognitive disturbances; (4) stress response; and (5) dissociation. The authors note that, in addition to the other identified advantages of the Rorschach for the evaluation of trauma, the Rorschach allows for individual variation in the symptoms and expression of PTSD and captures the often repetitive cognitive avoidance strategies that suppress trauma images or the breakdown of defensive cognitive operations. Also, the Rorschach, unlike self-report inventories, provides avenues for emotional, tactile, sensory, kinesthetic, and interpersonal imagery and expression. Five suggested areas, utilizing CS and R-PAS scores are:

1. Cognitive Constriction: One would expect fewer responses, more pure form responses, more responses with animal content, perseverations, card rejections, low scores on prompts in R-PAS, fewer Blends, and a low Complexity score on R-PAS.

2. Trauma-Related Imagery: This is captured in an organized fashion by the Trauma Content Index in the Exner CS, and in the Critical Content score in R-PAS. Viglione et al. (2012) note that the Critical Content score is highly correlated with the TCI but adds Explosion, Fire, X-ray and imaging contents. The authors reassert that these Trauma and Critical Contents involve the break-through of intrusive traumatic imagery, but idiosyncratic intrusive imagery may escape the broad net cast by these pre-conceived content categories.

3. Specific Trauma-Related Cognitive Disturbances: Individuals with PTSD often display disturbed thinking in their responses, measured by form quality and cognitive codes. Form Quality is a measure of reality testing, judgment, maturity, and adaptation. In the CS, these are captured in FQ- responses, X-%, low WDA%, unusual detail locations, and Cognitive Special Scores (SevCog, WSum6). In R-PAS, the Thought and Perceptual Composite and Ego Impairment Index capture the cognitive disarray seen in trauma. Unlike with other psychiatric disorders, the cognitive disruption is in response to trauma images.

4. Stress Response: There is a robust empirical relationship between environmental stress and elevations in inanimate movement (m) and diffuse shading (Y; Exner, 2003). Meta-analytic analysis supported a relationship between m and internal tension or stress and between Y and stress and distress in general (Mihura et al., 2013). These scores capture the psychological state of helplessness and feeling controlled by outside forces, both common in the experience of trauma.

5. Dissociation. Dissociation is suggested by dimensional and distancing responses scored FD in the CS, and a lower Afr, which reflects avoidance of color. The Labott et al. (1992) indicators of dissociation have received the best empirical support. These include: (a) forms seen through obscuring media such as veils, fog, or mist, so that the form seems blurry or unreal; (b) responses in which distance appears exaggerated such that objects or figures appear vague or far away; (c) objects are experienced as unstable, shifting, moving, or rapidly changing. Such responses in a record were found to correlate to scores on the Dissociative Experiences Scale (Leavitt & Labott, 1997).

Viglione et al. (2012) suggest these five guidelines as a framework for researching and assessing PTSD and trauma-related symptoms.

Malingering

Almost since its inception, and certainly in studies of trauma, the possibility of dissimulation on the Rorschach was raised. Ganellen (2008) reviews typical Rorschach Scores in defensive protocols: Low R, high Lambda, low Blends, Populars, and Personalizations. The susceptibility of the Rorschach to dissimulation sets of "faking good" or "faking bad" has received additional study, some of which has been inspired by the publication of a great deal of information about the Rorschach, including the actual cards, on Wikipedia (Smith, 2010; Hartmann & Hartmann, 2014). Sewell (2008; Sewell & Helle, 2018) notes that there are few studies on faking good, and for faking bad found that skilled practitioners often misclassify those faking bad as genuine patients. Strategies for faking have remained relatively constant, however. Those seeking to present a picture of health tend to give a brief form-based protocol, with Populars and few Blends. This resembles the constricted protocols of trauma survivors. Those seeking to malinger PTSD typically provide dramatic contents. Mihura (2012) notes that malingerers are more likely to focus on the content of the response versus other aspects like form quality or cognitive scores. These "dramatic contents," contain themes such as morbidity, sex, aggression, blood, fire, and explosions. However, no study compared malingerers of trauma with actual trauma patients, who are known to produce a high number of similar contents, which in the CS comprise the Trauma Content Index, and in R-PAS, Critical Contents. The implication from Mihura (2012) is to examine formal scores.

Overview of 50 Years of Research on the Rorschach and Trauma

The research from before and after 2005 on the Rorschach and trauma is quite consistent across trauma groups and across adults and children. The finding of utility for the Rorschach in the assessment of trauma has held firm – the Rorschach is a "screen" upon which patients project their unique trauma experience as well as the manner in which they cope with the disturbing memories evoked by the blots. The finding of a biphasic response to trauma has also held firm. The Rorschach captures the avoidant phase of PTSD in records that are constricted, and the re-experiencing and hyperaroused phase of PTSD in records that are flooded with trauma images and markers of reality distortion. These findings have continued with the emergence of the R-PAS. While the content of Rorschach responses will likely differ, depending on the type of trauma experienced and the stage of recovery at the time of testing, the Viglione et al. (2012) guidelines offer consistent signs for evaluating trauma protocols. The most fruitful method for evaluating trauma on the Rorschach is to survey the areas of: (1) cognitive constriction; (2) trauma-related imagery; (3) trauma-related cognitive disturbances; (4) stress response; and (5) dissociation.

Future research is needed particularly in the area of treatment: amenability to treatment, recommendations for treatment, and response to treatment. Both the CS and R-PAS systems offer scores that will assist in this endeavor. Rorschach trauma research might well inform us whether there is a difference in Rorschach responses as a result of the type of trauma, that is, interpersonal trauma versus natural catastrophe or accident. Would the former have more of an effect on relatedness? Given the new dimensional approach to diagnosis, hierarchical taxonomy of psychopathology (HITOP; Kotov et al., 2017), do the personality spectra of internalizing and externalizing produce different Rorschach results? The field will also benefit from additional R-PAS studies of trauma as more practitioners begin to employ this scoring system.

References

American Psychiatric Association (APA) (2013). *Diagnostic and statistical manual of mental disorders (DSM-5).*
Armstrong, J. G. (1991). The psychological organization of multiple personality disordered patients as revealed in psychological testing. *Psychiatric Clinics of North America, 14,* 533–546.

Armstrong, J. G. (2002). Deciphering the broken narrative of trauma: Signs of traumatic dissociation on the Rorschach. *Rorschachiana, 25*(1), 11–27. https://doi.org/10.1027/1192-5604.25.1.11

Armstrong, J. G., & Kaser-Boyd, N. (2003). Projective assessment of psychological trauma. In M. Hilsenroth & D. Segal (Eds.), *Objective and projective assessment of personality and psychopathology: Vol. 2. Comprehensive handbook of psychological assessment* (pp. 500–512). Wiley.

Armstrong, J. G., & Loewenstein, R. J. (1990). Characteristics of patients with multiple personality and dissociative disorders on psychological testing. *The Journal of Nervous and Mental Disease, 178*, 448–454.

Arnon, Z., Maoz, G., Gazit, T., & Klein, E. (2011). Rorschach indicators of PTSD: A retrospective study. *Rorschachiana, 35*, 5–26. https://doi.org/10.1027/1192-5604/a000013

Brand, B. L., Armstrong, J. G., & Loewenstein, R. J. (2006). Psychological assessment of patients with dissociative identity disorder. *Psychiatric Clinics of North America, 29*(1), 145–168. https://doi.org/10.1016/j.psc.2005.10.014

Brand, B. L., Armstrong, J. G., Loewenstein, R. J., & McNary, S. W. (2009). Personality differences on the Rorschach of Dissociative Identity Disorder, Borderline Personality Disorder, and Psychotic Inpatients. *Psychological Trauma: Theory, Research, Practice & Policy, 1*(3), 188–205. https://doi.org/10.1037/a0016561

Bremner, J. D. (1999). Alterations in brain structure and function associated with posttraumatic stress disorder. *Seminars in Clinical Neuropsychiatry, 4*, 249–255.

Brewster, J., Wickline, P. W., & Stoloff, J. L. (2010). Using the Rorschach Comprehensive System in police psychology. In P. A. Weiss (Ed.), *Personality assessment in police psychology: A 21st century perspective* (pp. 188–221). Charles C. Thomas Publishers.

Briere, J. (2001). *Detailed assessment of posttraumatic stress: Professional manual.* Psychological Assessment Resources.

Briere, J. (2011). *Trauma Symptom Inventory–2: Professional manual.* Psychological Assessment Resources.

Carlson, E. B., & Putnam, F. W. (1992). *Manual for the Dissociative Experiences Scale.* NIMH.

Cerney, M. (1990). The Rorschach and traumatic loss: Can the presence of traumatic loss be detected from the Rorschach? *Journal of Personality Assessment, 55*, 781–789.

DeBellis, M. D., Lefter, L., Trickett, P. K., & Putnam, F. W. (1994). Urinary catecholamine excretion in sexually abused girls. *Journal of the American Academy of Child and Adolescent Psychiatry, 33*, 320–327.

Ephraim, D. (2002). Rorschach trauma assessment of survivors of torture and state violence. *Rorschachiana, 25*, 58–76. https://doi.org/10.1027/1192-5604.25.1.58

Ephraim, D. (2020). Rorschach assessment of complex trauma in youth. *Rorschachiana, 41*(1), 19–41. https://doi.org/10.1027/1192-5604/a000122

Ephraim, D., & Kaser-Boyd, N. (2003, March). *A Rorschach index to assess preoccupation with danger.* Paper presented at the Annual Meeting of the Society for Personality Assessment, San Francisco, CA.

Evans, F. B. (2008). The Rorschach and immigration evaluations. In C. B. Gacono, F. B. Evans, N. Kaser-Boyd, & L. Gacono (Eds.), *The handbook of forensic Rorschach assessment* (pp. 489–504). Routledge.

Evans, F. B., & Hass, G. A. (2018). *Forensic psychological assessment in immigration court: A guidebook for evidence-based and ethical practice.* Routledge.

Exner, J. E. (1974). *The Rorschach: A comprehensive system*. Wiley.

Exner, J. E. (1993). *The Rorschach: A comprehensive system. Vol. 1: Basic foundations* (3rd ed.). Wiley.

Exner, J. E. (2003). *The Rorschach: A comprehensive system, Vol. 1: Basic foundations* (4th ed.). Wiley.

Foa, E. B., Keane, T. M., & Friedman, M. J. (2000). Guidelines for treatment of PTSD. *Journal of Traumatic Stress, 13*(4), 539–588. https://doi.org/10.1023/A:1007802031411

Franchi, V., & Andronikof-Sanglade, H. (1999). Methodological and epistemological issues raised by the use of the Rorschach Comprehensive System in cross-cultural research. *Rorschachiana, 23*(1), 118–134. https://doi.org/10.1027/1192-5604.23.1.118

Frueh, B. C., & Kinder, B. N. (1994). The susceptibility of the Rorschach inkblot test to malingering of combat-related PTSD. *Journal of Personality Assessment, 62*, 280–298. https://doi.org/10.1207/s15327752jpa6202_9

Ganellen, R. J. (2008). Rorschach assessment of malingering and defensive response sets. In C. B. Gacono, F. B. Evans, N. Kaser-Boyd, & L. A. Gacono (Eds.), *The handbook of forensic Rorschach assessment* (pp. 89–120). Routledge.

Gravenhorst, M. C. (2002). Rorschach psychodynamics of psychic trauma in sexually abused children. *Rorschachiana, 25*(1), 77–85. https://doi.org/10.1027/1192-5604.25.1.77

Hartman, W. R., Clark, M. E., Morgan, M. K., Dunn, V. K., Fine, A. D., Perry, G. G. Jr., & Winsch, D. L. (1990). Rorschach structure of a hospitalized sample of Vietnam veterans with PTSD. *Journal of Personality Assessment, 54*, 149–159. https://doi.org/10.1080/00223891.1990.9673982

Hartmann, E., & Hartmann, T. (2014). The impact of exposure to internet-based information about the Rorschach and the MMPI-2 on psychiatric outpatients' ability to simulate mentally healthy test performance. *Journal of Personality Assessment, 96*(4), 432–444. https://doi.org/10.1080/00223891.2014.882342

Holaday, M., & Whittenberg, T. (1994). Rorschach responding in children and adolescent who have been severely burned. *Journal of Personality Assessment, 62*, 269–279. https://doi.org/10.1207/s15327752jpa6202_8

Jay, J. (1991). Terrible knowledge. *Family Therapy Networker, 15*, 18–29.

Kamphuis, J. H., Kugeares, S. L., & Finn, S. E. (2000). Rorschach correlates of sexual abuse: Trauma content and aggression indices. *Journal of Personality Assessment, 75*, 212–224. https://doi.org/10.1207/S15327752JPA7502_3

Kamphuis, J. H., Trin, N., Timmermans, M., & Punamaki, R. (2008). Extending the Rorschach trauma content index and aggression indexes to dream narratives of children exposed to enduring violence: An exploratory study. *Journal of Personality Assessment, 90*, 578–584. https://doi.org/10.1080.00223890802388558

Kaser-Boyd, N. (1993). Rorschachs of women who commit homicide. *Journal of Personality Assessment, 60*, 458–470.

Kaser-Boyd, N. (2008). Battered woman syndrome: Assessment-based expert testimony. In C. B. Gacono, F. B. Evans, N. Kaser-Boyd, & L. A. Gacono (Eds.), *The handbook of forensic Rorschach assessment* (pp. 467–487). Routledge.

Kaser-Boyd, N., & Evans, F. B. (2008). Rorschach assessment of psychological trauma. In C. B. Gacono, F. B. Evans, N. Kaser-Boyd, & L. A. Gacono (Eds.), *The handbook of forensic Rorschach assessment* (pp. 255–278). Routledge.

Kotov, R., Krueger, R. F., Watson, D., Achenbach, T. M., Althoff, R. R., Bagby, R. M., Brown, T. A., Carpenter, W. T., Caspi, A., Clark, L. A., Eaton, N. R., Forbes, M. K., Forbush, K. T.,

Goldberg, D., Hasin, D., Hyman, S. E., Ivanova, M. Y., Lynam, D. R., Markon, K., ... Zimmerman, M. (2017). The hierarchical taxonomy of psychopathology (HITOP): A dimensional alternative to traditional nosologies. *Journal of Abnormal Psychology, 126*(4), 454–477. https://doi.org/10.1037/abn0000258

Labott, S. M., Leavitt, F., Braun, B. G., & Sachs, R. G. (1992). Rorschach indicators of multiple personality disorder. *Perceptual and Motor Skills, 75*(1), 147–158. https://doi.org/10.2466/pms.1992.75.1.147

Leavitt, F., & Labott, S. M. (1997). Criterion-related validity of Rorschach analogues of dissociation. *Psychological Assessment, 9*(3), 244–249. https://doi.org/10.1037/1040-3590.9.3.244

LeDoux, J. (1996). *The emotional brain: The mysterious underpinnings of emotional life.* Simon & Schuster.

LeDoux, J. (1998). Fear and the brain: Where have we been and where are we going? *Biological Psychiatry, 44,* 1229–1238. https://doi.org/10.1016/s0006-3223(98)00282-0

Leifer, M., Shapiro, J. P., Martone, M. W., & Kassem, L. (1991). Rorschach assessment of psychological functioning in sexually abused girls. *Journal of Personality Assessment, 56*(1), 14–28. https://doi.org/10.1207/s15327752jpa5601_2

Levin, P., & Reis, B. (1996). Use of the Rorschach in assessing trauma. In J. P. Wilson & T. Keane (Eds.), *Assessing psychological trauma and PTSD* (pp. 529–543). Guilford Press.

Meyer, G. J., Erdberg, P., & Shaffer, T. W. (2007). Toward international normative reference data for the Comprehensive System. *Journal of Personality Assessment, 89*(S1), 5201–5216. https://doi.org/10.1080/00223890701629342

Meyer, G. J., Shaffer, T. W., Erdberg, P., & Horn, S. L. (2015). Addressing issues in the development and use of the Composite International Reference Values as Rorschach norms for adults. *Journal of Personality Assessment, 97*(4), 330–347. https://doi.org/10.1080/00223891.2014.961603

Meyer, G. J., Viglione, D. J., & Mihura, J. L. (2017). Psychometric foundations of the Rorschach Performance Assessment System (R-PAS). In R. E. Erard & F. B. Evans (Eds.), *The Rorschach in multimethod forensic assessment: Conceptual foundations and practical applications* (pp. 23–91). Routledge.

Meyer, G. J., Viglione, D. J., Mihura, J. L., Erard, R. E., & Erdberg, P. (2011). *Rorschach performance assessment system: Administration,* coding, interpretation, and technical manual. Rorschach Performance Assessment System.

Mihura, J. L. (2012). The necessity of multiple test methods in conducting assessments: The role of the Rorschach and self-report. *Psychological Injury and Law, 5*(2), 97–106. https://doi.org/10.1007/s12207-012-9132-9

Mihura, J. L., Meyer, G. J., Dumitrascu, N., & Bombel, G. (2013). The validity of individual Rorschach variables: Systematic reviews and meta-analyses of the comprehensive system. *Psychological Bulletin, 139*(3), 548. https://doi.org/10.1037/a0029406

Morey, L. C. (1991). *The Personality Assessment Inventory: Professional manual.* Psychological Assessment Resources.

Mrevlje, T. P. (2018). Police trauma and Rorschach indicators: An exploratory study. *Rorschachiana, 39*(1), 1–19. https://doi.org/10.1027/1192-5604/a000097

Opaas, M., & Hartmann, E. (2013). Rorschach assessment of traumatized refugees: An exploratory factor analysis. *Journal of Personality Assessment, 95*(5), 457–470. https://doi.org/10.1080/00223891.2013.781030

Perry, G. G., & Kinder, B. N. (1992). The susceptibility of the Rorschach to malingering: A critical review. *Journal of Personality Assessment, 54*(1–2), 47–57.

Salley, R., & Teiling, P. (1984). Dissociated rage attacks in a Vietnam veteran: A Rorschach study. *Journal of Personality Assessment, 48*, 98–104.

Schachter, D. L. (1996). *Searching for memory: The brain, the mind, and the past.* Basic Books.

Sewell, H. W. (2008). Dissimulation on projective measures. In R. Rogers (Ed.), *Clinical assessment of malingering and deception* (3rd ed., pp. 207–217). Guilford Press.

Sewell, H. W., & Helle, A. C. (2018). Dissimulation on projective measures: An updated appraisal of a very old question. In R. Rogers & S. D. Bender (Eds.), *Clinical assessment of malingering and deception* (4th ed., pp. 301–313). Guilford Press.

Shalit, B. (1965). Effects of environmental stimulation on the M, FM, and m responses in the Rorschach. *Journal of Projective Techniques and Personality Assessment, 29*, 228–231.

Sloan, P., Arsenault, L., & Hilsenroth, M. (2002). Use of the Rorschach in the assessment of war-related stress in military personnel. *Rorschachiana, 25*(1), 86–122. https://doi.org/10.1027/1192-5604.25.1.86

Sloan, P., Arsenault, L., Hilsenroth, M., Harvill, L., & Handler, L. (1995). Rorschach measures of posttraumatic stress in Persia Gulf War veterans. *Journal of Personality Assessment, 64*(3), 397–414. https://doi.org/10.1207/s15327752jpa6403_1

Smith, B. (2010). The Rorschach – Wikipedia controversy. *SPA Exchange, 22*(1), 7.

Smith, J. M., Gacono, C. B., & Cunliffe, T. B. (2020). Using the Rorschach Trauma Content Index (TCI) with incarcerated women. *Journal of Projective Psychology and Mental Health, 27*, 12–20.

Swanson, G. S., Blount, J., & Bruno, R. (1990). Comprehensive system Rorschach data on Vietnam combat veterans. *Journal of Personality Assessment, 54*(1–2), 160–169.

Tori, C. D. (1989). Homosexuality and illegal residency status in relations to substance abuse and personality traits among Mexican nationals. *Journal of Clinical Psychology, 45*, 814–821.

Van der Kolk, B. A. (1987). *Psychological trauma.* American Psychiatric Press.

Van der Kolk, B. A., & Ducey, C. (1989). The psychological processing of traumatic experience: Rorschach patterns in PTSD. *Journal of Traumatic Stress, 2*, 259–263.

Van der Kolk, B. A., & Greenberg, M. S. (1987). The psychobiology of the trauma response: Hyperarousal, constriction, and addiction to traumatic reexposure. In B. A. Van der Kolk (Ed.), *Psychological trauma* (pp. 63–88). American Psychiatric Press.

Viglione, D. J., & Giromini, L. (2016). The effects of using the international versus Comprehensive System Rorschach norms for children, adolescents, and adults. *Journal of Personality Assessment, 98*(4), 391–397. https://doi.org/10.1080/00223891.2015.1136313

Viglione, D. J., & Meyer, G. J. (2008). An overview of Rorschach psychometrics for forensic practice. In C. B. Gacono, F. B. Evans, N. Kaser-Boyd, & L. Gacono (Eds.), *The handbook of forensic Rorschach assessment* (pp. 21–53). Routledge.

Viglione, D. J., Towns, B., & Lindshield, D. (2012). Understanding and using the Rorschach Inkblot Test to assess post-traumatic conditions. *Psychological Injury and Law, 5*, 135–144. https://doi.org/10.1007/s12207-012-9128-5

World Health Organization (2019). *The international classification of diseases (ICD-11).*

Yehuda, R., Southwick, S. M., Giller, E. L., Ma, C., & Mason, J. W. (1992). Urinary catecholamine excretion and severity of PTSD symptoms in Vietnam combat veterans. *Journal of Nervous and Mental Disease, 180*, 321–325.

Zivney, O. A., Nash, M. R., & Hulsey, T. L. (1988). Sexual abuse in early versus late childhood: Differing patterns of pathology as revealed on the Rorschach. *Psychotherapy – Theory, Research, and Practice, 25*, 99–106.

History

Received May 4, 2020
Revision received September 26, 2020
Accepted September 29, 2020
Published online September 15, 2021

ORCID

Nancy Kaser-Boyd
 https://orcid.org/0000-0002-4144-3110

Nancy Kaser-Boyd
Geffen School of Medicine
University of California Los Angeles
10833 Le Conte Avenue
Los Angeles, CA 90095
USA
nkbforensics@gmail.com

Summary

The Rorschach assesses psychological variables that self-report measures do not tap and creates a testing situation that allows the trauma patient to communicate trauma images and display the manner in which they cope with these intrusive images. Early research described two classic responses to Rorschach cards: emotionally constricted, characterized by a short, form-based record, and emotionally flooded, characterized by traumatic images and scores signaling cognitive disarray. This biphasic response to trauma has been supported by studies that now span 50 years and are seen in patients who have experienced a variety of traumas (torture, domestic violence, sexual abuse, rape, civilian disaster, and responding as a helper in traumas), and in children and adults. A decision to use the Rorschach to evaluate trauma should begin with a consideration of the fragility of the evaluee, since the Rorschach evokes traumatic memories. Viglione and colleagues (2012) combine findings from the Exner Comprehensive System and R-PAS to suggest five interpretive areas for evaluating trauma with the Rorschach: (1) cognitive constriction; (2) trauma-related imagery; (3) trauma-related cognitive disturbances; (4) stress response; and (5) dissociation. Individuals who attempt to malinger trauma will likely deliver dramatic contents similar to the Trauma Content Index in the Comprehensive System and Critical Contents in the R-PAS but are not likely able to produce the trauma-related cognitive disturbances and scores known to occur with stress.

Résumé

Le Rorschach évalue les variables psychologiques que les mesures d'auto-évaluation ne relèvent pas et crée une situation de test qui permet au patient traumatisé de communiquer des images de traumatisme et de mettre en avant la manière dont le patient fait face à ces images intrusives.

Les premières recherches décrivaient deux réponses classiques à la carte de Rorschach: Emotionnel resserré, caractérisé par une réponse courte basée sur une forme, et émotionnellement inondée, caractérisée par des images traumatiques et des scores signalant un désarroi cognitif. Cette réponse biphasique au traumatisme a été soutenue par des études qui s'étendent maintenant sur 50 ans et sont observées chez des patients qui ont subi une variété de traumatismes (torture, violence domestique, abus sexuels, viol, catastrophe civile et réponse en tant qu'aide dans les traumatismes) chez les enfants et les adultes. La décision d'utiliser le Rorschach pour évaluer un traumatisme doit commencer par une prise en compte de la fragilité de la personne évaluée, puisque le Rorschach évoque des souvenirs traumatiques. Viglione, Towns et Lindshield (2012) combinent les résultats de l'Exner Comprehensive System et du R-PAS pour suggérer cinq domaines d'interprétation pour évaluer le traumatisme avec le Rorschach : (1) constriction cognitive; (2) l'imagerie liée au traumatisme; (3) troubles cognitifs liés aux traumatismes; (4) réponse au stress; et (5) dissociation. Les personnes qui tentent de simuler un traumatisme fourniront probablement un contenu dramatique similaire à l'indice du contenu du traumatisme dans le CS et au contenu critique du R-PAS, mais ne sont probablement pas en mesure de produire les perturbations cognitives et les scores liés au traumatisme connus pour se produire avec le stress.

Resumen

El Rorschach evalua las variables psicológicas que las medidas de autoinforme no pueden valorar, facilitando una situación de prueba que permite al paciente con trauma comunicar imágenes del trauma y mostrar la forma en que se enfrenta a estas imágenes intrusivas. Las primeras investigaciones describieron dos respuestas clásicas a las láminas del Rorschach: Constricción emocional, caracterizado por un registro corto basado en la forma y con mucha carga emocional, caracterizado por imágenes traumáticas y puntuaciones que indican desorden cognitivo. Esta respuesta bifásica al trauma ha sido respaldada por estudios que ahora abarcan 50 años de trayectoria y se ven en pacientes que han experimentado una variedad de traumas (tortura, violencia doméstica, abuso sexual, violación, desastre civil y respuesta como ayudante en traumas), en niños y adultos. La decisión de utilizar el Rorschach para evaluar el trauma debia comenzar con una consideración de la fragilidad del evaluado, ya que el Rorschach evoca recuerdos traumáticos. Viglione, Towns y Lindshield (2012) combinan los hallazgos del Sistema Comprehensivo de Exner y R-PAS para sugerir cinco áreas interpretativas para evaluar el trauma con el Rorschach: (1) constricción cognitiva; (2) imágenes relacionadas con el trauma; (3) alteraciones cognitivas relacionadas con el trauma; (4) respuesta al estrés; y (5) disociación. Los individuos que intentan simular un trauma probablemente expresaran contenidos dramáticos similares al Índice de contenido de trauma en el CS y Contenido crítico en el R-PAS, pero probablemente no puedan producir alteraciones cognitivas relacionadas con el trauma ni puntuaciones originadas por el estrés.

要約

ロールシャッハは、自記式の検査では測定できない心理的変数を評価する。そして、トラウマ患者がトラウマのイメージを伝えたり、侵入的なイメージに対処する方法を表示できたりするようなテスト状況を作り出す。初期の研究では、ロールシャッハカードに対する2つの古典的な反応が記述されている。1つ目は、感情的に収縮していて、短く型にはまった記録によって特徴づけられている。2つ目は、感情的に溢れているもので、トラウマのイメージと認知の混乱を示すスコアによって特徴づけられている。トラウマに対してのこの二層性の反応は、これまで50年にわたる研究によって支持されており、さまざまなトラウマ（拷問、家庭内暴力、性的虐待、レイプ、市民災害、トラウマ援助者の二次的被害）を経験した患者や子ども、大人に

見られる。ロールシャッハを用いてトラウマを評価するかどうかの決定は、まず評定対象者の脆弱性を考慮することから始めるべきである。なぜなら、ロールシャッハテストはトラウマ記憶を惹起するからである。Viglioneら（2015）は、包括システムとR-PASから得られた知見を組み合わせて、ロールシャッハを用いてトラウマを評価する5つの解釈領域を提案している。(1) 認知的狭窄、(2)トラウマに関連したイメージ、(3) トラウマに関連した認知障害、(4) ストレス反応、(5) 解離 である。トラウマを麻痺させようとする人は、包括システムのトラウマコンテンツやR-PASのクリティカルコンテンツに似た劇的な内容を提供する可能性が高いが、ストレスに伴って起こることが知られているトラウマに関連した認知障害やスコアを出すことができない可能性が高い。

A Commentary on "The Rorschach and Trauma" (Kaser-Boyd, 2021)

Steven N. Gold

College of Psychology, Nova Southeastern University, Fort Lauderdale, FL, USA

Is the Rorschach Test a valid and useful instrument in assessing for traumatization? Variable by variable, Dr. Kaser-Boyd (2021) has done an impressive job of combing through and collating the relevant research literature to provide us with ample empirical findings to answer this question in the affirmative. And yet, there is a poignant irony entailed in the very asking of this question, let alone in painstakingly responding to it by consulting the fairly extensive studies on the topic. Clearly, it is precisely the territory of the quantitative and empirical that detractors of the Rorschach have set up as the guiding standard for measuring the validity and utility of the Rorschach. But the reality is that while Dr. Kaser-Boyd's paper substantiates the ability of the Rorschach to identify indicators of traumatization, I would strenuously argue that limiting our attention to this arena fails to capture some of the most advantageous attributes of the Rorschach, especially when our aim is to assess for the impact of traumatic events.

Just as is the case for any assessment instrument, there certainly is value, even necessity, in confirming the statistical validity of discrete Rorschach variables and indices in evaluating trauma-related reactivity. It is likely the singular approach seen as legitimate by those critical of the Rorschach. However, it is a tactic that in essential respects misses the forest for the trees. Proceeding in this way is akin to producing a Rorschach record exclusively consisting of isolated D and Dd percepts and totally lacking in "big picture" W responses. Unlike so-called objective measures, the Rorschach test differs from other commonly used psychological instruments designed to assess for the presence or absence of specific symptom patterns or personality traits of the respondent. While diagnostic and characterological information is attainable via the Rorschach, the total Gestalt that emerges, when the unique features of the content of a protocol are integrated with the constellation of locations chosen, response determinants, and other aspects of the record produced, is truly much greater than the sum of its parts. These factors can then coalesce to comprise a portrait of the idiosyncratic lens through which the respondent views the self, others, and their surrounding environment.

In the particular context of assessing for traumatization, the Rorschach helps us to capture the perceptual, cognitive, emotional, imaginal, impulsive, and behavioral inclinations and biases shaped by the individual's trauma history. This type of information, obviously, is radically more intricate and clinically useful than the comparatively limited data provided by categorial measures.

We find ourselves in an age when the standardization represented by structured objective assessment instruments, discrete diagnostic categories, and a priori intervention approaches codified in treatment manuals are frequently touted as the epitome of solid clinical work. In this professional context, the critical role of identifying, appreciating, and being responsive to a survivor's unique experience of traumatization is too often largely obscured or overlooked altogether. It is difficult to think of an assessment tool that captures this aspect of trauma better than the Rorschach, or that is more useful in augmenting the trauma practitioner's effectiveness by providing a glimpse into the particular survivor's experiential realm.

This unparalleled feature of the Rorschach is captured by Dr. Kaser-Boyd in the very first line of her paper: As any student of both Rorschach psychology and trauma psychology can affirm, Rorschach inkblot stimuli have the capacity to be *triggering*. They are not just a tool for detecting the presence of or enumerating types of traumatic reactions; they can actually *elicit* them. Rather than asking the respondent whether or not they experience various phenomena, or, at best, to what degree they experience them, the Rorschach provides a standardized situation within which the respondent's perceptual proclivities can be elicited and sampled.

In light of this somewhat unique property among assessment tools, the Rorschach is particularly well suited to the evaluation of the impact of trauma on an individual. The triggering potential of the test is a powerful indicator that the information it generates approximates a reproduction of the respondent's characteristic pattern of trauma-related reactivity. For example, traumatization primes those affected to perceive danger where it may not exist because stimuli associated with the original traumatic event in the mind of the respondent are likely to provoke reactions similar to those experienced at the time of the event. This attribute of trauma survivors endows seemingly harmless and inert ambiguous stimuli – reproductions of random inkblots – with the power to elicit the perceptual, emotional, and physiological qualities associated with the activating properties of posttraumatic stress and the inhibitory and disorienting aspects of trauma-induced dissociation.

The benefit of this particular feature of the Rorschach is hinted at in the remainder of the first paragraph of Dr. Kaser-Boyd's review. Unlike many other instruments, including those specifically designed to measure traumatization, the data provided by the Rorschach extend well beyond the identification of discrete trauma-relevant symptoms that can function as corroborative evidence that the respondent has been traumatized or be organized to reveal the presence of specific trauma-related diagnoses. Other, so-called objective measures can isolate these various dimensions of traumatization. But the Rorschach, rather than merely rendering the marks of traumatization detectable and tallying them, can furnish a multifaceted image, a fuller understanding, of how encounters with trauma have shaped the scope, limitations, and at times even the content of the patterns of perception, sensation, cognition, emotionality, imagination, and interpersonal style of the traumatized individual. Much more importantly, Rorschach data allow us to peer into the idiosyncratically wrought, trauma-tinged perceptual world as it appears through the distinct eyes of the particular survivor being examined. In doing so, the Rorschach can disclose subjective characteristics of the imprint of trauma on the survivor's view of self, others, and the world that more rigidly structured tools never could.

Given the triggering qualities of the perceptually indistinct, alternately menacingly dark and vividly colored splotches, one key and not at all surprising observation in the literature is that Rorschach inkblot stimuli can be extremely unsettling and even somewhat destabilizing to highly traumatized clients. Although Dr. Kaser-Boyd cites Brand et al. (2006) as specifically identifying those with complex dissociative disorders such as dissociative identity disorder as being at risk for exhibiting this vulnerability, it seems unlikely that this intense reactivity is exclusively exhibited by this limited subset of trauma survivors. While reactions such as these can certainly be disturbingly unwelcome, they do powerfully illustrate the potential for the Rorschach to dramatically elicit the very reactivity that is emblematic of traumatization.

However, there is yet another classic hallmark of traumatization in Rorschach protocols noted by Dr. Kaser-Boyd: oscillation between extreme over- and under-reactivity. The research literature repeatedly captures the fluctuation between these two excesses. Some examinees produce records with a paucity of responses, retreat from the more stimulating nuances of the inkblot images via over-reliance on restriction of attention to their form-based characteristics to describe relatively simple, if sometimes distorted percepts. Others veer in the opposite direction, formulating responses that combine several dimensions, such as color, shading, and the attribution of tactile qualities and dimensionality, into a single, if at times complex, image. And in still other instances, respondents amass Rorschach records that vacillate between these polar-opposite styles. In this way the Rorschach can provoke the range of expressiveness – from stark to effusive to an alternation between the two – actually observed among trauma survivors.

When the Rorschach data are interpreted, understood, and applied in this way, they take on a much fuller clinical utility than the mere enumeration of symptoms and identification of diagnoses. In conjunction with the empirical findings yielded by aggregate, nomothetic studies of the Rorschach, an idiographic viewpoint enables the therapist to grasp some degree of the lived experience of the trauma survivor. Identification of symptoms and syndromes tends to point us in the direction of determining which interventions may be relevant for optimizing treatment outcome. By contrast, an idiographic appreciation of the individual client's manner of making sense of the environment, others, and self lends itself to informing the practitioner of what, especially for those with severe and complex traumatization, can be an even more decisive contribution to the success of trauma therapy. I refer here to the provision of the evolution and maintenance of a treatment relationship that fosters a sense of safety, trust, predictability, and, ultimately, a capacity for connection – to one's surroundings, other people, and even one's own first-hand experience – that may previously have been entirely foreign and unknown to the trauma survivor, especially in instances of extensive childhood trauma.

As the sophistication of our understanding of trauma and its impact matures, and we increasingly come to appreciate the prevalence of dissociative modes of experience among the traumatized, the immense importance of the treatment alliance in promoting and enhancing the capacities for a sense of safety, trust, and connection is coming to be increasingly recognized. By offering a window into the survivor's experiential world, the Rorschach provides the practitioner with a map for navigating the landscape of the trauma survivor's intrapersonal and interpersonal world. Employed in this way, the Rorschach can be a matchless source of understanding and irreplaceable guide for understanding, relating to and joining forces with the survivor as a foundation for promoting release from the encumbrances of traumatization.

References

Brand, B. L., Armstrong, J. G., & Loewenstein, R. J. (2006). Psychological assessment of patients with dissociative identity disorder. *Psychiatric Clinics of North America, 29*(1), 145–168. https://doi.org/10.1016/j.psc.2005.10.014

Kaser-Boyd, N. (2021). The Rorschach and trauma – An update. *Rorschachiana, 42*(2), 118–138. https://doi.org/10.1027/1192-5604/a000133

Published online September 15, 2021

Steven N. Gold
College of Psychology
Nova Southeastern University
Fort Lauderdale, FL
USA
gold@nova.edu

Special Issue: The Rorschach Test Today: An Update on the Research
Research Article

Can Neuroscience Provide a New Foundation for the Rorschach Variables?

Koji Jimura[1], Tomoki Asari[2], and Noriko Nakamura[3]

[1]Department of Biosciences and Informatics, Keio University, Yokohama, Japan
[2]Madhyama Mental Clinic, Kawasaki, Japan
[3]Nakamura Psychotherapy Institute, Tokyo, Japan

Abstract: Recent progress in neuroscience has made it possible to use neurophysiological techniques to validate and deepen the interpretation of Rorschach variables. The aim of this article is to review the results from Rorschach studies using the neurophysiological approach to discuss the consistencies and inconsistencies between the different results, and then to consider the future direction of Rorschach research in this area. We also provide unpublished data to complement the picture from peer-reviewed studies. Two main approaches to neuropsychological studies on the Rorschach exist. One approach is to measure brain activities directly during the Rorschach administration; a series of studies using multiple neurophysiological methods revealed activation of the mirror neuron system with relation to human movement responses. Another possible approach is to investigate whether individual differences in Rorschach scores can be explained by neurophysiological measurements during the administration of another psychological task. This article reviews how these two approaches provide novel insights into the Rorschach Test.

Keywords: brain, cognition, emotion, functional MRI, individual differences

Although the Rorschach Test (Rorschach, 1921) is still considered a projective test, based on the influence of 20th century psychoanalytic theory, Hermann Rorschach himself was a psychiatrist working in a psychiatric hospital; the first individuals to whom Rorschach administered his test were mostly patients with psychosis or organic brain disease. He discovered that the "original" responses, in which the actual form of the inkblot is inadequately perceived, frequently appear in the records of schizophrenic patients. This observation led to the idea that an elevation in the number of responses with poor form quality is one of the signs of psychosis. Hence, since the onset of the test, Hermann Rorschach researched a connection between scores and brain functions.

Thirty-six years after the publication of the Rorschach Test, Piotrowski (1957) focused on the neuropsychological aspects of the test and developed the idea of "the organic signs," such as a small number of responses, longer reaction time, and a paucity of M responses. The standardization of the Rorschach Test by Exner

(2003) facilitated further research and accumulation of data in this field. A large number of Rorschach studies have been conducted on patients with neurological disorders (Muzio, 2016), including head injury (Exner et al., 1996), and dementia of the Alzheimer's type (Muzio et al., 2001), and have repeatedly demonstrated the usefulness of Rorschach indices to detect cognitive dysfunction in organic brain disease. In one of the newest attempts to use Rorschach indices as neurocognitive markers, it was also shown that some of the Rorschach indices correlate with the level of neurocognitive skills (Meyer, 2016), which are impaired in neurodevelopmental disorders. Meanwhile, with increasing awareness that psychosis is a neurobiological disorder, the poor reality testing and thought disorder shown in the records of schizophrenic patients gained more importance not only in diagnostics, but also in the neurobiological understanding of the disease, in which the disruption in neural networks is thought to be one of the etiologies of the disease (Weinberger & Berman, 1988).

By combining these trends from the neurobiological application of the Rorschach Test with the recent developments in neuroscience and cognitive psychology, Acklin and Wu-Holt (1996) proposed a neurocognitive model to explain the psychological processes occurring during the Rorschach administration, and presumed the following brain regions were involved in the different processes: prefrontal areas in maintaining attention, context information, and response inhibition; temporal cortex and hippocampus in memory processing; visual and associational cortex in retrieval and "goodness of fit" operation. In an article published in the same year, Zillmer and Perry (1996) developed the idea that "personality is dependent upon brain functions" (p. 213). On the basis of this idea, they conducted a factor analysis of the Rorschach and MMPI indices and extracted two Rorschach-related factors: "Rorschach Response Process" including Zf, W, F, M, and "Rorschach Perceptual Accuracy" including X-% and P, suggesting that different neural networks are separately involved in these two factors.

In the last century, numerous studies were conducted to verify the validity of Rorschach scores. However, most studies grounded their validity in the correlation of the Rorschach scores with behavioral measurements, the scores from other psychological tests including self-report questionnaires, or clinical diagnosis based on nosology (Exner, 2003; Mihura et al., 2013). Despite the proposal by Acklin and Wu-Holt (1996), few neurophysiological studies have been conducted to address the nature of neuronal processes during the performance of the Rorschach Test until the beginning of this century.

In the past decade, by utilizing the advancements of noninvasive neuroimaging techniques, researchers have explored neural mechanisms during Rorschach administration. The Rorschach cards were presented to healthy individuals while brain activity was measured using functional magnetic resonance imaging (fMRI; Asari et al., 2008; Giromini, Viglione, Pineda, et al., 2019; Mazhirina et al., 2020; Vitolo et al., 2020), electroencephalography (EEG; Giromini et al., 2010; Luciani et al., 2014), and near-infrared spectroscopy (NIRS; Hiraishi et al., 2012). One fMRI study focused on the human movement determinant (Giromini, Viglione, Pineda, et al., 2019), while another fMRI study focused on form quality (Asari et al., 2008), which provided helpful information about the interpretation of these response variables. fMRI scanning was also used while patients with mental disorders were presented with the Rorschach cards. A higher level of thought disorder during test administration is associated with decreased brain activity in multiple temporal and frontal regions, as indicated by literature on the neurobiology of thought processes (Kircher et al., 2000, 2001, 2002, 2003, 2004, 2005).

In this article, the results from neurophysiological research addressing the neuronal basis of the Rorschach Test in the past decade are summarized. The following individual sections of this article focused on the five major Rorschach response categories: movement determinants, achromatic determinants, chromatic determinants, form quality, and some other scores from R-PAS.

To perform the literature search, PubMed was used; we used the keywords, "Rorschach" and "neuroimaging," or "Rorschach" and "functional MRI" [https://pubmed.ncbi.nlm.nih.gov/?term=(Rorschach+AND+neuroimaging)+OR +(Rorschach+AND+functional+MRI)], and we found 30 articles. We included only the original research articles using neurophysiological methods such as fMRI, EEG, rTMS, etc. We excluded case reports. A total of 16 articles remained to be cited (see table in Electronic Supplementary Material 1). The consistencies and inconsistencies within the studies are discussed. When available, we also report previously unpublished results from reanalyses of previously collected data.

Movement Determinants

The M (Human Movement) response is one of the most important determinants in the interpretation of Rorschach data. There has been a lot of debate regarding the meaning of M responses, but a commonly shared view is that the M response is linked to social cognition, empathy, or mentalization (Exner, 2003; Meyer et al., 2011; Mihura et al., 2013). In neuroscience, there are two schools of thought about how human beings understand other people's minds. One theory originates from electrophysiological studies using macaque monkeys (di Pellegrino et al., 1992). Researchers discovered the neurons that are activated when the monkeys perform an action or observe another monkey perform the same action, and they named this kind of neuron a "mirror neuron," and hypothesized the mirror neuron system (MNS) is the neural basis of action recognition and imitation. Human experiments were also performed by many researchers to detect the analogous system in humans. EEG studies found "*mu* wave suppression" in the human sensorimotor cortex, which is considered to reflect human mirror neuron activities. fMRI studies found activation in the sensorimotor cortex (Dinstein et al., 2007), inferior parietal lobule (Chong et al., 2008), temporo-parietal junction (Mengotti et al., 2012), when humans performed a similar task to that of the monkeys. Another key concept in neuroscience regarding the mechanism of understanding other people's minds is the "theory of mind." This concept also originates from observations of the behavior of monkeys (Premack & Woodruff, 1978), but has been developed particularly to understand the pathology shown in autism (Frith & Frith, 1999). One of the typical behavioral tasks to detect abnormality in the theory of mind approach is the "false-belief task," which requires participants to discriminate between the facts they themselves understand and beliefs that the characters understand. fMRI experiments in which human participants performed false-belief tasks revealed activation in medial prefrontal regions and temporo-parietal regions (Fletcher et al., 1995; Rowe et al., 2001; Samson et al., 2004; Saxe & Kanwisher, 2003).

Starting with the pioneering work that detected *mu* wave suppression in relation to M responses, Giromini et al. (2010) carried out a series of subsequent neurophysiological studies focusing on M responses and mirror neuron systems. They confirmed the magnitude of *mu* suppression is significantly larger in M responses than in other types of responses including non-M human responses, non-human movement responses, and F responses (Porcelli et al., 2013). Their hypothesis was also confirmed by an rTMS study (Ando et al., 2015), which demonstrated a significant reduction in the number of M responses after inhibitory rTMS over the left inferior frontal gyrus (a putative MNS area).

Most recently, in experiments for an fMRI study (Giromini, Viglione, Pineda, et al., 2019), participants in the scanner were told to look at one of 10 Rorschach cards and just to think of one response each time. Each card was presented twice. The inquiry took place later outside the scanner. Regions of interest (ROIs) were defined on the basis of previous neuroimaging studies focusing on the mirror neuron system. For that purpose, a web-based platform was used called "Neurosynth" (Yarkoni et al., 2011), which automatically generates anatomical maps. It was demonstrated that significantly larger activation occurred in the seven ROIs including the middle temporal gyrus, superior parietal lobule, postcentral gyrus, superior temporal gyrus, and inferior frontal gyrus when participants gave M responses than when they gave other types of responses. These results demonstrated a robust relationship between M responses and MNS during the performance of the Rorschach Test at the individual level.

Another relevant question is whether individual differences in the total M score in each protocol can be explained by individual differences in brain activities. In one of the authors' previous studies (Jimura et al., 2010), a false-belief task was performed in the MRI scanner, and then brain activities related to understanding others' mental state (false-belief vs. control) were revealed in the medial prefrontal cortex, temporo-parietal junction, temporal pole, and precuneus. Interestingly, the location of the temporo-parietal activation (Brodmann area [BA] 22) shown in the study is very close to the ROI in the superior temporal gyrus, which showed high significance in the fMRI study by Giromini, Viglione, Vitolo, et al. (2019), suggesting that MNS might overlap with the neural network involving theory of mind. The participants were administered the Rorschach Test on a separate day from the fMRI experiment in the same procedure as is described in another report (Jimura, Konishi, Asari, et al., 2009). Following on from this published study, we have reanalyzed the imaging data to investigate whether movement determinants correlated with brain activity during understanding others' mental states (see Author Notes). Variables were classified along two dimensions: whether the variables involved movements and whether the variables involved human contents, entailing a 2 × 2 factorial design (Figure 1A). Technically, human and non-human movement variables are M and FM+m, respectively. A variable for human non-movement determinants was calculated as the difference between the human content variable and M variable, [H+(H) +Hd+(Hd)-M], and a variable for non-human non-movement determinants was calculated as the rest of the responses. Then, we explored correlations between brain activity across the whole brain during the understanding of others' mental states (false belief vs. control) and the four variables. Preliminary results showed that the human movement variable (M) had a negative correlation with the activity in mPFC, but not in TPJ (Figure 2B, second left). On the other hand, the non-human movement variable (FM+m) had a negative correlation with the activity in TPJ, but not in mPFC (Figure 2C, middle). Variables without movements did not correlate with these two brain regions (Figure 2B, fourth/fifth left). These preliminary as yet unpublished results demonstrate a functional–neuroanatomical double dissociation between the movement variables and the brain regions. Specifically, the results suggest that human and non-human movement variables are specifically associated with mPFC and TPJ activity, respectively. The negativity of the correlation suggests that individuals' low movement variables require greater cognitive demands due to insufficient psychological resources and/or premature thought processes to perform the task. This intriguing hypothesis should be considered tentatively and with caution since it derives from already existing data and did not undergo a peer-review process.

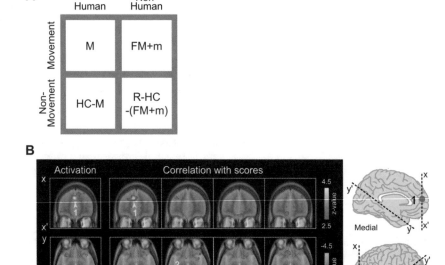

Figure 1. The variables for movement responses explain individual differences in neural mechanisms involved in social cognition. (A) Classification of responses to the Rorschach Test. One dimension classifies whether the response involved human contents, and the other dimension classifies whether the response involved movements, entailing a 2 × 2 factorial design. In Comprehensive System terminology, the numbers of human and non-human movement scores are M and FM+m variables, respectively (top two cells). The number of human non-movement responses (bottom left) is defined as the human content (HC) variables minus the M variable. The rest of the responses are classified as non-human non-movement (bottom right); all responses (R) minus HC minus (FM+m). Note that the sum of these four cells is equal to the total number of responses (R). (B) Brain regions showing prominent activation during understanding others' mental states, and correlation with the Rorschach Test scores. In activation maps (left), hot and cool colors indicate greater and lower activity, respectively, during understanding others' mental states. In correlation maps (middle), hot and cool colors indicate positive and negative correlation between the activity and the scores indicated on the bottom, respectively. The maps are overlaid onto 2D anatomical slices of the standard brain, as indicated by the sections (x-x' and y-y') on the schematic 3D illustrations of the brain on the right.

Achromatic Determinants

The achromatic response was first defined and coded by Klopfer (1938) and predicted to be associated with depressive features. This interpretation was also supported by Piotrowski (1957). In the Comprehensive System (Exner, 2003),

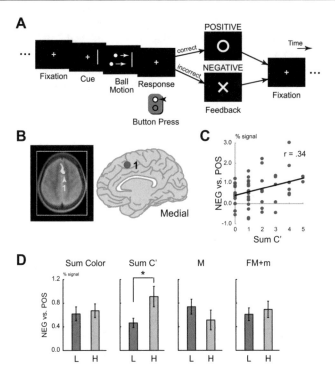

Figure 2. Figure 2. The variable for achromatic responses explains individual differences in brain activity during negative emotions. (A) Participants performed a behavioral task that required them to predict ball motions. Two balls moved in parallel from different starting points with different constant speeds toward a yellow finish line and then disappeared before actually reaching the finish line. The participants had to predict which ball would have reached the finish line first. The negative feedback or positive feedback was presented after incorrect or correct prediction, respectively. (B) Brain regions showing greater activity during exposure to negative feedback compared with positive feedback. Formats are similar to those in Figure 1A. (C) Brain activity in the medial part of the prefrontal cortex (Focus 1 in panel B) was greater in the higher score of the Sum C' (chromatic) variable. (D) Region of interest (ROI) analysis. The ROI was defined based on the activation map in the panel B, and activity during exposure to negative feedback was compared between individuals with high and low variables. Far left, Sum Color; second left, Sum C'; second right, M; far right, FM+m.

the cumulative frequency of achromatic responses (Sum C') was adopted as one of the variables constituting the depression index (DEPI). Also, the meta-analysis by Mihura et al. (2013) demonstrated the validity of achromatic color as an index of negative emotion was shown.

To investigate whether there is a correlation between Sum C' and the brain activity associated with negative emotion, an fMRI study was conducted (Jimura,

Konishi, Asari, et al., 2009) using the motion prediction task to evoke the brain activation associated with negative emotion. In this task, participants were required to predict whether a moving dot on the screen would reach the goal within the time limit. If their prediction was wrong, negative feedback was presented. This was one of the representative neuroscientific paradigms to induce depressive mood; that is, we feel depressed when we get negative feedback indicating that the behavioral goal could not be achieved due to our own failures (Derryberry, 1990; Kaplan & Zaidel, 2001).

The non-Rorschach literature indicates that the rostral part of the dorsal medial prefrontal cortex (rdmPFC) is activated when negative feedback is presented for a certain behavior (Monchi et al., 2001; Konishi et al., 2002; Ullsperger & Von Cramon, 2003), and rdmPFC activity is thought to reflect both the negative emotions and cognitive aspect of adaptive behavioral regulation triggered by feedback (Jimura et al., 2004; Ullsperger & Von Cramon, 2003). To test the hypothesis that SumC' is correlated with brain activation related to negative emotion, we measured brain activity while participants performed a motion prediction task, where positive or negative feedback was presented depending on success or failure of the prediction (Figure 2A; Jimura, Konishi, Asari, et al., 2009; Ullsperger & Von Cramon, 2003). When participants received negative feedback compared with positive feedback, rdmPFC showed greater activity (Figure 2B). The Rorschach Test was administered on a different day, and we found a positive correlation between Sum C' and rdmPFC activity (Figure 2C). We also compared the rdmPFC activity between high- versus low-variable individuals for other major determinants – M, FM+m and unweighted cumulative frequency of chromatic responses, but found no significant correlation. These results suggest that SumC' reflects the magnitude of brain activity related to negative emotion and might validate the interpretation of SumC' as a marker of depressive mood.

Chromatic Determinants

Rorschach proposed that chromatic responses are related to emotions, and the stability of the emotions is reflected in the dominance of the color or form referred to in the responses. He considered that form-dominant chromatic responses were related to a more controlled and regulated expression of emotions, whereas color-dominant chromatic responses were related to a more intense divergence of emotions. These interpretations have been adopted by the Comprehensive System, which evaluates emotional expression and cognitive mediation by inspecting the three variables of pure C, CF, and FC. More specifically, individuals with higher pure C and FC variables are characterized as emotionally impulsive and controlled, respectively, and CF variables reflect an intermediate emotional intensity and stability between the other two variables. Also in R-PAS, WSumC is retained as a marker of reactivity to emotional stimuli (Meyer et al., 2011).

There are as yet few neuroscientific studies dealing specifically with the chromatic responses in the Rorschach Test. Ishibashi et al. (2016) compared the brain activations when participants look at the chromatic cards with those when participants look at achromatic cards, and found significantly higher activation in the left lingual gyrus and the left orbitofrontal area. Considering that the orbitofrontal area is known to be involved in emotional processing, these results are consistent with the notion that chromatic determinants are markers of emotional reactivity. However, the limitation of this study is that they adopted a blocked-design analysis extracting sustained brain activity occurring throughout task performance instead of an event-related analysis enabling the extraction of transient activity time-locked to specific behavioral events; therefore, activity related to chromatic response generation was not discriminated from that related to achromatic response generation on the same card.

If there is a correlation between pure C and brain activity associated with emotional reactivity, it could provide neurobiological support for chromatic determinants as markers of emotional reactivity. The facial expression recognition task is a simple task, in which one of three types of facial expressions is presented, and participants are required to judge whether the presented face is happy, sad, or neutral. This task is thought to consist of two components; one is the reasoning about others' mental state (Frith & Frith, 1999), which is related to brain activation in the dorsal part of the medial prefrontal cortex (Fletcher et al., 1995; Rowe et al., 2001). The other component is the intuitive perception of emotional facial expressions (Blair et al., 1999), which is thought to be related to brain activation in the ventral part of the medial prefrontal cortex (Bush et al., 2000). If pure C or CF +C is a marker of emotional reactivity, people with higher pure C should show greater activation in the ventral medial prefrontal area, while people with lower pure C should show greater activation in the dorsal medial prefrontal area, in the same facial expression recognition task.

To test this hypothesis, we reanalyzed for this paper the data from our previous fMRI study (Jimura, Konishi, Asari, et al., 2009) using the facial expression recognition task (Figure 3A). The perception of emotional faces (happy and sad faces averaged) showed greater activity in the dorsal and ventral parts of the medial prefrontal cortex (dmPFC, vmPFC, respectively; Figure 3B, left), whereas such a prominent difference was not observed between the perception of happy and sad faces (Figure 3B, middle), suggesting that dmPFC and vmPFC are associated with the perception of emotion independently of its positive-negative direction.

The Rorschach Test was administered on a different day, similarly to the aforementioned study (Jimura, Konishi, Asari, et al., 2009). We focused on

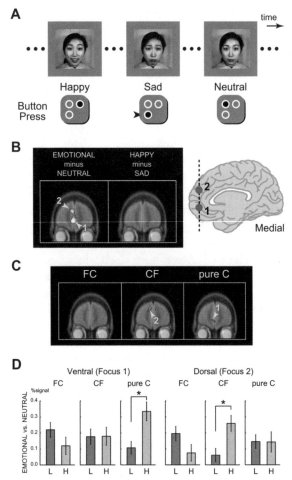

Figure 3. The variables for chromatic responses explain individual differences in neural mechanisms involved in the perception of social emotion. (A) Participants judged the expression in the presented face, and made a corresponding button press. (B) Brain regions showing prominent activity during the perception of emotional relative to neutral faces (left), and happy relative to sad faces (right). Formats are similar to those in Figure 1A. (C) Individuals with higher chromatic variables showed greater activity in distinct brain regions in the medial prefrontal cortex during the perception of emotional faces. Brain activity was compared between high- and low-variable individuals, and the difference was mapped on the 2D slices of the brain. The hot color indicates greater activity in high-variable individuals. Left, FC variable; middle, CF variable; right, pure C variable. (D) Regions of interest (ROI) analysis. Two ROIs were defined, ventral and dorsal medial prefrontal cortex (Foci 1 and 2, respectively), based on the activation map in Panel B. For each of the ROIs and chromatic variables, activity magnitude was compared between high- and low-variable individuals. *$p < .05$.

chromatic response variables (FC, CF, pure C). Preliminary results showed that the mean (± standard deviation) of these variances across participants was FC = 2.42 ± 1.70, CF = 2.24 ± 1.37, and pure C = 0.44 ± 0.78. The median of the pure C variable was 0 in our data set. The medians of the CF and FC variables were 2. The participants were divided into two groups based on the median of FC, CF, and pure C variables. The numbers of participants in the high- and low-variable groups were 19 and 23 for high and low FC, respectively; 24 and 18 for high and low CF, respectively; 11 and 31 for high and low pure C, respectively.

Then, we compared activity in dmPFC and vmPFC during the perception of others' emotional faces between the high- and low-variable groups for FC, CF, and pure C variables. Preliminary results showed that participants with high pure C and CF variables had greater activity in vmPFC (Figure 3C, right) and dmPFC (Figure 3C, middle), respectively. These results demonstrate a functional-neuroanatomical double-dissociation between chromatic variables and brain regions. Specifically, vmPFC and dmPFC activations are associated with pure C and CF variables, suggesting high pure C is related to more primitive emotion, while FC is related to more controlled emotion, consistent with the traditional view of the chromatic variables.

Form Quality

Form quality (FQ) is one of the most well-established variables that has important clinical significance. FQ reflects the degree of relevance of fit of the card image (external environment) to the selected/referenced memory (internal representation). It is well known that the proportion of low FQ responses (X-%) is high in patients with schizophrenia (Exner, 2003). An extensive meta-analysis performed by Mihura et al. (2013) also proved that Rorschach variables including FQ have the distinctive ability to differentiate patients with psychotic disorders from those with other disorders.

At the neurocognitive level, responses with higher FQ might recruit brain regions involved in reality testing, while responses with lower FQ might recruit brain regions involved in reality distortion, possibly through emotional interference. To address these issues, we designed an experiment in which the Rorschach Test was administered during fMRI scanning (Asari et al., 2008). During the experiment, participants were presented with the card on a projector screen in an MRI scanner; they responded aloud during continuous fMRI administration; and they were able to freely rotate the card, simulating a clinical setting as much as possible. The inquiry was performed outside the scanner. Each response of the fMRI participant was classified into one of three levels of frequency that was seen in the normative sample (unique: 0%; intermediate: less than 2%; frequent: not less than 2%; for more details, see Asari et al., 2008). Notably, the recording of vocal responses inside the scanner enabled the event-related analyses to be time-locked to the vocal onsets.

Generating unique responses exhibits greater brain activity in the right temporal cortex (TP; Figure 4A). Previous non-Rorschach studies suggested that the temporal pole might be involved in linking perceptive and emotional processes (Olson et al., 2007). On the other hand, the left anterior prefrontal cortex (aPFC) and occipitotemporal (OCT) regions were more active during generation of frequent responses (Asari et al., 2008, 2010b). The anterior prefrontal cortex is thought to be involved in higher functioning such as inhibition, inference, and the evaluation of internally generated representations (Christoff & Gabrieli, 2000). The occipitotemporal regions are thought to be involved in the retrieval of visual contents (Wheeler & Buckner, 2003). Interestingly, the anterior prefrontal cortex and the occipitotemporal regions identified in this study overlap with the activated regions shown in a previous blocked fMRI design study (Giromini et al., 2017), which contrasted the brain activities during passively viewing a Rorschach figure relative to a resting state. A near-infrared spectroscopy (NIRS) study showed consistent prefrontal involvement (Hiraishi et al., 2012). This is not surprising, assuming that the process of reality testing is expected to be occurring through the overall processes during the administration of the Rorschach. The laterality of the prefrontal activation associated with frequent responses is consistent with the study that showed that stimulating the left prefrontal cortex with excitatory anodal transcranial direct current stimulation increased the number of meaningful responses to a Rorschach figure (Bartel et al., 2020). It might be possible to say that the fronto-temporo-occipital network revealed here is the neural substrate for the "Rorschach Perceptual Accuracy" factor extracted by Zillmer and Perry (1996).

We also conducted a voxel-based morphometry analysis and found that participants who generated more unique responses had a larger anatomical volume of the amygdala (AMY; Figure 4B; Asari et al., 2010a). More specifically, across participants, we examined the correlation between the ratio of unique responses (corresponding to X-%) to total responses (R) and local gray matter volume, and found a positive correlation in the amygdala. It is well known that the amygdala is strongly related to emotion. In those individuals with a higher unique response ratio, excessive amygdala activation, which is possibly associated with enlarged amygdala volume at the anatomical level, may result in distorted perception of external stimuli at the behavioral level.

Because we failed to detect amygdalar activity time-locked to the response, we hypothesized the modulatory role of the amygdala on the neocortical network consisting of fronto-temporal-occipital regions identified in the event-related analyses

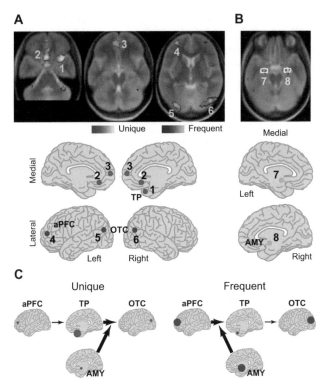

Figure 4. Neural mechanisms involved in the generation of responses during the Rorschach Test. (A) Brain regions showing prominent activity during response generation. Hot and cool colors indicate greater activity during the generation of unique and frequent responses, respectively (top). The activation maps are overlaid onto 2D anatomical slices of the standard brain. The activated regions are labeled in schematic 3D anatomical illustrations of the brain (bottom). The region labels correspond to the 2D and 3D maps. TP, temporal pole; aPFC, anterior prefrontal cortex; OTC, occipitotemporal cortex. (B) Individuals who made more unique responses showed a larger amygdala volume. A map of correlation between local anatomical volume and the ratio of unique responses is overlaid onto a 2D anatomical slice (top). The hot color indicates regions showing positive correlation between the ratio of unique responses and regional anatomical volume. The white outlines indicate the anatomically defined region of the amygdala. The activated regions are labeled in schematic 3D anatomical maps in the brain (bottom). (C) Schematic diagrams of neural mechanisms during the generation of a unique response (left) and a frequent response (right). When generating unique responses, TP activity is greater, whereas OTC activity is weaker; then, when AMY activity becomes smaller, functional coupling between these regions is enhanced. When frequent responses are generated, aPFC activity becomes greater, whereas TP activity is smaller; then, if tAMY activity is enhanced, functional coupling between these regions is also enhanced.

(Asari et al., 2008). Functional connectivity analyses were performed to investigate how the amygdalar activity modulates a top–down signal from the left anterior prefrontal cortex and the object recognition network connecting the right temporal pole and the occipitotemporal regions (Figure 4C; Asari et al., 2010b). We found the amygdalar activity put a positive modulation on the fronto-temporal network, suggesting the compensatory enhancement of the top–down regulatory signal to counterbalance the influence of an emotion-related signal, and at the same time we found the amygdalar activity put a negative modulation on the temporo-occipital regions, suggesting the interference from the emotion-related signal on the object recognition processes during the administration of the Rorschach.

Other Scores From R-PAS

The researchers promoting the R-PAS have begun to seek a foundation for newly defined variables not only in behavioral measurements, but also in neurobiological measurements. Their basic concept is that there is a parallelism between the behavioral dimension represented as Rorschach scores and the neurobiological dimension represented as brain activities measured by fMRI. On the basis of this concept, two of the major variables, Oral Dependent Language (ODL) and Complexity, have become the targets of the research.

ODL is coded when a respondent uses words with an oral or dependent connotation, and it is thought to reflect an implicit need or desire for dependency (Meyer et al., 2011). Giromini, Viglione, Vitolo et al. (2019) hypothesized that the brain regions involved with oral dependency are activated when an ODL response is generated. To test this hypothesis, they used the same data set obtained in the study for M responses (Giromini, Viglione, Pineda, et al., 2019). They entered two keywords, "dependence" and "oral," to Neurosynth, and then obtained the ROIs including cortical and subcortical regions involved in the reward system, and motor and premotor areas involved in various functions associated with language and with the movement of the mouth. The ROI analyses using the intersection of "dependence" and "oral" ROI showed a significant difference between the brain activation associated with ODL responses and non-ODL responses, consistent with their original hypothesis.

Most recently, the Complexity score has become the focus of their comprehensive research using the same dataset (Vitolo et al., 2020). The Complexity score is one of the most important scores in R-PAS. It was obtained as the "first factor" from the factor analysis of the Rorschach Test, and is defined by the sum of each score from three parameters: the complexity related to the location, space, and object quality of responses; the complexity related to the contents of responses; and the complexity related to the determinants of responses. This score is thought to reflect the level of psychological activity and effort that the test-taker makes during the Rorschach administration as well as in real-life situations. It might be possible to say that this score roughly corresponds to the "Rorschach Response Process" factor revealed by Zillmer and Perry (1996).

In previous non-Rorschach neuroimaging studies (Corbetta & Shulman, 2002; Vossel et al., 2014), the dorsal attentional network (DAN) consisting of the intraparietal sulcus, the precuneus, the posterior cingulate cortex, the supplementary eye fields, and the frontal eye fields has been associated with the top–down control of attention. Vitolo and colleagues (2020) hypothesized that the higher the complexity score, the more the test-taker is attentive to the stimuli, and the higher the engagement of the DAN. To test this hypothesis, they performed the ROI analyses using the DAN ROI defined by Neurosynth, in a similar way to their previous studies (Giromini, Viglione, Pineda, et al., 2019; Giromini, Viglione, Vitolo, et al., 2019). The responses when the Complexity score is more than 3 are defined as "complex responses," and activation related to complex responses and activation related to non-complex response were compared within the ROI. The ROI analyses were also conducted for the other variables from the Engagement and Cognitive Processing domain of R-PAS. Only Complexity and Sy (Synthesis) showed a significant difference in activation between target and non-target responses after applying the Bonferroni correction, and Complexity showed the highest Cohen's d value, consistent with their hypothesis.

Discussion

The series of neurophysiological studies starting from the study by Giromini et al. (2010) has repeatedly demonstrated the involvement of the mirror neuron system in the generation of human movement responses. Their fMRI study showed higher activation associated with M responses, compared with non-M responses, within the MNS including the superior temporal region. Our preliminary study investigated correlations between movement determinants and brain activities related to understanding others' mental state (false-belief vs. control), and found an inverse correlation of the FM score, not the M score, with brain activities in the temporo-parietal junction close to the superior temporal gyrus. We found an inverse correlation of the M score with brain activities in the medial prefrontal region. It should be noted that these two studies were based on totally different experimental paradigms; in the studies by Giromini, Viglione, Pineda, et al. (2019), the Rorschach Test was administered in the MRI scanner. In our study, the Rorschach Test was administered outside the scanner, and fMRI experiments using the false-belief task were performed with the same participants.

As said, our results are not peer-reviewed and therefore they should be considered tentatively and with caution, particularly when contrasted with peer-reviewed studies.

Previous studies suggest that the theory of mind has two components: a social-perceptive component involving judgment of mental states from facial and body expressions and a social-cognitive component involving language and theory building (Tager-Flusberg & Sullivan, 2000). Pineda and Hecht (2009) demonstrated that *mu* suppression is positively correlated with accuracy in the social-perceptual task but not in the social-cognitive task. Taking into account the results from the studies addressing the M responses and MNS, it is obvious that M has a social-perceptive component. However, these results do not necessarily rule out the possibility that M also has a social-cognitive component, as our preliminary results suggest. It might be interesting if the ROI analysis were conducted on the same dataset, using the ROI for theory of mind, including the medial prefrontal region.

Although the chromatic determinants are the important counterpart of M in the classic "Erlebnistypus" proposed by Hermann Rorschach (Rorschach, 1921), few neuroimaging studies have been conducted to investigate if there are neuronal activities specific to chromatic responses. Our preliminary results showed differential medial prefrontal activities during the performance of a facial expression recognition task, depending on the number of pure C and CF responses. However, this study provides no information about the brain activity during the Rorschach administration, to be more specific, the brain activity associated with chromatic responses, compared with non-chromatic responses to the same card. To address this issue, experiments with an event-related design may be required. Considering the relative paucity of pure C responses, a large sample size might be necessary.

Our studies focused on form quality showed that both the top-down signal from the anterior prefrontal cortex and the bottom-up signal from the occipitotemporal regions contribute to generate responses with good form quality, while the emotional modulation from the amygdalae on the fronto-temporo-occipital network through the temporal pole might result in generation of responses with poor form quality. These findings are consistent with the reduced cortical volume in the temporal cortex of patients with schizophrenia and perceptual disturbance identified by the Rorschach Test (Ota et al., 2011). These results are consistent with the neurocognitive model proposed by Acklin and Wu-Holt (1996) who considered the neuropsychological processes of the response phase during the administration of the Rorschach as the integration of the top–down processing and the bottom–up processing, in which the limbic structure plays an important role in generating responses through activating biographical or emotional memory.

Considering that the Rorschach Test is a multiscale method consisting of many variables, multiple comparisons across the variables are highly important to evaluate the statistical significance of the correlations between specific variables and the activity within the relevant brain regions. In that sense, the ongoing projects from R-PAS (Giromini, Viglione, Vitolo, et al., 2019; Vitolo et al., 2020) to extract the brain activities associated with the variables are promising in providing robust neurobiological foundations for the variables, because their studies are conducted in a systemic and comprehensive way on the same dataset. One of the limitations for their studies is, as the authors noted (Vitolo et al., 2020), their dependence on one specific web platform to define the relevant ROIs. To go beyond this limitation, exploratory analyses without a priori hypotheses might also be helpful in discovering unexpected aspects of the variables.

Acklin and Wu-Holt (1996, p. 177) wrote, "Emerging application of cognitive science to the Rorschach will deepen our understanding of the test as well as provide the basis for a new research." Their prophecy has partially been fulfilled in the past decade; however, there remains a lot to be done in this field, including the validation of less frequently coded variables such as shading and reflection.

Electronic Supplementary Material

The electronic supplementary material is available with the online version of the article at https://doi.org/10.1027/1192-5604/a000147
ESM 1. Table shows previous studies retrieved in literature search.

References

Acklin, M. W., & Wu-Holt, P. (1996). Contributions of cognitive science to the Rorschach technique: Cognitive and neuropsychological correlates of the response process. *Journal of Personality Assessment, 67*(1), 169–178.

Ando, A., Salatino, A., Giromini, L., Ricci, R., Pignolo, C., Cristofanelli, S., Ferro, L., Viglione, D. J., & Zennaro, A. (2015). Embodied simulation and ambiguous stimuli: The role of the mirror neuron system. *Brain Research, 1629*, 135–142.

Asari, T., Konishi, S., Jimura, K., Chikazoe, J., Nakamura, N., & Miyashita, Y. (2008). Right temporopolar activation associated with unique perception. *NeuroImage, 41*(1), 145–152.

Asari, T., Konishi, S., Jimura, K., Chikazoe, J., Nakamura, N., & Miyashita, Y. (2010a). Amygdalar enlargement associated with unique perception. *Cortex, 46*(1), 94–99.

Asari, T., Konishi, S., Jimura, K., Chikazoe, J., Nakamura, N., & Miyashita, Y. (2010b). Amygdalar modulation of frontotemporal connectivity during the inkblot test. *Psychiatry Research: Neuroimaging, 182*(2), 103–110.

Bartel, G., Marko, M., Rameses, I., Lamm, C., & Riečanský, I. (2020). Left prefrontal cortex supports the recognition of meaningful patterns in ambiguous stimuli. *Frontiers in Neuroscience, 14*, Article 152.

Blair, R. J. R., Morris, J. S., Frith, C. D., Perrett, D. I., & Dolan, R. J. (1999). Dissociable neural responses to facial expressions of sadness and anger. *Brain, 122*(5), 883–893.

Bush, G., Luu, P., & Posner, M. I. (2000). Cognitive and emotional influences in anterior cingulate cortex. *Trends in Cognitive Sciences, 4*(6), 215–222.

Chong, T., Cunningham, R., Williams, M., Kanwisher, N., & Mattingly, J. (2008). MRI adaption reveals mirror neurons in human inferior parietal cortex. *Current Biology, 18*, 1576–1580.

Christoff, K., & Gabrieli, J. D. (2000). The frontopolar cortex and human cognition: Evidence for a rostrocaudal hierarchical organization within the human prefrontal cortex. *Psychobiology, 28*(2), 168–186.

Corbetta, M., & Shulman, G. L. (2002). Control of goal-directed and stimulus-driven attention in the brain. *Nature Reviews Neuroscience, 3*(3), 201–215.

Derryberry, D. (1990). Right hemisphere sensitivity to feedback. *Neuropsychologia, 28*(12), 1261–1271.

Dinstein, I., Hasson, U., Rubin, N., & Heeger, D. J. (2007). Brain areas selective for both observed and executed movements. *Journal of Neurophysiology, 98*(3), 1415–1427.

di Pellegrino, G., Fadiga, L., Fogassi, L., Gallese, V., & Rizzolatti, G. (1992). Understanding motor events: a neurophysiological study. *Experimental Brain Research, 91*(1), 176–180.

Exner, J. E. (2003). *The Rorschach: A comprehensive system: Vol. 1. Basic foundations* (4th ed.). Wiley.

Exner, J. E. Jr., Colligan, S. C., Boll, T. J., Stischer, B., & Hillman, L. (1996). Rorschach findings concerning closed head injury patients. *Assessment, 3*(3), 317–326.

Fletcher, P. C., Happe, F., Frith, U., Baker, S. C., Dolan, R. J., Frackowiak, R. S., & Frith, C. D. (1995). Other minds in the brain: A functional imaging study of "theory of mind" in story comprehension. *Cognition, 57*(2), 109–128.

Frith, C. D., & Frith, U. (1999). Interacting minds – a biological basis. *Science, 286*(5445), 1692–1695.

Giromini, L., Porcelli, P., Viglione, D. J., Parolin, L., & Pineda, J. A. (2010). The feeling of movement: EEG evidence for mirroring activity during the observations of static, ambiguous stimuli in the Rorschach cards. *Biological Psychology, 85*(2), 233–241.

Giromini, L., Viglione, D. J., Jr., Pineda, J. A., Porcelli, P., Hubbard, D., Zennaro, A., & Cauda, F. (2019). Human movement responses to the Rorschach and mirroring activity: An fMRI study. *Assessment, 26*(1), 56–69.

Giromini, L., Viglione, D. J., Vitolo, E., Cauda, F., & Zennaro, A. (2019). Introducing the concept of neurobiological foundation of Rorschach responses using the example of oral dependent language. *Scandinavian Journal of Psychology, 60*(6), 528–538.

Giromini, L., Viglione, D. J., Jr., Zennaro, A., & Cauda, F. (2017). Neural activity during production of Rorschach responses: An fMRI study. *Psychiatry Research: Neuroimaging, 262*, 25–31.

Hiraishi, H., Haida, M., Matsumoto, M., Hayakawa, N., Inomata, S., & Matsumoto, H. (2012). Differences of prefrontal cortex activity between picture-based personality tests: A near-infrared spectroscopy study. *Journal of Personality Assessment, 94*(4), 366–371.

Ishibashi, M., Uchiumi, C., Jung, M., Aizawa, N., Makita, K., Nakamura, Y., & Saito, D. N. (2016). Differences in brain hemodynamics in response to achromatic and chromatic cards of the Rorschach. *Rorschachiana, 37*(1), 41–57. https://doi.org/10.1027/1192-5604/a000076

Jimura, K., Konishi, S., Asari, T., & Miyashita, Y. (2009). Involvement of medial prefrontal cortex in emotion during feedback presentation. *NeuroReport, 20*(9), 886–890.

Jimura, K., Konishi, S., Asari, T., & Miyashita, Y. (2010). Temporal pole activity during understanding other persons' mental states correlates with neuroticism trait. *Brain Research, 1328*, 104–112.

Jimura, K., Konishi, S., & Miyashita, Y. (2004). Dissociable concurrent activity of lateral and medial frontal lobe during negative feedback processing. *NeuroImage, 22*(4), 1578–1586.

Jimura, K., Konishi, S., & Miyashita, Y. (2009). Temporal pole activity during perception of sad faces, but not happy faces, correlates with neuroticism trait. *Neuroscience Letters, 453*(1), 45–48.

Kaplan, J. T., & Zaidel, E. (2001). Error monitoring in the hemispheres: The effect of lateralized feedback on lexical decision. *Cognition, 82*(2), 157–178.

Kircher, T. T., Brammer, M. J., Levelt, W., Bartels, M., & McGuire, P. K. (2004). Pausing for thought: Engagement of left temporal cortex during pauses in speech. *NeuroImage, 21*(1), 84–90.

Kircher, T. T., Brammer, M. J., Williams, S. C., & McGuire, P. K. (2000). Lexical retrieval during fluent speech production: An fMRI study. *Neuroreport, 11*(18), 4093–4096.

Kircher, T. T., Liddle, P., Brammer, M., Murray, R., & McGuire, P. (2003). Neural correlates of "negative" formal thought disorder. *Der Nervenarzt, 74*(9), 748–754.

Kircher, T. T., Liddle, P. F., Brammer, M. J., Williams, S. C., Murray, R. M., & McGuire, P. K. (2001). Neural correlates of formal thought disorder in schizophrenia: Preliminary findings from a functional magnetic resonance imaging study. *Archives of General Psychiatry, 58*(8), 769–774.

Kircher, T. T., Liddle, P. F., Brammer, M. J., Williams, S. C. R., Murray, R. M., & McGuire, P. K. (2002). Reversed lateralization of temporal activation during speech production in thought disordered patients with schizophrenia. *Psychological Medicine, 32*(3), 439.

Kircher, T. T., Oh, T. M., Brammer, M. J., & McGuire, P. K. (2005). Neural correlates of syntax production in schizophrenia. *The British Journal of Psychiatry, 186*(3), 209–214.

Klopfer, B. (1938). The shading responses. *Rorschach Research Exchange, 2*(3), 76–79.

Konishi, S., Hayashi, T., Uchida, I., Kikyo, H., Takahashi, E., & Miyashita, Y. (2002). Hemispheric asymmetry in human lateral prefrontal cortex during cognitive set shifting. *Proceedings of the National Academy of Sciences, 99*(11), 7803–7808.

Luciani, M., Cecchini, M., Altavilla, D., Palumbo, L., Aceto, P., Ruggeri, G., Vecchio, F., & Lai, C. (2014). Neural correlate of the projection of mental states on the not-structured visual stimuli. *Neuroscience Letters, 573*, 24–29.

Mazhirina, K. G., Dzhafarova, O. A., Kozlova, L. I., Pervushina, O. N., Fedorov, A. A., Bliznyuk, M. V., Khoroshilov, B. M., Savelov, A. A., Petrovskii, E. D., & Shtark, M. B. (2020). The relationships between cortical activity while observing images featuring different degrees of ambiguity and ambiguity tolerance. *Bulletin of Experimental Biology and Medicine, 169*(4), 421–425.

Mengotti, P., Corradi-Dell'Acqua, C., & Rumiati, R. I. (2012). Imitation components in the human brain: An fMRI study. *NeuroImage, 59*(2), 1622–1630.

Meyer, G. J. (2016). Neuropsychological factors and Rorschach performance in children. *Rorschachiana, 37*(1), 7–27. https://doi.org/10.1027/1192-5604/a000074

Meyer, G. J., Erard, R. E., Erdberg, P., Mihura, J. L., & Viglione, D. J. (2011). *Rorschach Performance Assessment System: Administration, coding, interpretation, and technical manual*. Rorschach Performance Assessment Systems LLC.

Mihura, J. L., Meyer, G. J., Dumitrascu, N., & Bombel, G. (2013). The validity of individual Rorschach variables: systematic reviews and meta-analyses of the comprehensive system. *Psychological Bulletin, 139*(3), 548–605.

Monchi, O., Petrides, M., Petre, V., Worsley, K., & Dagher, A. (2001). Wisconsin Card Sorting revisited: Distinct neural circuits participating in different stages of the task identified by event-related functional magnetic resonance imaging. *Journal of Neuroscience, 21*(19), 7733–7741.

Muzio, E. (2016). Inkblots and neurons: Correlating typical cognitive performance with brain structure and function. *Rorschachiana, 37*(1), 1–6. https://doi.org/10.1027/1192-5604/a000073

Muzio, E., Andronikof, A., David, J. P., & Di Menza, C. (2001). L'intérêt du test du Rorschach (Système Intégré) dans l'évaluation psychométrique en gériatrie: Exemple de la démence de type Alzheimer [The advantage of the Rorschach Test (Comprehensive System) in the psychometric assessment in geriatrics: The example of dementia of the Alzheimer type]. *La Revue de Gériatrie, 26*(2), 121–130.

Olson, I. R., Plotzker, A., & Ezzyat, Y. (2007). The enigmatic temporal pole: A review of findings on social and emotional processing. *Brain, 130*(7), 1718–1731.

Ota, M., Obu, S., Sato, N., & Asada, T. (2011). Neuroimaging study in subjects at high risk of psychosis revealed by the Rorschach Test and first-episode schizophrenia. *Acta Neuropsychiatrica, 23*(3), 125–131.

Pineda, J. A., & Hecht, E. (2009). Mirroring and mu rhythm involvement in social cognition: Are there dissociable subcomponents of theory of mind? *Biological Psychology, 80*(3), 306–314.

Piotrowski, Z. A. (1957). *Perceptanalysis: A fundamentally reworked, expanded, and systematized Rorschach method*. Macmillan.

Porcelli, P., Giromini, L., Parolin, L., Pineda, J. A., & Viglione, D. J. (2013). Mirroring activity in the brain and movement determinant in the Rorschach test. *Journal of Personality Assessment, 95*(5), 444–456.

Premack, D., & Woodruff, G. (1978). Does the chimpanzee have a theory of mind? *Behavioral and Brain Sciences, 1*(4), 515–526.

Rorschach, H. (1921). *Psychodiagnostik: Methodik und Ergebnisse eines warhrnehmungsdiagnostischen Experiments (Deutenlassen von Zufallsformen)* (Vol. 2) [Psychodiagnostics: Methodology and results of a perception diagnostic experiment (allowing random forms to be interpreted)]. Ernst Bircher Verlag.

Rowe, A. D., Bullock, P. R., Polkey, C. E., & Morris, R. G. (2001). 'Theory of mind' impairments and their relationship to executive functioning following frontal lobe excisions. *Brain, 124*(3), 600–616.

Samson, D., Apperly, I. A., Chiavarino, C., & Humphreys, G. W. (2004). Left temporoparietal junction is necessary for representing someone else's belief. *Nature Neuroscience, 7*(5), 499–500.

Saxe, R., & Kanwisher, N. (2003). People thinking about thinking people: The role of the temporo-parietal junction in "theory of mind". *NeuroImage, 19*(4), 1835–1842.

Tager-Flusberg, H., & Sullivan, K. (2000). A componential view of theory of mind: Evidence from Williams syndrome. *Cognition, 76*(1), 59–90.

Ullsperger, M., & Von Cramon, D. Y. (2003). Error monitoring using external feedback: Specific roles of the habenular complex, the reward system, and the cingulate motor area revealed by functional magnetic resonance imaging. *Journal of Neuroscience, 23*(10), 4308–4314.

Vitolo, E., Giromini, L., Viglione, D. J., Cauda, F., & Zennaro, A. (2020). Complexity and cognitive engagement in the Rorschach Task: An fMRI Study. *Journal of Personality Assessment*, 1–11. Advance online publication.

Vossel, S., Geng, J. J., & Fink, G. R. (2014). Dorsal and ventral attention systems: Distinct neural circuits but collaborative roles. *The Neuroscientist, 20*(2), 150–159.

Weinberger, D. R., & Berman, K. F. (1988). Speculation on the meaning of cerebral metabolic hypofrontality in schizophrenia. *Schizophrenia Bulletin, 14*(2), 157–168.

Wheeler, M. E., & Buckner, R. L. (2003). Functional dissociation among components of remembering: Control, perceived oldness, and content. *Journal of Neuroscience, 23*(9), 3869–3880.

Yarkoni, T., Poldrack, R. A., Nichols, T. E., Van Essen, D. C., & Wager, T. D. (2011). Large-scale automated synthesis of human functional neuroimaging data. *Nature Methods, 8*(8), 665–670.

Zillmer, E. A., & Perry, W. (1996). Cognitive-neuropsychological abilities and related psychological disturbance: A factor model of neuropsychological, Rorschach, and MMPI indices. *Assessment, 3*(3), 209–224.

History
Received February 9, 2021
Revision received March 29, 2021
Accepted April 10, 2021
Published online September 15, 2021

Acknowledgments
We thank Arianna Antonelli for manuscript edits.

Authorship
The first author, Koji Jimura, and the second author, Tomoki Asari, share first authorship and contributed equally to the manuscript.

Author Note
The results of our reanalysis in the sections "Movement determinants" (Figure 1), and "Chromatic responses" (Figure 3) are not yet available in a peer-reviewed publication; those results should therefore be considered as preliminary. We will make the details of our re-analyses available to the interested reader upon application to the main author. The results of the original analysis are available in our previous studies (Jimura, Konishi, & Miyashita, 2009; Jimura, Konishi, Asari, & Miyashita, 2010). The assessment procedures for the Rorschach Test were similar to those in our previous study (Jimura, Konishi, Asari, et al., 2009).

ORCID
Koji Jimura
ⓘ https://orcid.org/0000-0003-1991-3371

Koji Jimura
Department of Biosciences and Informatics
Keio University
3-14-1 Hiyoshi, Kohoku-ku
Yokohama, 223-0061
Japan
jimura@bio.keio.ac.jp

Summary

Since the birth of the Rorschach Test, numerous empirical studies have been conducted mainly by confirming the correlation of the Rorschach variables with behavioral measurements or with the scores from other psychological tests. Recent progress in neuroscience has made it possible to use neurophysiological techniques to validate and to deepen the interpretation of Rorschach variables. The aim of this article is to review the results from Rorschach studies using the neurophysiological approach, including the reanalyses of our data, to discuss the consistency and inconsistency within the studies, and to explore the future direction of Rorschach research. One approach is to directly measure brain activity during administration of the Rorschach Test; a series of studies using multiple neurophysiological methods revealed activation of the mirror neuron system with relation to human movement responses. Another possible approach is to investigate whether the individual differences in the Rorschach score can be explained by neurophysiological measurements during the administration of another psychological task. This article offers an overview of the novel insights about the Rorschach Test provided by these two approaches.

要約

ロールシャッハテストの誕生以来，テスト変数と，行動の尺度，または他の心理検査との関係を調べる実証的研究が数多く行われてきた．そして最近の神経科学の進歩により，神経生理学的手法を使ってロールシャッハテストの解釈と検証が可能になってきた．本論文の目的は，神経生理学的手法を用いたロールシャッハテストに関連する研究を総括し，再分析を含めて一連の研究の一貫性について議論して，ロールシャッハ研究の将来を展望することである．神経生理学的手法を用いた枠組みの1つは，ロールシャッハテストの実施中に脳活動を計測することであり，多様な脳活動計測手法を使った一連の研究により，人間運動反応に関連する脳機構が解明されてきた．一方で，ロールシャッハスコアと心理行動課題の遂行中の脳活動の個人差を調べることにより，スコアと脳機能の関係を評価することも可能である．本論文では，これらの2つの枠組みによって提供されてきたロールシャッハテストに関する知見の概要を解説する．

Résumé

Depuis la naissance du test de Rorschach, de nombreuses études empiriques ont été menées, principalement en confirmant la corrélation des variables de Rorschach avec des mesures comportementales ou avec les scores d'autres tests psychologiques. Les progrès récents en neurosciences ont permis d'utiliser des techniques neurophysiologiques pour valider et approfondir l'interprétation des variables du Rorschach. L'objectif de cet article est de passer en revue les résultats des études du Rorschach utilisant l'approche neurophysiologique, y compris les ré-analyses de nos données, de discuter de la cohérence et de l'incohérence des études, puis d'explorer la direction future de la recherche sur le Rorschach. Une approche consiste à mesurer directement les activités cérébrales pendant l'administration du Rorschach; une série d'études utilisant de multiples méthodes neurophysiologiques a révélé une activation du système des neurones miroirs en relation avec les réponses aux mouvements humains. Une autre approche possible est d'étudier si les différences individuelles dans le score du Rorschach peuvent être expliquées par des mesures neurophysiologiques pendant l'administration d'une autre tâche psychologique. Cet article donne un aperçu de ce que ces deux approches apportent de nouveau sur le test de Rorschach.

Resumen

Desde el nacimiento del test de Rorschach, se han realizado numerosos estudios empíricos, principalmente confirmando la correlación de las variables de Rorschach con las mediciones conductuales o con las puntuaciones de otros tests psicológicos. Los recientes avances en neurociencia han permitido utilizar técnicas neurofisiológicas para validar y profundizar en la interpretación de las variables del Rorschach. El objetivo de este artículo es revisar los resultados de los estudios del Rorschach utilizando el enfoque neurofisiológico, incluyendo los reanálisis de nuestros datos, para discutir la consistencia e inconsistencia dentro de los estudios, y luego explorar la dirección futura de la investigación del Rorschach. Un enfoque es medir directamente las actividades cerebrales durante la administración del Rorschach; una serie de estudios que utilizan múltiples métodos neurofisiológicos revelaron la activación del sistema de neuronas espejo con relación a las respuestas de movimiento humano. Otro enfoque posible es investigar si las diferencias individuales en la puntuación del Rorschach pueden explicarse mediante mediciones neurofisiológicas durante la administración de otra tarea psicológica. En este artículo se describe lo que estos dos enfoques aportan de nuevo sobre el test de Rorschach.

A Commentary on "Can Neuroscience Provide a New Foundation for the Rorschach Variables?" (Jimura et al., 2021)

L. Andre van Graan

Institute of Neurology, University College London, UK
Private Practice, London, UK

The neurosciences span multiple disciplines that have benefited from new technologies and development in data analytic methods. Despite these advances, psychiatric and psychological disorders are still usually diagnosed based on behavioral indicators only, even though current neurophysiological methods can contribute to intervention by the modulation of brain networks (Sambataro et al., 2019; Zhuo et al., 2021) and provide biomarkers for diagnosis, prognosis, and clinical trial outcome measures. Such biomarkers are established with circumstantial evidence, in line with the tools in clinical neuropsychology that rely on construct validity rather than etiology. Neurophysiological studies represent an opportunity to deepen the understanding of the Rorschach and brain function, helping to inform the clinical picture.

Scientific enquiry of observed physiological brain activity during and associated with Rorschach responses is set out in a review of studies over the past decade that investigate neural correlates. The review by Jimura, Asari, and Nakamura (2021) provides a conceptual framework for neurophysiological investigation and provides an opportunity to elaborate the construct validity and clinical application of Rorschach variables.

The article contributes to a relatively small body of work. While repetitive transcranial magnetic stimulation (rTMS) and near-infrared spectroscopy (NIRS) are relatively new therapeutic and imaging techniques, electroencephalography (EEG) is long-established. Most of the reported neural correlates constitute results from functional magnetic resonance imaging (fMRI) studies, which have proliferated since the introduction of this method in the 1990s. One reason for the relative dearth of Rorschach investigation in this context may lie in the simple technical demands of many tasks that are more often employed to study responses associated with perceptual, cognitive, emotional, motor, and language functions and these simpler tasks are more readily accessible to the neuroscientific community compared with the scarcity of expertise in the Rorschach.

Rorschachiana (2021), *42*(2), 166–174
https://doi.org/10.1027/1192-5604/a000149

Our understanding of brain function and the Rorschach is advanced by findings that show that the test provides unique information about the relationship between discrete brain areas and specific mental functions. Selected Rorschach response categories are helpfully presented in a systematic fashion. Only a few studies have addressed the neuroscientific validation of nonhuman movement determinants and chromatic determinants (Jimura, Konishi, Asari, et al., 2009; Jimura, Konishi, & Miyashita, 2009) and the authors have included new hypotheses and preliminary results from re-analyses of their previously published research.

Neurophysiological validation of Rorschach variables in the context of the multiple perceptual and cognitive facets engaged in giving responses to the test is not straightforward and the authors discuss studies within a framework of hypotheses derived from related theory and data, in line with nomological networks (Cronbach & Meehl, 1955) as well as recommendations for predictions in Rorschach validation research (Atkinson et al., 1986; Kleiger, 1992; Viglione & Tanaka, 1997; Weiner, 1996, 1999).

Brief descriptions of methodology during the acquisition of neurophysiological data are provided. The visualizations in the article are excellent and the intuition behind the presented results, including the use of a color spectrum to represent the location and statistical values of neurophysiological activity, is not obscured by technical details. Further description of the technical details for the acquisition protocols and data analytic methods will widen its impact beyond a niche audience familiar with both neuroscientific investigation and the Rorschach. While many cited studies employed a selected region of interest (ROI) analysis that aids in the comparison of results, important differences and limits provide the context for elaborating hypotheses with these methods. Of note is that NIRS and scalp EEG observations are limited to below the cortical surface and, along with rTMS, provide limited brain coverage compared with fMRI. The advantage of EEG, with a spectrum of electrical frequency ranges, taken from an array of electrodes on the scalp that represent large areas of cortex, and rTMS, which delivers pulses from an electromagnetic coil to a selected cortical area, is that they both effectively constitute real-time, direct observation of changes in neural electrical activity. The fMRI and the NIRS signal, a measure of refracted light, provides greater anatomical accuracy with a spatial resolution of millimeters, but it is an indirect and delayed measure of neuronal activity, derived from differential properties of oxygen-rich and oxygen-deprived blood.

The article's contribution would benefit from further discussion as to what neurophysiological validity of Rorschach variables would entail. One form of empirical support, effectively a cause-and-effect observation, has long been employed in postmortem and neuropsychological lesion studies to characterize the relevant anatomy for a wide range of behaviors. Empirical inference as to functional anatomical specialization is based on identifying a correlation between the most active anatomy or change in electrical correlates and the specific behavior during recordings, which is a time-locked correlation, or related to observations away from the scanner or recordings. Identifying functional specialization and validation for tasks such as language and motor function is implicit and relatively simple, once the elicitation of neurophysiological activity by non-relevant cognitive or motor processes in responses is controlled for. Functional imaging methods are now widely used to identify or confirm the eloquent areas and risks to such functions posed by planned surgical resection. The identification of a neuroanatomical double dissociation for human and nonhuman movement variables, involving the brain regions of the medial prefrontal cortex (mPFC) and temporoparietal junction (TPJ), suggests that Rorschach variables may yet, in this context, have a role to play. That is, potential clinical utility is subsumed in the identification of functional specialization, which may serve to help predict psychologically relevant effects of major interventions such as surgery (Duncan, 2011; Rosenow & Luders, 2001; Roux et al., 2003) and medication (Wandschneider et al., 2017; Yasuda et al., 2013).

Differences and changes in Rorschach scores are, however, for the most part not likely to be associated with changes in identified functional specialization. The authors elaborate on the nature of the relationship between Rorschach variables and localized neurophysiological activity. The report of a positive correlation reflects the association of an increased score/value with increased activation, or a decreased value with decreased activation, whereas a negative correlation reflects decreased neurophysiological activation with an increase in a behavioral value and vice versa – characterizing not only the presence but also the direction of correlation. However, realization of the Rorschach's potential contribution requires that the intensity of neurophysiological activity be related to the greater or lesser degree of a psychological characteristic, as reflected in the values of the coded Rorschach variables. This principle is illustrated in fMRI studies of language (Trimmel et al., 2018) and working memory (Karlsgodt et al., 2006), which showed that both hyper- and hypoactivation occur along a continuum of behavioral performance so that greater fMRI activations were associated with higher scores and ability. The authors creatively compared high- and low-variable groups for FC, CF, and pure C variables, using neurophysiological data from an fMRI experiment that tapped emotional responses. The preliminary results include demonstration of an activation–behavioral continuum in that high pure C and CF variables showed greater activity in the ventromedial (vm)PFC and dorsomedial (dm)PFC, respectively. Interestingly, the authors' work on form quality using voxel-based morphometry (a form analysis that measures structure rather than function) showed an association between the ratio of unique responses (corresponding to X-%) to total responses (R) and local gray matter volume in the amygdala. These results indicate that an association between Rorschach responses also reflects a structure–behavioral continuum, consistent with the well-established literature on the relationship between brain structure/volume and function (Davies et al., 2020; O'Neill & Frodl, 2012; Rolls, 2019), suggesting avenues for further study.

The attribution of the negative correlation specifically between low movement variables and the most active anatomy, to low psychological resources in the demonstrated double dissociation of mPFC and TPJ in relation to movement responses, is consistent with the notion that greater cognitive load manifests in higher activation. However, it also introduces the conundrum of anatomical reorganization and neuronal adaptation, respectively; localization that has been established in healthy individuals may not be valid for individuals in whom injury or disease may result in reorganization. Relevant to repeated Rorschach administration is the observation that practice with familiar stimuli may result in an increase or a decrease in activation in the brain areas involved in task performance (Chein & Schneider, 2005; Kelly & Garavan, 2005). Caution and the need for a careful history and psychological assessment when making inferences in individual cases are necessary, given that variance between individual brains is no less than variance between individual psychologies!

The patterns of neural organization related to personality features and psychological and psychiatric disability are still poorly understood. Studies that link the Rorschach Movement response to processes that can be encapsulated by the rubric of executive cognition, and the mirror neuron system (MNS) that has putative overlap with the neural network involving theory of mind, represent an important development. One implication relates to the well-known relationship between executive cognition and adaptive behavior, which could usefully be elaborated to provide a new complimentary approach to address the current limitations in the ecological validity of the psychometric evaluation of executive function.

Our understanding has shifted from discrete brain regions to the recognition that distributed networks of functionally coupled brain regions underpin psychological and cognitive processes (Friston, 1994; Smith et al., 2009). A number of studies exploit these connectivity networks, canonical insofar they are observed across subjects, and their behavioral characteristics (Laird et al., 2011) in an ROI approach. Findings related to form quality that link Zillmer and Perry's (1996) "Rorschach Perceptual Accuracy" factor to a fronto-temporo-occipital network include network characterization and a factor analytic approach, both of which are employed experimentally in the work of Vitolo et al. (2020) linking the dorsal attention network (DAN) to the RPAS complexity score. This approach demonstrates the relevance of factor analytic validity and nomological networks to construct validity and suggests the potential value of large-scale data-driven methods for investigation of the neural correlates of personality (Kunisato et al., 2011). While canonical networks studied at rest (Cristofanelli et al., 2016) and during task will be advantageous for a standardized approach to the neurophysiological characterization of Rorschach variables, the use of native connectivity analysis across the whole brain relevant to the study of personality (Adelstein et al., 2011) with either existing or constructed variables (as demonstrated in the authors' work on understanding others' mental states) is likely to capture networks that are uniquely correlated with Rorschach variables or those derived from cluster or factor studies. Successful task execution relies on the interplay of both task-positive and task-negative responses (Raichle et al., 2001; Seghier & Price, 2012) that emphasizes the need for attention to the functional relevance of deactivation networks (i.e., areas with significant decrease in oxygenated blood) in Rorschach processing.

A major challenge to the design of neurophysiological experiments arises from the nature of the Rorschach, which contains multiple variables and the limitations imposed by a blocked design employed in several studies. Standardized Rorschach administration includes the sequence of card presentation that introduces caveats relevant to the conclusions of neurophysiological studies. Blocked design refers to the allocation of discrete periods during which either stimuli or a baseline such as rest is presented in a continuous series so that the brain's response is cumulated over the entire block and contrasted with a baseline. It assumes that a different cognitive process can be "inserted" without affecting active processes in the baseline task (Friston et al., 1996) and that the baseline task does not activate processes contained in the task being studied. Thus the authors' recommendation for event-related designs that employ one-off or brief exposure to stimuli, suited to unique stimuli, and those that require subjective interpretation such as spontaneous transitions in perception of an ambiguous visual stimulus (Kleinschmidt et al., 1998). Rather than averaged data, responses can post hoc be contrasted individually (Wagner et al., 1998) by statistical subtraction, or better, by statistical conjunction, which avoids the criteria for pure insertion, so that the neural correlates of two or more distinct task pairs are associated with common areas of activation and each share a common processing difference (Price & Friston, 1997). It allows for a factorial design such that the individual main effects of two or more variables can be calculated as well as the effect of one variable on another, for the observation of interactions (Friston et al., 1996) as is evident in the authors' work in social cognition. Standard administration of the Rorschach cards and an event-related design can be employed, to better meet the criteria of ecological and construct validity.

Concordance in the neurophysiological literature has been hampered by a plethora of differences in the experimental methods. In the context of fMRI, this has to some extent been overcome by meta-analysis afforded by very large image data banks; although the findings are not unique to the Rorschach, and are robust, given the error introduced by inter-study conversion algorithms. The article introduces many exciting potential contributions to a range of research questions and clinical applications for the Rorschach. There are also many challenges that are unique to neurophysiological research and this highlights a need for concordance in methods across a very limited number of labs.

The complexity of the brain still baffles science such that basic questions as to how structure and function are related, as well as where and how information is stored, retrieved, and processed, remain unresolved. Neuroscientific contributions to construct validity in neuropsychology include a better understanding of memory systems (Budson & Price, 2005), new concepts such as salience (Menon, 2011), and the neurophysiological impact associated with successful psychotherapy (Collerton, 2013). The article demonstrates the potential value of the Rorschach in this developing field of study.

References

Adelstein, J. S., Shehzad, Z., Mennes, M., Deyoung, C. G., Zuo, X.-N., Kelly, C., Margulies, D. S., Bloomfield, A., Gray, J. R., Castellanos, F. X., & Milham, M. P. (2011). Personality is reflected in the brain's intrinsic functional architecture. *PLoS One, 6*(11), Article e27633. https://doiorg/10.1371/journal.pone.0027633

Atkinson, L., Cyr, J. J., Quarrington, B., & Alp, I. E. (1986). Rorschach validity: An empirical approach to the literature. *Journal of Clinical Psychology, 42*(2), 360–362. https://doi.org/10.1002/1097-4679(198603)42:2<360::AID-JCLP2270420225>3.0.CO;2-R

Budson, A. E., & Price, B. H. (2005). Memory dysfunction. *The New England Journal of Medicine, 352*(7), 692–699. https://doi.org/10.1056/NEJMra041071

Chein, J. M., & Schneider, W. (2005). Neuroimaging studies of practice-related change: fMRI and meta-analytic evidence of a domain-general control network for learning. *Cognitive Brain Research, 25*(3), 607–623. https://doi.org/10.1016/j.cogbrainres.2005.08.013

Collerton, D. (2013). Psychotherapy and brain plasticity. *Frontiers in Psychology, 4*, 548–548. https://doi.org/10.3389/fpsyg.2013.00548

Cristofanelli, S., Pignolo, C., Ferro, L., Ando', A., & Zennaro, A. (2016). Rorschach nomological network and resting-state large scale brain networks: Introducing a new research design. *Rorschachiana, 37*(1), 74–92. https://doi.org/10.1027/1192-5604/a000078

Cronbach, L. J., & Meehl, P. E. (1955). Construct validity in psychological tests. *Psychological Bulletin, 52*(4), 281–302. https://doi.org/10.1037/h0040957

Davies, G., Hayward, M., Evans, S., & Mason, O. (2020). A systematic review of structural MRI investigations within borderline personality disorder: Identification of key psychological variables of interest going forward. *Psychiatry Research, 286*, 112864–112864. https://doi.org/10.1016/j.psychres.2020.112864

Duncan, J. (2011). Epilepsy & behavior selecting patients for epilepsy surgery: Synthesis of data. *Epilepsy & Behavior, 20*(2), 230–232. https://doi.org/10.1016/j.yebeh.2010.06.040

Friston, K. J. (1994). Functional and effective connectivity in neuroimaging: A synthesis. *Human Brain Mapping, 2*(1–2), 56–78. https://doi.org/10.1002/hbm.460020107

Friston, K. J. J., Price, C. J. J., Fletcher, P., Moore, C., Frackowiak, R. S. J. S., & Dolan, R. J. J. (1996). The trouble with cognitive subtraction. *NeuroImage, 4*(2), 97–104. https://doi.org/10.1006/nimg.1996.0033

Jimura, K., Asari, T., & Nakamura, N. (2021). Can neuroscience provide a new foundation for the Rorschach variables? *Rorschachiana, 42*(2), 143–165. https://doi.org/10.1027/1192-5604/a000147

Jimura, K., Konishi, S., Asari, T., & Miyashita, Y. (2009). Involvement of medial prefrontal cortex in emotion during feedback presentation. *Neuroreport, 20*(9), 886–890. https://doi.org/10.1097/WNR.0b013e32832c5f4d

Jimura, K., Konishi, S., & Miyashita, Y. (2009). Temporal pole activity during perception of sad faces, but not happy faces, correlates with neuroticism trait. *Neuroscience Letters, 453*(1), 45–48. https://doi.org/10.1016/j.neulet.2009.02.012

Karlsgodt, K. H., Glahn, D. C., van Erp, T. G., Therman, S., Huttunen, M., Manninen, M., Kaprio, J., Cohen, M. S., Lönnqvist, J., & Cannon, T. D. (2006). The relationship between performance and fMRI signal during working memory in patients with schizophrenia, unaffected co-twins, and control subjects. *Schizophrenia Research, 89*(1), 191–197. https://doi.org/10.1016/j.schres.2006.08.016

Kelly, A. M. C., & Garavan, H. (2005). Human functional neuroimaging of brain changes associated with practice. *Cerebral Cortex, 15*(8), 1089–1102. https://doi.org/10.1093/cercor/bhi005

Kleiger, J. H. (1992). A conceptual critique of the EA:es Comparison in the comprehensive rorschach system. *Psychological Assessment, 4*(3), 288–296. https://doi.org/10.1037/1040 3590.4.3.288

Kleinschmidt, A., Buchel, C., Zeki, S., & Frackowiak, R. S. (1998). Human brain activity during spontaneous reversing perception of ambiguous figures. *Proceedings of the Royal Society of London B: Biological Sciences, 265*(1413), 2427–2433. https://doi.org/10.1109/SSBI.2002.1233971

Kunisato, Y., Okamoto, Y., Okada, G., Aoyama, S., Nishiyama, Y., Onoda, K., & Yamawaki, S. (2011). Personality traits and the amplitude of spontaneous low-frequency oscillations during resting state. *Neuroscience Letters, 492*(2), 109–113. https://doi.org/10.1016/j.neulet.2011.01.067

Laird, A. R., Fox, P. M., Eickhoff, S. B., Turner, J. A., Ray, K. L., McKay, D. R., Glahn, D. C., Beckmann, C. F., Smith, M. N., & Fox, P. T. (2011). Behavioral interpretations of intrinsic connectivity networks. *Journal of Cognitive Neuroscience, 23*(12), 4022–4037. https://doi.org/10.1162/jocn_a_00077

Menon, V. (2011). Large-scale brain networks and psychopathology: A unifying triple network model. *Trends in Cognitive Sciences, 15*(10), 483–506. https://doi.org/10.1016/j.tics.2011.08.003

O'Neill, A., & Frodl, T. (2012). Brain structure and function in borderline personality disorder. *Brain Structure & Function, 217*(4), 767–782. https://doi.org/10.1007/s00429-012-0379-4

Price, C. J., & Friston, K. J. (1997). Cognitive conjunction: A new approach to brain activation experiments. *NeuroImage, 5*(4 Pt. 1), 261–270. https://doi.org/10.1006/nimg.1997.0269

Raichle, M. E., MacLeod, A. M., Snyder, A. Z., Powers, W. J., Gusnard, D. A., & Shulman, G. L. (2001). A default mode of brain function. *Proceedings of the National Academy of Sciences of the United States of America, 98*(2), 676–682. https://doi.org/10.1073/pnas.98.2.676

Rolls, E. T. (2019). The cingulate cortex and limbic systems for emotion, action, and memory. *Brain Structure & Function, 224*(9), 3001–3018. https://doi.org/10.1007/s00429-019-01945-2

Rosenow, F., & Luders, H. (2001). Presurgical evaluation of epilepsy. *Brain: A Journal of Neurology, 124*(Pt 9), 1683–1700. https://doi.org/10.1093/brain/124.9.1683

Roux, F.-E. E., Boulanouar, K., Lotterie, J.-A. A., Mejdoubi, M., LeSage, J. P., & Berry, I. (2003). Language functional magnetic resonance imaging in preoperative assessment of language areas: Correlation with direct cortical stimulation. *Neurosurgery, 52*(6), 1335–1347. https://doi.org/10.1227/01.NEU.0000064803.05077.40

Sambataro, F., Thomann, P. A., Nolte, H. M., Hasenkamp, J., Hirjak, D., Kubera, K. M., Hofer, S., Seidl, U., Depping, M. S., Stieltjes, B., Maier-Hein, K., & Wolf, R. C. (2019). Transdiagnostic modulation of brain networks by electroconvulsive therapy in schizophrenia and major depression. *European Neuropsychopharmacology, 29*(8), 925–935. https://doi.org/10.1016/j.euroneuro.2019.06.002

Seghier, M. L., & Price, C. J. (2012). Functional heterogeneity within the default network during semantic processing and speech production. *Frontiers in Psychology, 3.* https://doi.org/10.3389/fpsyg.2012.00281

Smith, S. M., Fox, P. T., Miller, K. L., Glahn, D. C., Fox, P. M., Mackay, C. E., Filippini, N., Watkins, K. E., Toro, R., Laird, A. R., & Beckmann, C. F. (2009). Correspondence of the brain's functional architecture during activation and rest. *Proceedings of the National Academy of Sciences of the United States of America, 106*(31), 13040–13045. https://doi.org/10.1073/pnas.0905267106

Trimmel, K., van Graan, A. L., Caciagli, L., Haag, A., Koepp, M. J., Thompson, P. J., & Duncan, J. S. (2018). Left temporal lobe language network connectivity in temporal lobe epilepsy. *Brain: A Journal of Neurology, 141*(8), 2406–2418. https://doi.org/10.1093/brain/awy164

Viglione, D. J. Jr., & Tanaka, J. (1997). Problems in Rorschach research and what to do about them. *Journal of Personality Assessment, 68*(3), 590–599. https://doi.org/10.1207/s15327752jpa6803_7

Vitolo, E., Giromini, L., Viglione, D. J., Cauda, F., & Zennaro, A. (2020). Complexity and cognitive engagement in the Rorschach Task: An fMRI study. *Journal of Personality Assessment*, 1–11. https://doi.org/10.1080/00223891.2020.1842429

Wagner, A., Schacter, D., Rotte, M., Koutstaal, W., Maril, A., Dale, A. M., Rosen, B. R., & Buckner, R. L. (1998). Building memories: Remembering and forgetting of verbal experiences as predicted by brain activity. *Science, 281*(5380), 1188–1191. https://doi.org/10.1126/science.281.5380.1188

Wandschneider, B., Burdett, J., Townsend, L., Hill, A., Thompson, P. J., Duncan, J. S., & Koepp, M. J. (2017). Effect of topiramate and zonisamide on fMRI cognitive networks. *Neurology, 88*(12), 1165–1171. https://doi.org/10.1212/WNL.0000000000003736

Weiner, I. B. (1996). Some observations on the validity of the Rorschach inkblot method. *Psychological Assessment, 8*(2), 206–213.

Weiner, I. B. (1999). What the Rorschach can do for you: Incremental validity in clinical applications. *Assessment, 6*(4), 327–340. https://doi.org/10.1177/107319119900600404

 Rorschachiana (2021), *42*(2), 166–174

Yasuda, C. L., Centeno, M., Vollmar, C., Stretton, J., Symms, M., Cendes, F., Mehta, M. A., Thompson, P., Duncan, J. S., & Koepp, M. J. (2013). The effect of topiramate on cognitive fMRI. *Epilepsy Research, 105*(1–2), 250–255. https://doi.org/10.1016/j.eplepsyres.2012.12.007

Zhuo, C., Fang, T., Chen, C., Chen, M., Sun, Y., Ma, X., Li, R., Tian, H., & Ping, J. (2021). Brain imaging features in schizophrenia with co-occurring auditory verbal hallucinations and depressive symptoms – implication for novel therapeutic strategies to alleviate the reciprocal deterioration. *Brain and Behavior, 11*(2), Article e01991. https://doi.org/10.1002/brb3.1991

Zillmer, E. A., & Perry, W. (1996). Cognitive-neuropsychological abilities and related psychological disturbance: A factor model of neuropsychological, Rorschach, and MMPI indices. *Assessment, 3*(3), 209–224. https://doi.org/10.1177/1073191196003003003

Published online September 15, 2021

L. Andre van Graan
Institute of Neurology
University College London
UK
dravangraan@aol.com

Special Issue: The Rorschach Test Today: An Update on the Research
Original Article

The Rorschach and Violent Crime

A Literature Review and Case Illustration

Corine de Ruiter

Faculty of Psychology & Neuroscience, Maastricht University, The Netherlands

Abstract: Over the years, a significant number of Rorschach studies have been conducted with forensic adult and adolescent samples, partly motivated by the use of the test in forensic psychological evaluations. Could the Rorschach, as a performance-based personality assessment tool, provide unique information that is not as vulnerable to distortion on the part of the examinee as self-report measures are? This article provides a review of Rorschach studies on relevant Rorschach variables, including those with different forensic samples. Empirical findings are mixed; there is not a one-on-one relationship between certain Rorschach variables and forensically relevant traits, such as psychopathy or hostility. This does not mean the Rorschach cannot provide useful information in answering psychological questions before the court. A case illustration of a male college student, who committed a (first) violent offense, illustrates the unique contribution of the Rorschach for understanding the psychological dynamics behind a violent act that was seemingly out of character.

Keywords: Rorschach inkblot method, forensic assessment, aggression coding, incremental validity, case study

Hermann Rorschach's monograph *Psychodiagnostik* was first published in 1921 and included around 30 case examples, none of which involved patients with a "forensic profile" (Rorschach, 1942). Some of the coding categories he created were relevant to forensic populations, such as white Space-responses, which he related to oppositional tendencies (p. 39) and C-responses, which represented impulsiveness (p. 99), according to Rorschach (1942).

It would take until 1994 for the study of Rorschach responses in forensic patients to take a leap forward, with the publication of Gacono and Meloy's book, *The Rorschach Assessment of Aggressive and Psychopathic Personalities* (Gacono & Meloy, 1994). At that time, Exner's Comprehensive System had become the predominant coding and interpretation system, at least in Anglo-Saxon countries. Meloy and Gacono (1992) introduced four additional aggression scoring categories, developed from the work of Schafer (1954) and Rapaport (Rapaport et al., 1946/1948) among others. One of these four scoring categories, Aggressive Content (AgC), has been extensively studied over the past decades, resulting in the inclusion of this thematic code in the Rorschach Performance Assessment

System (R-PAS; Meyer et al., 2011) on grounds of good empirical support in the literature.[1] This review discusses studies that (1) examined the validity of specific Rorschach variables, such as Gacono and Meloy's aggression codes, which may be particularly relevant for use in forensic psychological assessment in criminal cases, and (2) applied the Rorschach to study forensic samples. A brief discussion of the value of performance-based personality assessment, including assessment using the Rorschach, in forensic evaluations is followed by a case illustration of the incremental validity of the Rorschach in forensic psychological assessment of a violent offender case.

Forensic Psychological Assessment

Forensic psychological assessment is performed to assist the trier of fact in answering a legal question that has a psychological dimension. Examples of such questions are: criminal responsibility, termination of parental rights, and personal injury under worker's compensation (Heilbrun et al., 2009). A few notable differences between forensic and clinical assessment should be acknowledged. Most importantly, distorted response styles (both faking good and faking bad) are more common among forensic examinees, both as a consequence of the adversarial legal context and because of a higher prevalence of cluster B personality traits (American Psychiatric Association, 2013), which may serve as a cause for defensive and distorted responding (De Ruiter & Kaser-Boyd, 2015). To control for problematic response styles, forensic assessors use self-report instruments containing response style scales, such as the MMPI or the PAI, and/or special symptom validity testing tools (Rogers, 2008). Performance-based personality tests, such as the Rorschach, can contribute uniquely to forensic assessment because they are somewhat less transparent to the examinee, although still not impervious to distortion (Sewell, 2008). For instance, it was shown that psychiatric outpatients instructed to fake good mental health on the Rorschach were unable to reduce perceptual and cognitive disturbances, but did successfully limit the level of aggressive and disturbing content (Hartmann & Hartmann, 2014). In addition, forensic psychological assessment requires use of collateral information, such as interviews with informants, medical and criminal records, and behavioral

---

1   It should be noted that the Aggressive Content (AGC) variable in R-PAS differs slightly from the original AgC coding as well as from the Baity et al. (2000) list of aggressive contents (see Meyer et al., 2011, p. 138).

observation. Ideally, forensic psychological assessment is multimethod and evidence-based (Gacono et al., 2008; Hopwood & Bornstein, 2014).

Research on Rorschach Aggression-Related Codes

Obviously, all Rorschach codes are of relevance in a forensic psychological evaluation, as they provide insight into the examinee's psychological functioning in many domains. Still, there are Rorschach variables that provide information on personality characteristics that are of particular importance in forensic assessment, such as aggression and impulsivity. We will briefly review validity research on the measurement of these personality traits using various Rorschach codes. This review will be limited to empirical studies published in English.

Aggression Codes

Before Exner's Comprehensive System (CS) became the dominant coding and interpretation system in many countries (Exner, 2003), several scholars had developed criteria for coding aggression in Rorschach responses. Examples are Elizur's Hostility Scale and Holt's Primary (A1) and Secondary Process (A2) Aggression (Elizur, 1949; Holt, 1977). Exner did not include aggressive content codes in the CS, but only included a code for aggressive movement (AG, now AGM in the R-PAS system). This was seen as limiting the utility of the Rorschach with forensic clients (Meloy & Gacono, 1992) and resulted in the introduction of aggressive content scores, such as AgC, AgPot, and AgPast, which have been studied quite extensively (Baity & Hilsenroth, 2002; Baity et al., 2000; Mihura et al., 2003). Mihura and colleagues (2013) conducted meta-analyses of the criterion validity of CS variables and found a small but significant association ($r = .10$) between AGM and criterion measures of anger and aggressive behavior, either expressed or experienced.

However, the association between the aggressive content scores (e.g., those developed by Gacono and Meloy, and by Holt) and real-life aggression and experienced anger, appears to be stronger than associations with AGM. Baity and Hilsenroth (1999) were the first to examine the relation between seven different Rorschach aggression variables (AGM, MOR, AgC, AgPast, AgPot, and Holt's A1 and A2) in a sample of 78 patients with mixed personality disorders. Stepwise regression analyses revealed that AgC was a positive predictor of the number of Antisocial Personality Disorder criteria these patients met and AgC also predicted patients' scores on the Antisocial Practices (ASP) Scale of the MMPI. AgPast was a significant predictor of scores on the MMPI Anger (ANG) scale. Interestingly,

MOR was a significant predictor of the number of Borderline Personality Disorder criteria (Baity & Hilsenroth, 1999). In a subsequent study, Baity and Hilsenroth (2002) evaluated the relation between AgC, MOR, and AGM and real-world aggressive behavior, as derived from chart material of 94 psychiatric patients. Real-world aggressiveness was predicted by all three variables, but AgC was the only nonredundant predictor of aggressiveness.

Mihura and colleagues examined the associations between AGM, AgC, AgPot, AgPast, and self-reported aggression as measured by several scales of the Personality Assessment Inventory (PAI) in a sample of 70 college students (Mihura et al., 2003). Note that AGM was unrelated to self-reported physical aggression in this study. Self-reported physical aggression potential was significantly associated with AgC ($r = .26$), AgPot ($r = .29$), and AgPast ($r = .24$); self-reported self-destructive behaviors were significantly related to AgPast ($r = .30$). A recent study failed to find significant correlations between self-reports of three possible anger responses to stress and AgC ($r = -.006$) and AgPast ($r = -.013$) in a sample of 416 medical students (Meyer et al., 2018).

AgPast responses are believed to represent internal representations of past victimization (Gacono & Meloy, 1994). Kamphuis and colleagues (2000) hypothesized that AgPast would be able to differentiate between three groups of psychiatric outpatients: those with histories of (a) definite sexual abuse ($n = 22$), (b) suspected but unconfirmed sexual abuse ($n = 13$), or (c) no sexual abuse ($n = 43$), but this hypothesis was not supported. In a post hoc analysis, they found a significant association between AgPast and sexual abuse that was violent or sadistic.

By means of principal components analysis, the structure of nine Rorschach variables related to aggression (AGM, MOR, A1, A2, AgC, AgPast, and Elizur's Strong and Lesser Hostility) was examined in a sample of 225 medical students. The first component was defined by AgC, A2, and Lesser Hostility; the second component included AgPast, MOR, A1, and Stronger Hostility (Katko et al., 2010). Katko and colleagues (2010) conclude that to simplify Rorschach coding of aggression, assessors could limit themselves to AgC and AgPast. A recent study by Joubert and Webster (2017) examined the latent structure of Rorschach aggression scores in a sample of 108 children and adolescents who had been placed in foster care because of maltreatment from caregivers. Three classes were distinguishable: The first latent class showed little evidence of aggression on the Rorschach, except for one AgC response. The other two were characterized by aggression directed at others (AgC, AGM) and at the self (AgPast, MOR). Interestingly, the authors did not find isomorphic associations between these classes and psychological symptoms (internalizing or externalizing symptoms) in abused children (Joubert & Webster, 2017).

In an experimental study, Benjestorf and colleagues (2013) instructed participants (half were violent offenders; half were nonoffenders) to either suppress or not suppress aggressive content on the Rorschach. Findings indicate that both subgroups gave significantly fewer aggression responses in the suppression condition, with a large effect size (ES) for AgC and a small ES for AgPast. AG did not show a difference, probably due to a low prevalence of AG. The suppression instruction was meant to simulate the context of forensic evaluations, in which an offender may wish to convince the examiner or court that he or she is no longer dangerous. As such, the study provides evidence that offenders and nonoffenders alike are able to screen out aggressive content when motivated to do so (Benjestorf et al., 2013).

Although there has been a substantial amount of research on the different Rorschach aggression codes, the findings presented above do not provide a clear picture. Research into the interpretive meaning of the different aggression codes is compounded by the confluence of victimization/trauma and aggressive behaviors in the same subjects (Lang et al., 2002; Weiler & Widom, 1996). It is unclear to what extent elevations in aggression scores on the Rorschach are indicative of actual aggressive and antisocial behaviors or are reflecting a preoccupation with or fear of violent victimization (Baity & Hilsenroth, 2002; Liebman et al., 2005).

White Space (S) Response

Hermann Rorschach (1921/1942) already mentioned a theoretical link between stubbornness and oppositionality and S responses. However, in their meta-analyses, Mihura et al. (2013) found no evidence ($r = .01$) for an association between S and oppositionality, neither as an outward behavior nor as an internally experienced emotion. In a subsequent, exploratory study (Rosso et al., 2015), three different subtypes of S responses (reversal, figure-ground integration, and figure-ground fusion) were related to self-reported feelings and expressions of anger in a sample of 50 students. The authors did not find associations in the expected direction between subtypes of S responses and self-reported feelings of wanting to express anger verbally or physically (Rosso et al., 2015).

FC: CF + C or Form Color Ratio

The degree to which Rorschach responses that contain Chromatic color are not form-dominated is thought to reflect an examinee's degree of emotional impulsivity. This construct is termed "Form Color Ratio" (Mihura et al., 2013) or "Color Form Level" (Mihura et al., 2003), calculated using the formula: (FC × 0.5) − (CF × 1.0) − (C × 1.5) − (Cn × 1.5). In the Mihura et al. (2013) meta-analyses, the Form Color ratio was significantly related to emotional impulsivity ($r = .32$). What was striking about this finding is that the 14 studies on which this finding was based used external criterion measures for impulsivity, such as acute stress reactions, child-abusing fathers [substantiated], and violent offending (Mihura et al., 2013).

Rorschach Research in Forensic Samples

Gacono and Meloy's (1994) work served as an impetus for studies that used the Rorschach in forensic samples. This review aims to shed light on the question of incremental validity of the Rorschach in forensic psychological assessment. In other words: Can the Rorschach provide insights into forensically relevant psychological traits of the examinee that other psychological tools cannot? Can the Rorschach add to the evidence base in a forensic evaluation by providing data that strengthen the evaluator's conclusions?

The Rorschach is not a diagnostic test in a strict sense; its outcome is not a psychiatric diagnosis, but rather a multifaceted picture of an examinee's personality, including (Weiner & Greene, 2008):

> Adaptive strengths and weaknesses in how people manage stress, how they attend to and perceive their surroundings, how they form concepts and ideas, how they experience and express feelings, how they view themselves, and how they relate to other people. (p. 347)

Attempts to validate the Rorschach as a tool to discriminate between certain types of diagnostic categories (e.g., psychopathic offenders vs. nonpsychopathic offenders) have largely failed, likely for the simple reason that the Rorschach is not fit for this purpose. For example, in persons with the same diagnostic label (e.g., borderline personality disorder), we will find different ways of coping with stress and different views of self and others. Still, studies on different subgroups of forensic patients can provide insights into structural and thematic features of their Rorschach profiles.

Since the early 1990s, a number of studies examined the ability of the Rorschach to detect psychopathy as defined by the Hare Psychopathy Checklist (PCL, PCL-R; Hare, 2003). This research was summarized in a meta-analytic review (Wood et al., 2010) of 22 studies including 780 forensic subjects. All these studies used the CS (Exner, 2003) for Rorschach coding and the PCL(-R) (Hare, 2003) to categorize psychopathy. The only medium-sized ($r = .23$) association was found for psychopathy and Aggressive Potential (AgPot) responses. Smaller but still significant associations were found for COP = 0, SumT, and PER. Many

Rorschach variables for which associations with psychopathy have been hypothesized (Gacono & Meloy, 2009), such as Reflections, pure H, SumV, Space, and AgC, did not yield significant findings. The authors conclude that the Rorschach is not a useful instrument for discriminating psychopaths from nonpsychopaths in forensic settings, which does not preclude the possibility that, "the greatest value of the Rorschach in criminal assessments is not to discriminate psychopaths from nonpsychopaths but to provide a richer picture of personality dynamics" (Wood et al., 2010; p. 346).

Weizmann-Henelius and colleagues (2006) compared a Finnish sample of incarcerated violent female offenders with a sample of female nonoffenders on nine CS (Exner, 2003) variables and three of the aggressive content variables developed by Gacono and Meloy (1994). Female offenders had significantly higher scores on the Coping Deficit Index (CDI) and on other indicators of coping difficulties (low EA, high F%). Unexpectedly, the offender sample did not show higher scores on any of the aggressive content variables. In an exploratory analysis, the authors found significant and medium-sized correlations between AgC and physical abuse in childhood, sexual abuse in childhood, and violence in the family of origin for the total sample. The authors hypothesize that AgC scores may point at identification with the aggressor in response to victimization experiences (Weizmann-Henelius et al., 2006), but this interpretation needs to be investigated further.

A high percentage (72%) of positive CDIs was also found in a sample ($N = 63$) of male adjudicated youth (Talkington et al., 2013). In general, the Rorschach CS records obtained from these youth reflected cognitive and emotional impoverishment (e.g., mean Lambda = 1.77; 75% COP = 0), which can perhaps at least partially be linked to their low average IQ (mean IQ = 77). Another study examined five Rorschach aggression variables (AGM, A1, A2, AgC, and AgPast) in relation to a measure of aggressive potential (measured with a self-report scale) and real-world aggression/violence (the Violence Rating Scale-Revised [VRS-R], rated from intake forensic reports) in 150 adjudicated adolescents (75 M, 75F; Liebman et al., 2005). Interestingly, there were no gender differences in mean number of aggression variables. AgC was the only variable that was significantly related to both the self-report aggressive potential scale and the clinician-rated VRS-R. Liebman et al. (2005) caution against interpreting the meaning of AgC responses as an indicator of violence potential:

> The AgC response may in part reflect the day-to-day experience of violence in the lives of these adolescents. (p. 38)

Like any Rorschach finding, it should be reviewed in the context of other diagnostic information (interview, self-report, collateral data; Baity & Hilsenroth, 2002).

A descriptive study of 45 violent prisoners with a PCL-R score of 30 or higher echoed a number of the aforementioned findings (Franks et al., 2009). Overall, 61% of their sample had a positive CDI, mean Lambda was 1.45, mean EA = 3.4, 73% had COP = 0, and 86% had AGM = 0. Interestingly, Franks et al. (2009) noted the similarity between the avoidant and constricted Rorschach profiles of these psychopathic prisoners and the Banality profile developed to describe the Rorschach responses of Nazi War criminals (Zillmer et al., 1995).

A few studies have investigated female forensic examinees' Rorschachs. Smith and colleagues (2020) studied Rorschach aggression codes in a sample of female psychopathic ($n = 84$) and nonpsychopathic offenders ($n = 39$). They found that female psychopathic offenders had significantly more AgC, AgPot, and AgPast in their Rorschachs compared with the nonpsychopathic female offenders, although the ESs were relatively small. No differences were found for AG. The authors speculate that the female psychopathic offender identifies both with the victim (AgPast) as well as the aggressor (AgPot), and aggressive behavior (AgC; Smith, Gacono, & Cunliffe, 2020). In another study, Smith et al. (2018) compared female ($n = 46$) and male ($n = 44$) psychopathic offenders on a selected set of Rorschach CS variables. The authors hypothesized that male psychopathic offenders would have significantly more Fr + rF and PER, while their female counterparts would produce more Pairs, MOR, SumV, SumT, and SumY. Most of these hypotheses received no support, but female psychopathic offenders did produce more SumT than their male counterparts (Smith et al., 2018).

Huprich and colleagues (2004) examined Rorschach Oral Dependency (ROD) scores and Gacono and Meloy's (1994) aggressive content scores, and their co-occurrence, in psychopathic violent offenders, sexual homicide perpetrators, and nonviolent sexual offenders against children (Huprich et al., 2004). ROD scores, expressed as a percentage of R, were significantly lower in psychopathic offenders compared with the other two offender groups. For sexual homicide perpetrators, almost 50% of ROD scores were accompanied by an aggression score. There were no meaningful differences between the three groups on AgC; however, sexual homicide perpetrators consistently gave the highest number of AgPast and AgPot scores of the three groups. The authors conclude that the ROD scale provides an implicit assessment of dependency needs that allows evaluators to better understand the underlying dynamics of offending behavior (Huprich et al., 2004).

In summary, the empirical research literature on the use of the Rorschach in forensic populations and forensically relevant Rorschach codes provides a mixed picture. The most consistent finding appears to be the high prevalence of Rorschach protocols with high Lambda and positive CDI, illustrating the maladaptive problem-solving style of individuals who are in conflict with the law. The aggression codes (AgC, AgPot, and AgPast) proposed by Meloy and

Gacono (1992) show inconsistent results, and it remains unclear whether these three codes indicate different intrapsychic mechanisms. In some studies, the three codes show high correlations, in others not at all. Additionally, the correlations with external criteria (e.g., behavioral aggression ratings, self-reported aggression, victimization) are inconsistent. Likely, all three codes indicate a preoccupation with aggressive imagery, but the manner in which this preoccupation plays a role in the individual's life (e.g., extreme fear of aggression, violent victimization, violence perpetration, denial of aggression) will have to be gauged from a thorough investigation of the individual's life history, other psychological test data, and collateral information.

As already mentioned, all Rorschach codes can provide meaningful information in a forensic evaluation. A pertinent example is the Rorschach's ability to provide information about a person's perception and thinking that is indicative of an underlying psychotic process, even before actual symptoms of psychosis have surfaced (Ilonen et al., 2010; Metsanen et al., 2004). The Rorschach, more specifically the Perceptual Thinking Index (PTI), is a highly sensitive measure of the presence of perceptual and thought disturbance, which makes it useful in the forensic assessment of psychosis, which may be relevant for both assessment of legal insanity and competency to stand trial (Acklin, 2008; Gray & Acklin, 2008). The meta-analyses by Mihura et al. (2013) found that the PTI had one of the highest validity coefficients of all Rorschach CS variables ($r = .39$) as an indicator of disturbed thinking and distorted perception. A recent study found that the PTI is unaffected by antipsychotic medication in a sample of 114 psychotic patients (Biagiarelli et al., 2017), which again suggests the PTI measures the underlying perceptual and thought processes, and not the symptoms of psychosis. Rorschach responses of patients with schizophrenia could be successfully simulated using a neural network model, which proposed lack of context integration, caused by an altered noise-to-signal ratio at the level of the single neuron, as the cause of distorted perception and thinking on the Rorschach (Peled & Geva, 2000). The following case example illustrates how the R-PAS coding system was used in a criminal responsibility evaluation. A number of studies and a meta-analysis have demonstrated that R-PAS keeps the response process of the Rorschach task, as reflected in coded variables, similar to that found in the CS, while optimizing interpretability by controlling R (Hosseininasab et al., 2019; Pianowski et al., 2021).

Forensic Criminal Case Example

Criminal responsibility assessment aims to assess a defendant's mental state at the time of the offense (MSO; Melton et al., 2007). By its nature, it is a task of retrospective reconstruction of the defendant's behavior and mental state leading up to, during, and in the aftermath of the offense. Various tools may help the assessor with this reconstruction: interviews with the defendant, eyewitness observations, reports of other informants, police reports, reports of treating mental health professionals, but also psychological tests (Acklin, 2008).

Peter has just turned 20 and has been in jail for nearly 2 months on a charge of attempted manslaughter against a female student, Melanie. He and the victim were living in the same student house. Peter is described by his student friends as shy and unassertive; he does not talk about his feelings. When he has had a few bottles of beer, he loosens up, but they also say he can become "annoying." On several occasions, Peter and Melanie have kissed and had sex after a long night of drinking and partying. Melanie stated before the police that about 3 weeks prior to the offense, she told Peter that she liked him, but not enough for her to want a relationship with him. Peter, on the other hand, told her he did want a relationship with her. On the following day, they talked about this again, and Melanie had the impression he was hiding his true feelings behind a veneer of coolness. Melanie says he went to see her in her room twice, but she sent him away. They did not have sexual intercourse during these 3 weeks.

The Saturday before the offense, the students in the house went out on the town and Peter saw Melanie kissing another guy. Peter left the group. One of the friends called him up and Peter said he was on the train, going home. The next day, his friends found Peter at around 5 p.m., sitting by himself in front of the student house, clearly drunk, a set of beer cans beside his chair. Around 5:30 p.m. Melanie, Peter, and another housemate went out to buy groceries for dinner and Peter bought a bottle of wine just for himself. The three watched a movie and Peter kept on drinking wine. After the movie, Melanie asked him why he left the previous night, which resulted in an argument. Melanie told the police she went to sleep around midnight.

Childhood

Peter grew up as the oldest son in a middle-class family with two sisters. His parents describe him as a reticent child, who cried a lot as a baby and had severe separation anxiety. Up until age 4 he had difficulty going to sleep in his own bed and he cried when his mother left him at daycare or with his grandparents. He played soccer in his free time and finished high school without much difficulty. However, his adjustment to college life did not run smoothly; he felt belittled and taken advantage of by his fraternity brothers to such an extent that he wanted to quit the fraternity. When one of the brothers found out about this, he started a conversation with Peter, who shared his experiences and dislikes. This cleared the air for a while and Peter got a set of new responsibilities in the fraternity.

Peter drank his first beer when he was 12, although the legal drinking age at the time was 16. He says he drank at parties because everyone did so but also to muster up the courage to talk to a girl. He says he mostly drinks when he goes out with his friends, sometimes to a point that he does not know his whereabouts anymore and friends have to take him home. During the last weeks before the offense, he also started to drink during the day, to forget about everything. On the day before the offense, he drank continually between 2 in the afternoon and 10 at night, added up it was around 500 ml of pure alcohol within 8 hr. He says this was the only day that he consciously tried to drown out his feelings by drinking alcohol. Peter does not use drugs.

The Offense

Before the offense, Peter wanted to kill himself. He took the stairs to the rooftop: "I wanted this misery to stop." The assessor asked him what he means by "this misery"? He said he did not feel happy, a kind of blockage inside, which started around age 14. He said it came out of the blue, nothing in particular triggered it. This is when he started to have a lot of conflicts with his parents, he felt disadvantaged, "a feeling that life is no longer for you." Peter said he had always tried to deny this feeling and to not let himself get distracted by it: "I find it hard to accept that there may be something wrong with me. I blame others, I blame myself. I want to change that but I cannot. At some point, it just goes away again."

His father said he recognizes Peter's depressive moods. Similar to Peter, he failed at college and felt he had disappointed his parents, and wished he was dead. This depressive period lasted for a number of years; sometimes it returns in the form of rumination, but he can deal with it nowadays by jogging. He also has compulsive behaviors, such as walking the stairs in a fixed way; he says Peter told him he also has to do things like that. His father noticed Peter's depressed mood for the first time, about 6 months before the offense, when Peter told him he had failed an exam. His father has worried that Peter might attempt suicide, but he never thought his son would hurt someone else. Both parents describe their son as "closed as an oyster," as someone who does not share his feelings with anyone else.

Peter says he could not fall asleep after his quibble with Melanie: "I felt awful, I started to walk up and down the hallway, with my phone and a knife in my hands. I was going to end my own life. That Sunday, when I woke up, I felt: 'This is my last day.' I had already started writing a farewell letter." He says he wanted to take Melanie with him, to have her for himself. The wish to kill himself was stronger than ever before and he thinks the alcohol made him go from thinking to acting. He went up to Melanie who was sleeping in her bed and caused serious injuries in her neck. He remembers her screaming: "I don't want to die, Peter," which led him to stop and to say he was sorry. He went to the rooftop, called the emergency services, and wanted to jump off the roof, but he was afraid to. In a state of frenzy, he crossed rooftops, and ran to the train station to go to his parents. He saw that it would take another hour before the first train would arrive. He was in his underwear and with blood on his hands; he was arrested by two policemen.

Clinically, Peter impresses the assessor as tense and much younger than his actual age. Quite remarkably, Peter does not show much emotion when the offense, and everything that led up to it, are discussed. The MMPI-2 validity scales reveal consistent responding without over- or underreporting of symptoms.[2] Peter is experiencing psychological distress. This distress is chronic and relates to issues with identity and self-efficacy. Instead of dealing with his problems, he denies and avoids them. Peter's MMPI-2 is a 07-profile, with scales 8 and 5 also clinically elevated. His self-esteem is so low that it causes confusion, guilt, and extreme tension. His sense of inadequacy results in obsessive rumination and compulsive behaviors. Rumination gives rise to sleep problems and suicidal ideation. Peter feels extremely uncomfortable around women. Excessive alcohol use is the result of an inadequate attempt to relax and manage the problems he feels. Suicide risk is still elevated at the time of testing.

The Rorschach was administered using R-Optimized administration and yielded 20 responses, which were coded using R-PAS (Meyer et al., 2011). The Engagement and Cognitive Complexity cluster (Page 1 Summary Scores) yielded highly normative scores, the only exception being a somewhat low F% (25%). The most remarkable findings on Page 1 are in the Perceptual and Thinking domain: Ego Impairment Index, Thought & Perception Composite (similar to PTI in the CS), WSumCognitive codes and SevereCognitive codes and WD−% are all elevated by one or two standard deviations above the mean T-score. He gives only three Popular responses. Thus, Peter's Rorschach reveals a lot of perceptual and thought distortion, a somewhat unexpected finding, given the lack of obvious psychotic symptoms in his clinical presentation or his MMPI-2.

Responses with Cognitive Special scores were examined. The first one is to Card III and relatively benign: "A frog with a red bowtie on" [smiling]. His smile shows Peter is aware of the incongruence. The next Cognitive Special score comes in his first response to Card VIII, where he sees a cross section of a volcano and a lake in

---

2   Peter's MMPI-2 profile was interpreted using: Friedman, A., Lewak, R., Nicholls, D., & Webb, D. (2001). *Psychological assessment with the MMPI-2*. Mahwah, NJ: Erlbaum.

front of it, revealing boundary diffusion. Similar boundary diffusion occurs in his last response to the test where he sees both the spine (inside the body), the neck, and a face on top of it. The Stress and Distress cluster does not reveal elevations; on the contrary, his scores tend to be below the mean on these variables. Peter's representations of others are immature and maladaptive (PHR/GHR = 64% and M− = 1). On the other hand, his AgC, COP, and H are normative. On Page 2 Summary Scores, Peter's R-PAS demonstrates an extremely high Dd percentage (50%), which could relate to his obsessive-compulsiveness. He has 1 Vista and 2 FD responses, revealing painful introspection. His emotion regulation is poor (pure C = 2) and he may try to run from his problems by passive daydreaming (Mp/Ma + Mp = 75%). Again, the Stress and Distress cluster does not show problematic functioning, although he experiences above average irritability because of holding back negative feelings (C' = 3). Finally, in the Self/Other Representations cluster, he has three AGM responses, which is remarkably high. Given the violence in his offense, we examined the responses in which either AGM and/or AgC were present:

Card III: "A crab because of the claws" (AgC)
Card IV: "A bull with horns. It also has something dark, a bit menacing, as if it is snarling at you." (AgC, AGM)
Card VIII: "A tiger, he is leaning forward, like the head of a tiger, sneaking through the jungle with its head facing forward." (AgC, AGM)
Card IX: "Two male deer, walking in on each other, with the antlers into each other." (AGM)

Interestingly, in the response to Card IV, Peter projects himself as the victim of the bull's threat, which appears to align with his real-life tendency to experience others as rejecting of him.

Diagnostic Conclusion

The life history, as stated by Peter's parents and Peter himself, indicates he had a difficult temperament, that is, a high level of emotional reactivity. Highly emotionally reactive children experience elevated levels of anxiety, frustration, anger, and sadness, and they are at risk of developing internalizing and externalizing behavioral disorders (Morris et al., 2007; Stifter & Spinrad, 2002). Because these children experience strong emotions, they need effective emotion regulation strategies to cope with internal tensions. They need parents who can help them contain their emotions (Goldsmith et al., 2004), including cognitive strategies to think differently about their feelings. Adolescence is the period when emotion regulation becomes of paramount importance, because this is when strong feelings related to loss of romantic relationships and sexual experiences arise for the first time. To get a grip on these emotions and experiences, adolescents need parents who are warm and responsive (Gottman et al., 1996). In contrast with this, some parents feel uncomfortable when their child expresses strong emotions and fail to use these moments as opportunities for intimacy and teaching problem-solving with their child.

Peter tends to deny and suppress negative emotions; his parents have been unable to help him develop more effective emotion-coping skills. Peter is still very dependent on his parents for his emotion regulation: When he failed his first exam, he immediately called his father. He also thought of calling his parents on the Sunday before the offense. In fact, he dialed his parents' number just before he dialed the emergency services for Melanie. Adolescents low in emotional autonomy are vulnerable to developing depressive and anxiety disorder symptoms, as we see in Peter (Allen et al., 1994). The (extreme) alcohol intoxication in the 24 hr before the offense appears to have been motivated by an attempt to numb his feelings. Most collateral informants (his student-friends, his parents) note Peter's young emotional age, even though he is 20 years old.

Peter's clinical presentation and his MMPI-2 results indicate serious depressive and obsessive-compulsive symptoms, as well as suicidal ideation. In addition, his Rorschach results indicate a possible underlying vulnerability for psychotic symptoms. The attack on Melanie was motivated by a wish to be with her in suicide, which could be seen as both a wish for fusion and a failure of his reality testing. When she tells him during the attack that she wants to live, the "spell" is broken and he helps her call the emergency services.

On the basis of the findings of this evaluation, I advised the court to apply juvenile law, because Peter's personality and emotional autonomy are comparable to that of an adolescent.[3] Application of juvenile law has a pedagogical basis and provides a lot more opportunities to assist Peter in his future development towards

---

3   On April 1, 2014, so-called adolescent criminal law was implemented in The Netherlands. One of the important changes is that adolescents between the age of 18 and 23 may now be tried under juvenile law, instead of adult criminal law, if deemed appropriate. The Netherlands Institute for Forensic Psychology and Psychiatry developed a set of criteria for forensic psychologists: https://www.nifp.nl/binaries/implementatie-van-de-wegingslijst-adolescentenstrafrecht-bij-het-nifp_tcm106-275345.pdf

becoming a socially and emotionally stable adult. Adjudication according to adult criminal law would merely serve a punitive purpose.

References

Acklin, M. W. (2008). The Rorschach test and forensic psychological evaluation: Psychosis and the insanity defense. In C. B. Gacono & F. B. Evans (Eds.), *The handbook of forensic Rorschach assessment* (pp. 157–174). Taylor & Francis.

Allen, J. P., Hauser, S. T., Eickholt, C., Bell, K. L., & O'Connor, T. G. (1994). Autonomy and relatedness in family interactions as predictors of expressions of negative adolescent affect. *Journal of Research on Adolescence, 4*, 535–552.

American Psychiatric Association (2013). *Diagnostic and statistical manual of mental disorders* (5th ed.).

Baity, M. R., & Hilsenroth, M. J. (1999). Rorschach aggression variables: A study of reliability and validity. *Journal of Personality Assessment, 72*(1), 93–110. https://doi.org/10.1207/s15327752jpa7201_6

Baity, M. R., & Hilsenroth, M. J. (2002). Rorschach Aggressive Content (AgC) variable: A study of criterion validity. *Journal of Personality Assessment, 78*(2), 275–287. https://doi.org/10.1207/S15327752JPA7802_04

Baity, M. R., McDaniel, P. S., & Hilsenroth, M. J. (2000). Further exploration of the Rorschach Aggressive Content (AgC) variable. *Journal of Personality Assessment, 74*(2), 231–241. https://doi.org/10.1207/S15327752JPA7402_5

Benjestorf, S. T., Viglione, D. J., Lamb, J. D., & Giromini, L. (2013). Suppression of aggressive Rorschach responses among violent offenders and nonoffenders. *Journal of Interpersonal Violence, 28*(15), 2981–3003. https://doi.org/10.1177/0886260513488688

Biagiarelli, M., Curto, M., Di Pomponio, I., Comparelli, A., Baldessarini, R. J., & Ferracuti, S. (2017). Antipsychotic treatment and the Rorschach Perceptual Thinking Index (PTI) in psychotic disorder patients: Effects of treatment. *Psychiatry Research, 251*, 294–297. https://doi.org/10.1016/j.psychres.2017.02.032

De Ruiter, C., & Kaser-Boyd, N. (2015). *Forensic psychological assessment in practice: Case studies*. Routledge.

Elizur, A. (1949). Content analysis of the Rorschach with regard to anxiety and hostility. *Rorschach Research Exchange and Journal of Projective Techniques, 13*, 247–287.

Exner, J. E. (2003). *The Rorschach: A comprehensive system: Vol 1. Basic foundations* (2nd ed.). Wiley.

Franks, K. W., Sreenivasan, S., Spray, B. J., & Kirkish, P. (2009). The mangled butterfly: Rorschach results from 45 violent psychopaths. *Behavioral Sciences and the Law, 27*, 491–506. https://doi.org/10.1002/bsl.866

Gacono, C. B., Evans, F. B., & Viglione, D. J. (2008). Essential issues in the forensic use of the Rorschach. In C. B. Gacono & F. B. Evans (Eds.), *The handbook of forensic Rorschach assessment* (pp. 3–20). Taylor & Francis.

Gacono, C. B., & Meloy, J. R. (1994). *The Rorschach assessment of aggressive and psychopathic personalities*. Lawrence Erlbaum Associates.

Gacono, C. B., & Meloy, J. R. (2009). Assessing antisocial and psychopathic personalities. In J. N. Butcher (Ed.), *Oxford handbook of personality assessment* (pp. 567–581). Oxford University Press.

Goldsmith, H. H., Lemery, K. S., & Essex, M. J. (2004). Temperament as a liability factor for childhood behavioral disorders: The concept of liability. In L. F. DiLalla (Ed.), *Behavior genetics principles: Perspectives in development, personality, and psychopathology* (pp. 19–39). American Psychological Association.

Gottman, J. M., Katz, L. F., & Hooven, C. (1996). Parental meta-emotion philosophy and the emotional life of families: Theoretical models and preliminary data. *Journal of Family Psychology, 10*(3), 243–268. https://doi.org/10.1037/0893-3200.10.3.243

Gray, B. T., & Acklin, M. W. (2008). The use of the Rorschach inkblot method in trial competency evaluations. In C. B. Gacono & F. B. Evans (Eds.), *The handbook of forensic Rorschach assessment* (pp. 141–155). Taylor & Francis.

Hare, R. D. (2003). *Manual for the Revised Psychopathy Checklist*. Multi-Health Systems.

Hartmann, E., & Hartmann, T. (2014). The impact of exposure to Internet-based information about the Rorschach and the MMPI-2 on psychiatric outpatients' ability to simulate mentally healthy test performance. *Journal of Personality Assessment, 96*(4), 432–444. https://doi.org/10.1080/00223891.2014.882342

Heilbrun, K., Grisso, T., & Goldstein, A. M. (2009). *Foundations of forensic mental health assessment*. Oxford University Press.

Holt, R. R. (1977). A method for assessing primary process manifestations and their control in Rorschach responses. In Rickers-Ovsiankina.(Ed.), *Rorschach psychology* (2nd ed., pp. 375–420). Krieger.

Hopwood, C. J., & Bornstein, R. F. (Eds.). (2014). *Multimethod clinical assessment*. Guilford Press.

Hosseininasab, A., Meyer, G. J., Viglione, D. J., Mihura, J. L., Berant, E., Resende, A. C., Reese, J., & Mohammadi, M. R. (2019). The effect of CS administration or an R-Optimized alternative on R-PAS Variables: A meta-analysis of findings from six studies. *Journal of Personality Assessment, 101*(2), 199–212. https://doi.org/10.1080/00223891.2017.1393430

Huprich, S. K., Gacono, C. B., Schneider, R. B., & Bridges, M. R. (2004). Rorschach Oral Dependency in psychopaths, sexual homicide perpetrators, and nonviolent pedophiles. *Behavioral Sciences and the Law, 22*, 345–356. https://doi.org/10.1002/bsl.585

Ilonen, T., Heinimaa, M., Korkeila, J., Svirskis, T., & Salokangas, R. K. (2010). Differentiating adolescents at clinical high risk for psychosis from psychotic and non-psychotic patients with the Rorschach. *Psychiatry Research, 179*(2), 151–156. https://doi.org/10.1016/j.psychres.2009.04.011

Joubert, D., & Webster, L. (2017). Aggressive drive derivatives in the Rorschachs of maltreated children and adolescents: Latent structure and clinical correlates. *Journal of Personality Assessment, 99*(6), 626–636. https://doi.org/10.1080/00223891.2016.1259168

Kamphuis, J. H., Kugeares, S. L., & Finn, S. E. (2000). Rorschach correlates of sexual abuse: Trauma content and aggression indexes. *Journal of Personality Assessment, 75*(2), 212–224.

Katko, N. J., Meyer, G. J., Mihura, J. L., & Bombel, G. (2010). A principal components analysis of Rorschach aggression and hostility variables. *Journal of Personality Assessment, 92*(6), 594–598. https://doi.org/10.1080/00223891.2010.513309

Lang, S., af Klinteberg, B., & Alm, P.-O. (2002). Adult psychopathy and violent behavior in males with early neglect and abuse. *Acta Psychiatrica Scandinavica, 106*(Suppl. 412), 93–100. https://doi.org/10.1034/j.1600-0447.106.s412.20.x

Liebman, S. J., Porcerelli, J., & Abell, S. C. (2005). Reliability and validity of Rorschach Aggression variables with a sample of adjudicated adolescents. *Journal of Personality Assessment, 85*(1), 33–39. https://doi.org/10.1207/s15327752jpa8501_03

Meloy, J. R., & Gacono, C. B. (1992). The aggression response and the Rorschach. *Journal of Clinical Psychology, 48*(1), 104–114. https://doi.org/10.1002/1097-4679(199201)48:1 %3C104::AID-JCLP2270480115 %3E3.0.CO;2-1

Melton, G. B., Petrila, J., Poythress, N. G., & Slobogin, C. (2007). *Psychological evaluations for the courts: A handbook for mental health professionals and lawyers* (3rd ed.). Guilford Press.

Metsanen, M., Wahlberg, K. E., Saarento, O., Tarvainen, T., Miettunen, J., Koistinen, P., Läksy, K., & Tienari, P. (2004). Early presence of thought disorder as a prospective sign of mental disorder. *Psychiatry Research, 125*(3), 193–203. https://doi.org/10.1016/j.psychres.2004.01.002

Meyer, G. J., Katko, N. J., Mihura, J. L., Klag, M. J., & Meoni, L. A. (2018). The incremental validity of self-report and performance-based methods for assessing hostility to predict cardiovascular disease in physicians. *Journal of Personality Assessessment, 100*(1), 68–83. https://doi.org/10.1080/00223891.2017.1306780

Meyer, G. J., Viglione, D. J., Mihura, J. L., Erard, R. E., & Erdberg, P. (2011). *Rorschach Performance Assessment System: Administration, coding, interpretation, and technical manual.* Rorschach Performance Assessment System.

Mihura, J. L., Meyer, G. J., Dumitrascu, N., & Bombel, G. (2013). The validity of individual Rorschach variables: Systematic reviews and meta-analyses of the Comprehensive System. *Psychological Bulletin, 139*(3), 548–605. https://doi.org/10.1037/a0029406

Mihura, J. L., Nathan-Montano, E., & Alperin, R. J. (2003). Rorschach measures of aggressive drive derivatives: A college student sample. *Journal of Personality Assessment, 80*(1), 41–49. https://doi.org/10.1207/S15327752JPA8001_12

Morris, A. S., Silk, J. S., Steinberg, L., Myers, S. S., & Robinson, L. R. (2007). The role of the family context in the development of emotion regulation. *Social Development, 16*(2), 361–388. https://doi.org/10.1111/j.1467-9507.2007.00389.x

Peled, A., & Geva, A. B. (2000). The perception of Rorschach inkblots in schizophrenia: A neural network model. *International Journal of Neuroscience, 104*, 49–61. https://doi.org/10.3109/00207450009035008

Pianowski, G., Meyer, G. J., de Villemor-Amaral, A. E., Zuanazzi, A. C., & do Nascimento, R. S. G. F. (2021). Does the Rorschach Performance Assessment System (R-PAS) differ from the Comprehensive System (CS) on variables relevant to interpretation? *Journal of Personality Assessment, 103*(1), 132–147. https://doi.org/10.1080/00223891.2019.1677678

Rapaport, D., Gill, M., & Schafer, R. (1946/1948). *Diagnostic psychological testing.* International Universities Press.

Rogers R. (Ed.). (2008). *Clinical assessment of deception and malingering.* Guilford Press.

Rorschach, H. (1942). *Psychodiagnostik* [Psychodiagnostics]. Bircher. (Original published in 1921)

Rosso, A. M., Chiorri, C., & Denevi, S. (2015). Rorschach Space responses and anger. *Psychological Reports, 117*(1), 117–132. https://doi.org/10.2466/03.02.PR0.117c10z4

Schafer, R. (1954). *Psychoanalytic interpretation in Rorschach testing.* Grune Stratton.

Sewell, K. W. (2008). Dissimulation on projective measures. In R. Rogers (Ed.), *Clinical assessment of malingering and deception* (pp. 207–217). Guilford Press.

Smith, J. M., Gacono, C. B., & Cunliffe, T. B. (2018). Comparison of male and female psychopaths on select CS Rorschach variables. *SIS Journal of Projective Psychology and Mental Health, 25*, 138–155.

Smith, J. M., Gacono, C. B., & Cunliffe, T. B. (2020). Female psychopathy and aggression: A study with incarcerated women and Rorschach aggression scores. *Journal of Aggression,*

Maltreatment & Trauma, 29(8), 936–952. https://doi.org/10.1080/10926771.2020.
1738614

Stifter, C. A., & Spinrad, T. L. (2002). The effect of excessive crying on the development of
emotion regulation. Infancy, 2(2), 133–152. https://doi.org/10.1207/
S15327078IN0302_2

Talkington, V., Hughes, T. L., & Gacono, C. B. (2013). Vulnerabilities in a school-based
conduct disorder sample as identified by the Rorschach and PCL: YV. Rorschachiana,
34(1), 83–110. https://doi.org/10.1027/1192-5604/a000041

Weiler, B. L., & Widom, C. S. (1996). Psychopathy and violent behaviour in abused and
neglected young adults. Criminal Behaviour and Mental Health, 6(3), 253–271.

Weiner, I. B., & Greene, R. L. (2008). Handbook of personality assessment. Wiley.

Weizmann-Henelius, G., Ilonen, T., Viemero, V., & Eronen, M. (2006). A comparison of
selected Rorschach variables of violent female offenders and female non-offenders.
Behavioral Sciences and the Law, 24(2), 199–213. https://doi.org/10.1002/bsl.680

Wood, J. M., Lilienfeld, S. O., Nezworksi, M. T., Garb, H. N., Allen, K. H., & Wildermuth, J. L.
(2010). Validity of Rorschach inkblot scores for discriminating psychopaths from
nonpsychopaths in forensic populations: A meta-analysis. Psychological Assessment,
22(2), 336–349. https://doi.org/10.1037/a0018998

Zillmer, E., Harrower, M., Ritzler, B. A., & Archer, R. P. (1995). The quest for the Nazi
personality: A psychological investigation of Nazi war criminals. Erlbaum.

History
Received July 8, 2020
Revision received October 9, 2020
Accepted October 20, 2020
Published online September 15, 2021

ORCID
Corine de Ruiter
 https://orcid.org/0000-0002-0135-9790

Corine de Ruiter
Faculty of Psychology & Neuroscience
Maastricht University
PO Box 616
6200 Maastricht
The Netherlands
corine.deruiter@maastrichtuniversity.nl

Summary

Forensic psychological assessment in criminal cases is performed to assist the trier of fact in answering legal questions that have a psychological dimension. Examples are criminal responsibility, violence risk assessment, and need for treatment. Performance-based personality tests, such as the Rorschach, can contribute uniquely to forensic assessment because they are somewhat less transparent to the examinee than self-report measures are. This paper reviews Rorschach studies on forensically relevant Rorschach variables, including those with different forensic samples. Empirical findings are mixed; there is not a one-on-one relationship between certain Rorschach variables, such as aggression codes, and forensically relevant traits, such as psychopathy, hostility, or aggressive behavior. Likely, all aggression codes indicate a preoccupation with aggressive imagery, but the manner in which this preoccupation plays a role in the examinee's life (e.g., extreme fear of aggression, violent victimization, violence perpetration, denial of aggression) needs to be determined on the basis of other data. A large number of Rorschach protocols with high Lambda and positive Coping Deficit Index, demonstrating coping and problem-solving difficulties, characterizes many offender samples.

Rorschach codes can provide meaningful and unique information in a forensic evaluation. A pertinent example is the Rorschach's ability to provide information about a person's perception and thinking that is indicative of an underlying psychotic process, even before actual symptoms of psychosis have surfaced. The incremental validity of the Rorschach is illustrated with a case example of a 20-year-old male college student, who committed a (first) violent offense, an assault with a knife on a female student, who had recently refused to have an intimate relationship with him. Data obtained from the defendant, his parents, his friends, and the victim were used to reconstruct the mental state at the time of the offense. Psychological test data, including the MMPI-2, but especially the Rorschach, provided insight into the psychological dynamics that motivated the attack, which was very much out of character for this timid and emotionally immature young adult.

Samenvatting

Forensisch psychologisch onderzoek in strafzaken wordt uitgevoerd om de rechter te helpen bij het beantwoorden van rechtsvragen die een psychologische dimensie hebben. Voorbeelden zijn strafrechtelijke verantwoordelijkheid, geweldsrisico-inschatting en behoefte aan behandeling. Prestatie-gebaseerde persoonlijkheidstests, zoals de Rorschach, kunnen een unieke bijdrage leveren aan forensisch onderzoek omdat ze minder transparant zijn voor de onderzochte dan zelfrapportage instrumenten. Dit artikel geeft een overzicht van Rorschach onderzoek naar forensisch relevante Rorschach variabelen, inclusief die met verschillende forensische steekproeven. De empirische bevindingen zijn gemengd; er is geen één-op-één relatie tussen bepaalde Rorschach variabelen, zoals agressiecodes, en forensisch relevante kenmerken, zoals psychopathie, vijandigheid, of agressief gedrag. Waarschijnlijk wijzen alle agressiecodes op een preoccupatie met agressie, maar de manier waarop deze preoccupatie een rol speelt in het leven van de onderzochte (b.v. extreme angst voor agressie, gewelddadig slachtofferschap, geweldpleging, ontkenning van agressie) moet worden vastgesteld op basis van andere gegevens. Een groot aantal Rorschach-protocollen met een hoge Lambda en een positieve Coping Deficit Index, waaruit blijkt dat er problemen zijn met coping en probleemoplossing, is kenmerkend voor veel dadersteekproeven.

Rorschach-codes kunnen zinvolle en unieke informatie opleveren in een forensische evaluatie. Een relevant voorbeeld is het vermogen van de Rorschach om informatie te verschaffen over de perceptie en het denken van een persoon die indicatief is voor een onderliggend psychotisch proces, zelfs voordat de echte symptomen van de psychose aan de oppervlakte zijn gekomen. De incrementele validiteit van de Rorschach wordt geïllustreerd aan de hand van een casus van een 20-jarige mannelijke student, die een (eerste) geweldsdelict pleegde, een aanval met een mes op een mede-studente, die kort daarvoor had geweigerd een intieme relatie met hem aan te gaan. Gegevens verkregen van de verdachte, zijn ouders, zijn vrienden en het slachtoffer werden gebruikt om de mentale toestand ten tijde van het delict te reconstrueren. Psychologische testgegevens, waaronder de MMPI-2, maar vooral de Rorschach, verschaften inzicht in de psychologische dynamiek die ten grondslag lag aan de aanval, die zeer ongewoon was voor deze timide en emotioneel onrijpe jongvolwassene.

Résumé

L'évaluation psychologique médico-légale dans les affaires pénales est effectuée pour aider le juge des faits à répondre aux questions juridiques qui ont une dimension psychologique. Il s'agit par exemple de la responsabilité pénale, de l'évaluation du risque de violence et de la nécessité d'un traitement. Les tests de personnalité basés sur les performances, tels que le Rorschach, peuvent contribuer de manière unique à l'évaluation médico-légale car ils sont un peu moins transparents pour la personne que les mesures d'auto-évaluation. Cet article passe en revue les études de Rorschach sur les variables de Rorschach pertinentes sur le plan médico-légal, y compris celles qui concernent différents échantillons médico-légaux. Les résultats empiriques sont mitigés ; il n'y a pas de relation individuelle entre certaines variables de Rorschach, telles que les codes d'agression, et des traits pertinents sur le plan médico-légal, tels que la psychopathie, l'hostilité ou le comportement agressif. Il est probable que tous les codes d'agressivité indiquent une préoccupation pour l'image de l'agressivité, mais la manière dont cette préoccupation joue un rôle dans la vie de la personne (par exemple, peur extrême de l'agression, victimisation violente, perpétration de violence, déni de l'agressivité) doit être déterminée sur la base d'autres données. Un grand nombre de protocoles de Rorschach avec un indice Lambda élevé et un indice positif de déficit d'adaptation (CDI), démontrant des difficultés d'adaptation et de résolution de problèmes, caractérise de nombreux Rorschachs de délinquants.

Les codes Rorschach peuvent fournir des informations significatives et uniques dans une évaluation médico-légale. Un exemple pertinent est la capacité du Rorschach à fournir des informations sur la perception et la pensée d'une personne, qui sont révélatrices d'un processus psychotique sous-jacent, avant même que les symptômes réels de la psychose n'apparaissent. La validité progressive du Rorschach est illustrée par le cas d'un étudiant de 20 ans, qui a commis un (premier) délit violent, une agression au couteau sur une étudiante, qui avait récemment refusé d'avoir une relation intime avec lui. L'information obtenues de l'accusé, de ses parents, de ses amis et de la victime ont été utilisées pour reconstruire l'état mental au moment de l'infraction. Les resultats des tests psychologiques, y compris le MMPI-2, mais surtout le Rorschach, ont permis de comprendre la dynamique psychologique qui a motivé l'attaque, ce qui était tout à fait inhabituel pour ce jeune adulte timide et émotionnellement immature.

Resumen

La evaluación psicológica forense en los casos penales se lleva a cabo para ayudar al juez a responder a las preguntas legales que tienen una dimensión psicológica. Algunos ejemplos son la responsabilidad penal, la evaluación del riesgo de violencia y la necesidad de tratamiento. Los tests de personalidad basados en el rendimiento, como el Rorschach, pueden contribuir de forma única a la evaluación forense porque son algo menos transparentes para el examinado que las medidas de autoinforme. Este artículo revisa los estudios de Rorschach sobre las variables de Rorschach de relevancia forense, incluyendo aquellos con diferentes muestras forenses. Los hallazgos empíricos son mixtos; no existe una relación de uno a uno entre ciertas variables de Rorschach, como los códigos de agresión, y los rasgos forenses relevantes, como la psicopatía, la hostilidad o el comportamiento agresivo. Es probable que todos los códigos de agresión indiquen una preocupación por las imágenes agresivas, pero la forma en que esta preocupación desempeña un papel en la vida del examinado (por ejemplo, miedo extremo a la agresión, victimización violenta, perpetración de violencia, negación de la agresión) debe determinarse sobre la base de otros datos. Un elevado número de protocolos de Rorschach con un Lambda alto y un índice de déficit de afrontamiento

(CDI) positivo, que demuestran dificultades de afrontamiento y de resolución de problemas, caracteriza a muchas protocolos de Rorschachs de delincuentes.

Los códigos de Rorschach pueden proporcionar información significativa y única en una evaluación forense. Un ejemplo pertinente es la capacidad del Rorschach para proporcionar información sobre la percepción y el pensamiento de una persona que es indicativa de un proceso psicótico subyacente, incluso antes de que los síntomas reales de la psicosis hayan aflorado. La validez incremental del Rorschach se ilustra con un ejemplo de caso de un estudiante universitario de 20 años, que cometió un (primer) delito violento, una agresión con un cuchillo a una estudiante, que recientemente se había negado a tener una relación íntima con él. Los datos obtenidos del acusado, sus padres, sus amigos y la víctima se utilizaron para reconstruir el estado mental en el momento del delito. Los datos de las pruebas psicológicas, entre ellas el MMPI-2, pero sobre todo el Rorschach, permitieron conocer la dinámica psicológica que motivó el ataque, muy fuera de lo habitual en este joven adulto tímido y emocionalmente inmaduro.

要約

刑事事件における法医学的な心理学的評価は、心理学的側面を持つ法的質問に答える際に、事実を求める裁判官を支援するために実行される。例としては、刑事責任、暴力リスク評価、治療の必要性などがある。ロールシャッハのようなパフォーマンスベースのパーソナリティ検査は、自記式の検査と比べて受検者に対する透明性がやや低いため、法医学的な評価に独自の貢献をすることができる。本論文では、法医学的に関連性のあるロールシャッハ変数に関するロールシャッハ研究を異なる法医学的サンプルを用いたものも含めてレビューする。経験的な知見はまちまちである。例えば、攻撃性のコードのような特定のロールシャッハ変数と、サイコパシー、敵意、攻撃的の行動のような法医学的に関連性のある特性との間に一対一の関係は存在しない。

おそらく、すべての攻撃性のコードは、攻撃的なイメージの先入観を示しているが、この先入観が被検者の生活の中でどのような役割を果たしているか（例えば、極端な攻撃性への恐怖、暴力的な犠牲、暴力の加害、攻撃性の否定など）については、他のデータに基づいて判断する必要がある。コーピングや問題解決の困難さを示す高いラムダと対処力不全指標がチェックされている多くのロールシャッハプロトコルは、犯罪者サンプルを特徴づけている。

ロールシャッハコードは、法医学的な評価において、意味のあるユニークな情報を提供することができる。適切な例として、精神病の症状が実際に表面化する前であっても、ロールシャッハは、その人の知覚や思考に関する情報を提供する力がある。ロールシャッハのさらなる有効性は、20歳の男子大学生の例で示されている。この学生の（最初の）暴力的な犯罪の内容は、犯罪の直近で親密な関係を持つことを拒否した女子学生へのナイフによる暴行であった。被告人、彼の両親、友人、および被害者から得られたデータは、犯罪時の精神状態を再構築するために使用された。MMPI-2と特にロールシャッハを含む心理テストデータによって、この臆病で感情的に未熟な若者の性格からはかけ離れた、攻撃の動機となった心理的ダイナミクスについての洞察が得られた。

A Commentary on "The Rorschach and Violent Crime" (de Ruiter, 2021)

Anita L. Boss

Independent Practice, Alexandria, VA, USA

One individual's violence and its origins can be as unique as his or her Rorschach responses. Dr. de Ruiter's succinct review (2021) demonstrates that the Rorschach provides a wealth of information about cognition and personality, and that at this time there are no reliable Rorschach correlates for the prediction of future violence. The nuances of personality features gleaned from a performance-based measure, while clinically informative, cannot predict whether or not an individual will act violently.

When considering cases of violence, forensic psychologists most often focus on the question of prediction of future violence and how to mitigate risk. What is lost in an approach focused solely on risk assessment/risk management is the amenability to using a theory-driven approach to clinical assessment in a context that relies on the evaluator to provide clinical information about an *individual*. As Dr. de Ruiter's case illustrates, using a performance-based measure of cognition and personality assessment can generate important incremental information to assist the court in determining whether a case involving a violent offense should be heard in juvenile or adult court. The Rorschach can also be a powerful tool for clinical intervention and treatment planning posttrial.

Any test used in a forensic context must meet the controlling court's rules for the admissibility of scientific evidence, as well as professional standards for reliability and validity. The criticisms of the Rorschach that were raised in the literature, beginning with Wood, Lilienfeld, and others (e.g., Lilienfeld et al., 2000; Wood et al., 1996) changed the course for the Rorschach in the United States (US). One of the results was a statement issued by the Board of Trustees of the Society of Personality Assessment (2005) that presented a wealth of literature on the Rorschach's reliability and validity. While some practitioners, particularly those in the Society for Personality Assessment, maintained that the Rorschach could be used appropriately in forensic assessment, the larger body of forensic psychologists and forensic training programs in the US has trended away from the Rorschach after these criticisms. This controversy is being mentioned for context, but further discussion is beyond the bounds of this commentary.

Rorschachiana (2021), 42(2), 196–201
https://doi.org/10.1027/1192-5604/a000144

In his 2008 survey of how the Rorschach is received in US courts, Reid Meloy found that when the data from the Rorschach are integrated into an unbiased and useful assessment, the courts most often accept the scientific foundation and incremental value. Meloy found that when Rorschach data are rejected by a court, it is usually related to misuse of the test or use of the test in a context in which it is not informative.

Forensic evaluators need to be intimately familiar with both the reliability and validity of the Rorschach variables relied upon, and the nature of the criticisms. While many variables do meet stringent forensic standards, not all are equally relevant and reliable in this context. This places the psychologist in the difficult but achievable position of explaining how selected variables add incremental validity to their assessment of the psycho-legal question, and which ones are extraneous or red herrings.

As described in the American Psychological Association's "Specialty Guidelines for Forensic Psychology" (2013), which grew from years of discussion and development of principles of forensic evaluation and standards of practice, forensic psychologists seek to rely upon multiple sources of data when conducting evaluations. Opinions should be unbiased and focused on the psycho-legal issue. Procedures employed should be useful in answering the specific referral questions.

Juvenile courts, with their focus on rehabilitation, provide a unique forensic context in which a broader comprehensive evaluation of the individual is more common and of greater utility. In The Netherlands, where Dr. de Ruiter's evaluation took place, laws were set up in 2014 to expand the age for hearing a case in juvenile court to 23, depending on a mental health professional's assessment of the individual's level of development. This is in line with the current science regarding adolescent brain development (e.g., see amicus briefs by American Medical Association et al., 2012; American Psychological Association et al., 2010, 2012; and Steinberg, 2017). By contrast, the US moved to a more punitive approach to juvenile offending in the early 1990s that made it easier to try children as adults. Depending on the jurisdiction, many juveniles sentenced to adult prisons in the US have limited resources for rehabilitation, and fewer resources for age-appropriate rehabilitation and treatment (Bonnie et al., 2013). This trend has been difficult to reverse, although as social sciences research has accumulated, the courts are beginning to respond, following US Supreme Court cases addressing the death penalty and life imprisonment of people who were under 18 at the time of the offense (*Graham v. Florida, 2010; Miller v. Alabama, 2012; Montgomery v. Louisiana, 2016; Roper v. Simmons, 2005*).

Comprehensive forensic assessment of juveniles in the US court system can inform the court as to whether transfer to adult court is appropriate; however, the Rorschach is not mentioned in the current American literature for this purpose. For example, in a foundational text published by the American Psychological Association (APA), chapters addressing the evaluation of developmental maturity, transfer to adult court, treatment, rehabilitation, and the forensic assessment of adolescents in general are silent about performance-based measures, except intelligence or neuropsychological tests when necessary (APA, 2016). In a chapter describing the importance of personality assessment and the forensic use of clinical assessment instruments, only self-report measures and checklists are discussed, with passing mention of the Wechsler intelligence scales (Archer & Baum, 2016). This illustrates the movement away from the Rorschach in a critical part of the US forensic psychology community. The omission does a disservice by not mentioning when and how this test can be relevant, reliable, and informative, and it limits the ability of forensic psychologists to defend its use when practicable.

As Heilbrun and Locklair (2016) noted, there is more overlap between clinical and forensic assessment of juveniles because of the focus on rehabilitation. In some US jurisdictions, as well as in some countries outside the US, the referral questions are broader, and the psychologist is expected to provide a comprehensive evaluation that addresses multiple questions. In Dr. de Ruiter's case, the standard requests from the court include present mental status, mental state at the time of the offense/criminal responsibility, recidivism risk, and treatment recommendations for risk management (de Ruiter, personal communication, January 12, 2021). Clearly, there are benefits to integrating the forensic approach with the broader clinical approach in this context. The forensic approach allows for more consistency, and theoretically more impartiality and fairness when principles and control of biases are carefully followed. The clinical approach facilitates more latitude for the clinician to focus on therapeutic or collaborative assessment, which are models that keep the goals of individual treatment and rehabilitation in mind.

One of the prominent questions to be answered in consideration of transferring a juvenile to adult court is the potential for recidivism. Research in adolescence-limited and life-course persistent (LCP) juvenile delinquent behavior would not suggest that the Rorschach has much utility in predicting which individuals will continue to commit criminal acts in adulthood. Early-onset, chronic aggressive behavior is the most salient factor to suggest LCP offending. Moffitt's (1997, 2015) theory assumes that LCP individuals have a convergence of individual vulnerability (e.g., low verbal intelligence, hyperactivity, and neuropsychological problems) and familial/environmental risk factors (Russell & Odgers, 2016). Following the range of etiological factors for early-onset aggressive behavior noted above, predictive factors for LCP antisocial behavior and aggression include high levels of early childhood aggression, chronic aggression, and both violent and nonviolent delinquency. Many of the other factors of relevance to LCP are environmental and/or socioeconomic (Russell & Odgers, 2016), which would not require psychological testing to assess.

Setting aside recidivism potential, when a case is presented in juvenile court, treatment planning is critical, which creates more room for clinical assessment. While the Rorschach will not assist in determining the likelihood of desistance versus life course persistence, it can help with risk reduction strategies when there are sufficient resources for treatment planning and wrap-around services. For example, using the Rorschach in the Collaborative Therapeutic Assessment (CTA) model in a residential treatment center for adolescents, Aschieri and Vetere (2020) demonstrated its utility as an intervention for both staff and an adolescent charged with a violent crime. The Rorschach used in the CTA context benefited the individual adolescent in treatment by enhancing the staff's empathy and understanding, helping to avoid frequent residential treatment pitfalls, and creating space for the staff to tailor treatment approaches to fit the adolescent.

The ability to integrate a wide range of information, including test data, into a coherent and accurate whole is a skill that is not only difficult to master, but difficult to teach. Dr. de Ruiter's article demonstrates the integration of test data with other collateral sources in an effort to address the court's questions. The robust Rorschach variables regarding thinking and perception provided a clearer understanding of the subject's distorted thinking as well as his immaturity, which were key factors in the recommendation for hearing the case in juvenile court. It was a benefit to the case that these variables were quantified by the Rorschach. There is depth to the final opinions with integrated data, and the recommendations are based on the confluence of information from multiple sources.

The Rorschach can be effectively used in a forensic setting, and with violent offenders, although its utility is limited by the referral question. In forensic settings where the examiner has broad referral questions, the Rorschach can be useful to enrich the forensic analysis when the data are corroborated by other information. Forensic personality assessment focused on social/emotional maturity, ruling in or out psychosis when the presentation is subtle, or the ability to manage stress are situations where the Rorschach potentially has incremental value. If the psycho-legal question is narrow, then the evaluator should take extra care to ascertain whether a Rorschach is necessary to answer it. It is incumbent upon the evaluator to understand the requirements of the court or referring entity. The Rorschach is best used when it adds incremental information, and not used as an exploratory device to provide more clinical material that, while interesting, has the potential to introduce information beyond the referral question that might be distracting, biasing, or not useful to the trier of fact.

References

American Medical Association and the American Academy of Child Adolescent Psychiatry as Amici Curiae in Support of Neither Party, *Miller v. Alabama*, 567 U.S. 460 (2012). Nos. 10-9646 & 10-9647. https://www.aacap.org/App_Themes/AACAP/docs/Advocacy/amicus_curiae/miller_v_alabama.pdf

American Psychological Association (2013). Specialty guidelines for forensic psychology. *American Psychologist, 68*(1), 7–19. https://doi.org/10.1037/a0029889

American Psychological Association (2016). *APA handbook of psychology and juvenile justice*.

American Psychological Association, American Psychiatric Association, and National Association of Social Workers as Amici Curiae in Support of Petitioners, *Graham v. Florida* and *Sullivan v. Florida*, 130 S. Ct. 2011 (2010). Nos. 08-7412, 08-7621. https://www.apa.org/about/offices/ogc/amicus/graham-v-florida-sullivan.pdf

American Psychological Association, American Psychiatric Association, and National Association of Social Workers as Amici Curiae in Support of Petitioners, *Miller v. Alabama* and *Jackson v. Hobbs*, 132 S. Ct. 2455 (2012). Nos. 10-9646, 10-9647. https://www.apa.org/about/offices/ogc/amicus/miller-hobbs.pdf

Archer, R. P., & Baum, L. J. (2016). Forensic uses of clinical assessment measures. In K. Heilbrun (Ed.), *APA handbook of psychology and juvenile justice* (pp. 425–443). American Psychological Association.

Aschieri, F., & Vetere, C. (2020). Using the Rorschach as a group intervention to promote the understanding of adolescents by staff members in inpatient residential programs. *Rorschachiana, 41*(2), 120–143. https://doi.org/10.1027/1192-5604/a000127

Bonnie, R. J., Johnson, R. L., Chemers, B. M., & Schuck, J. (2013). *Reforming juvenile justice: A developmental approach*. National Academies Press.

de Ruiter, C. (2021). The Rorschach and violent crime: A literature review and case illustration. *Rorschachiana, 42*(2), 175–195. https://doi.org/10.1027/1192-5604/a000134

Graham v. Florida, 560 U.S. 48 (2010). https://www.oyez.org/cases/2009/08–7412

Heilbrun, K., & Locklair, B. (2016). Forensic assessment of juveniles. In K. Heilbrun (Ed.), *APA handbook of psychology and juvenile justice* (pp. 345–363). American Psychological Association.

Lilienfeld, S. O., Wood, J. M., & Garb, H. N. (2000). The scientific status of projective techniques. *Psychological Science in the Public Interest, 1*(2), 27–66. https://doi.org/10.1111/1529-1006.002

Meloy, J. R. (2008). The authority of the Rorschach: An update. In C. B. Gacono & F. B. Evans (Eds.), *The handbook of forensic Rorschach assessment* (pp. 79–87). Routledge.

Miller v. Alabama, 567 U.S. 460 (2012). https://www.oyez.org/cases/2011/10-9646

Moffitt, T. E. (1997). Adolescence-limited and life-course persistent offending: A complimentary pair of developmental theories. In T. Thornberry (Ed.), *Advances in criminological theory: Developmental theories of crime and delinquency* (pp. 11–54). Routledge.

Moffitt, T. E. (2015). Life-course persistent versus adolescence-limited antisocial behavior. In D. Ciccetti & D. J. Cohen (Eds.), *Developmental psychopathology* (2nd ed., pp. 570–598). Wiley.

Montgomery v. Louisiana, 136 S. Ct. 718 (2016). https://www.oyez.org/cases/2015/14-280

Roper v. Simmons, 543 U.S. 551 (2005). https://www.oyez.org/cases/2004/03-633

Russell, M. A., & Odgers, C. L. (2016). Desistance and life-course persistence: Findings from longitudinal studies using group-based trajectory modeling of antisocial behavior. In K. Heilbrun (Ed.), *APA handbook of psychology and juvenile justice* (pp. 159–175). American Psychological Association.

Society for Personality Assessment (2005). The status of the Rorschach in clinical and forensic practice: An official statement by the Board of Trustees of the Society for Personality Assessment. *Journal of Personality Assessment, 85*(2), 219–237. https://doi. org/10.1207/s15327752jpa8502_16

Steinberg, L. (2017). Adolescent brain science and juvenile justice policymaking. *Psychology, Public Policy & Law, 23*(4), 410–420. https://doi.org/10.1037/law0000128

Wood, J. M., Nezworski, M. T., & Stejskal, W. J. (1996). The comprehensive system for the Rorschach: A critical examination. *Psychological Science, 7*(1), 3–10. https://doi.org/ 10.1111/j.1467-9280.1996.tb00658.x

Published online September 15, 2021

Acknowledgments
I gratefully acknowledge the assistance of Julie Gallagher, PsyD, ABPP, for her helpful review and comments in the final preparation of this article.

Anita L. Boss
Independent Practice
1200 Prince St.
Alexandria, VA 22314
USA
albosspsyd@comcast.net

Special Issue: The Rorschach Test Today: An Update on the Research
Research Article

Eating Disorders and the Rorschach

A Research Review From the French School and the Comprehensive System

Silvia Monica Guinzbourg de Braude[1,2], Sarah Vibert[3,4], Tommaso Righetti[5], and Arianna Antonelli[6]

[1]Department of Psychiatry, Hospital Italiano, Buenos Aires, Argentina
[2]Department of Psychology, Salvador University, Buenos Aires, Argentina
[3]Department of Psychology, Université Paris René Descartes, Paris, France
[4]Institut Mutualiste Montsouris, Paris, France
[5]Department of Psychology, Università Cattolica del Sacro Cuore, Milan, Italy
[6]Scuola di Psicoterapia Integrata – Sanicare, Massa, Italy

Abstract: In this article we review research on eating disorders with the Rorschach. In this field there are two main lines of research involving two specific methodologies: the Comprehensive System and the French school. We present the main results of the different studies separately and then comment on some similarities and differences in the findings. We find that the results of these studies are complementary on certain aspects of functioning found in anorexia nervosa as compared with other categories of eating disorders. Both sets of studies underline the self-centeredness of anorexic patients with their difficulty in communicating their feelings and thoughts. In both types of study, treatment is understood as relying on an integrative and multidisciplinary model that seeks to modify the eating behaviors and to improve ego functions in order to moderate the patient's distress. In addition, both types of research show that secure attachment would be the first priority for the therapist in psychological treatment, which should increase the patient's confidence in others. They also both stress the importance of the restoration of self-esteem and a sense of identity through the support offered by the relationship to the therapist.

Keywords: Rorschach, Comprehensive System, The French School, eating disorders, assessment

Eating Disorders

The prevalence of eating disorders (EDs) among adolescents and young adults is notable in Western countries due to the particular cultural framework (Selvini-Palazzoli, 1965). Epidemiological studies report that, in 2003, the average prevalence of anorexia and bulimia was 0.3% and 1%, respectively (Hoek & van Hoeken, 2003) and in 2016 these EDs were the sixth most prevalent mental disease with around 10.5 million cases worldwide (Ritchie & Roser, 2019).

Rorschachiana (2021), 42(2), 202–224
https://doi.org/10.1027/1192-5604/a000136

© 2021 Hogrefe Publishing

Many studies have investigated the genetic, physiological, familial, psychological, and cultural factors in the onset of these symptoms (Fairburn & Harrison, 2003). Researchers agree on the multidimensional nature of the etiological processes involved in EDs, and the multidisciplinary approach to treatment due to the need to address somatic, behavioral, cognitive, emotional, and intrapsychic issues (Gonzalez et al., 2007; Striegel-Moore & Bulik, 2007). However, differences exist between contradictory and competing theories about the underlying causal processes, reflecting the complexity of these disorders (Rothschild et al., 2008).

Today, the *Diagnostic and Statistical Manual of Mental Disorders* (5th ed. [DSM-5]; American Psychiatric Association, 2013) defines anorexia and bulimia and distinguishes between different types of EDs: anorexia nervosa (AN), which includes on the one hand a restrictive form (AN-R) and on the other hand another form with bulimia/vomiting or laxative intake (AN-B), bulimia nervosa (BN), pica, rumination disorder, avoidant/restrictive food intake disorder, binge-eating disorder (BED), unspecified eating disorders, and other specified feeding or eating disorders (OFSED).

In this classification, obesity is excluded because it is not considered a mental disorder; excluding obesity has been criticized (Cuzzolaro, 2013; Day et al., 2009). Other critics to the categorization of the DSM diagnoses in its different versions were: (1) EDs are more similar than different because they share a patho-logical core based on excessive preoccupation with weight, the body, and control of feeding (Fairburn et al., 2003). (2) DSM-5 diagnoses do not consider the role of personality in functioning, the clinical course of the illness, the treatment out-come, and the etiology of ED (Farstad, et al., 2016), which was found to be more central than the specific ED diagnosis (Thompson-Brenner et al., 2008; Westen & Harnden-Fischer, 2001; Wildes et al., 2011; Wonderlich et al., 2005). Moreover (3) some researchers state that personality is more closely associated with specific symptoms (e.g., binge eating) than to a specific ED (Farstad et al., 2016).

Regarding this point, Westen and Harnden-Fischer (2001) proposed three personality profiles to describe EDs: high functioning, constricted, and emotionally dysregulated. The high functioning profile includes healthy characteristics, such as consciousness and consistent emotionality, as well as anxiety, self-criticism, and perfectionism; this profile included significant obsessive-compulsive personality traits. The constricted profile is characterized by a lower level of functioning and by constriction of emotions and self-awareness, and difficulties in interper-sonal relationships and mentalization about himself/herself and others; these patients usually feel empty inside and bored and obtain elevated scores on measures relating to schizoid, schizotypal, and avoidant personality disorders. By contrast, patients with the emotionally dysregulated profile feel intense emotions, behave impulsively, and are constantly looking for relationships as a

© 2021 Hogrefe Publishing　　　　　　　　　*Rorschachiana* (2021), 42(2), 202–224 means of self-soothing. Patients with this profile obtain higher scores in paranoid and cluster B (antisocial, borderline, histrionic, and narcissistic) personality disorders, especially borderline personality disorder. We will apply this framework, noting that it is empirically derived (Thompson-Brenner & Westen, 2005) and that it has been replicated by several other researchers (Lavender et al., 2013; Steiger et al., 2010; Strober, 1983; Turner et al., 2014; Wildes et al., 2011; Wonderlich et al., 2005).

The Rorschach Test

The Rorschach test is a projective, performance-based instrument, with different approaches to its coding, scoring, and interpretation (Meyer, 2004; Mihura et al., 2019; Weiner, 1996). The studies using the Rorschach test with EDs are widely dispersed, with 24 articles published over the past 20 years (Piotrowski, 2017). In this article we focus on those studies that used the Comprehensive System (Exner, 2003) and the French School (Verdon & Azoulay, 2020) with EDs, in particular those referring to anorexia and bulimia.

The Comprehensive System (CS) provided the Rorschach test with a solid psychometric structure with good reliability and validity on which to base its clinical utility. Adherence to administration and scoring rules ensures that data are obtained in a standardized way for all examinees. Detailed guidelines for scoring test responses are followed to obtain high interrater agreement. Standardization of the CS method also means that norms can be collated.

The French School interprets projective test results with reference to the psychoanalytic theory of psychic functioning, according to the approach developed by Nina Raush de Traubenberg (de Traubenberg, 1970) and Catherine Chabert (Chabert, 1997). This interpretive system explores four factors: *thought* (the evaluation of whether there is any effective differentiation between inside and outside, and thought meaning investment); *narcissism* (identity development, differentiation of primary identifications, boundaries between self and the other, and access to sexual differentiation); *relationships with others and objective relationships* (representations of others and the quality of object relations); *impulse and affect* (expression of impulses and affects and level of anxiety). Results from these factors identify the main problems and the defensive organization in order to come to a hypothesis concerning the patient's psychic functioning.

Studies using the CS mainly focused on diagnosis and treatment and those referring to the French School focused more on diagnosis and an in-depth understanding of personality functioning. We present these different studies separately, but our goal is to consider the findings from both schools in the light of Westen and Harnden-Fischer's conceptualization of EDs in order to see which characteristics emerged in the Rorschach protocols in both systems to inform clinical work with patients who have an ED.

Comprehensive System Studies

Research on the use of the CS in ED is mainly composed of quantitative analyses that use both within-subjects and between-groups study designs. These studies aim to better understand samples of ED patients, comparing different types of disorders and different stages of the ED (acute phase vs. stabilization phase). The main results are shown in Table 1. A case study of anorexia is also presented.

Rothschild et al. (2008) argued that ED symptoms constitute a defensive coping mechanism against psychic pain. They hypothesized that weight stabilization and the reduction of disordered eating behavior will be associated on discharge with (1) a reduction in defensiveness and better contact with inner and external reality and (2) an increase in affective distress.

The sample consisted of 53 female adolescents aged 13–18 years who were hospitalized between 2002 and 2005 – 26 with restrictive anorexia (AN-R) and 27 with bulimia and anorexia (12 from AN B/P and 15 BN purgative subtype) – and who fulfilled diagnostic criteria for an ED. Patients were assessed at admission and discharge. Body mass index (BMI) and self-report tests (the Eating Attitude Test [EAT-26]; Garner et al., 1982; the Beck Depression Inventory [BDI]; Beck et al., 1961; and the State-Trait Anxiety Inventory [STAI]; Spielberger et al., 1970) were included along with the Rorschach.

Regarding Rorschach protocols, both subgroups showed high responsiveness to emotional stimuli (Afr > .46), low introspective capacities (FD < 1), and disorganized thinking (WSum6). This last marker indicated a serious thought disorder in the AN-R subgroup (11 < Wsum6 < 17), while the B/P patients showed severely disorganized thinking (WSum6 > 18).

The first hypothesis that stabilization of weight and disordered eating behaviors would be associated with a reduction in defensiveness and an increase in contact with reality in both groups was partially confirmed. Regarding defensiveness, the openness to experience measure (Form%) had not improved at discharge; the measure of responsiveness to emotional stimuli (Afr) decreased among the B/P group in the second phase, whereas the AN-R group presented only a minor elevation. The reduction in affective responsiveness in the B/P group may relate to the avoidant tendency, such that they become more defensive against emerging distress in the second phase, indicating this subgroup's decreased difficulties in

Table 1. Quantitative studies (CS)

Author(s)	Sample	Age	Comparison	Variable(s) that differentiate samples	p
Rothschild, L., Lacoua, L., Eshel, Y., & Stein, D. (2008)	A) Anorexia Nervosa (26)	15.19	Acute phase*		
	B) Bulimic/anorexic (27)	16.29	A > B	X+%	.353
			B > A	F%	.122
				Afr	.634
				WSum 6	.053
				M−	.233
				FD	.371
				DEPI	.422
				D	.961
			Stabilization of ED phase**		
			A > B	Afr	.163
				WSum 6	.614
				FD	.142
				DEPI	.811
			B > A	F%	.191
				X + %	.372
				M−	.201
				D	.804
Rothschild, L., Lacoua, L., & Stein, D. (2009)	A) Restricting anorexia nervosa (31)	15.51	Acute phase*		
	B) Bingeing/purging spectrum (25)	16.20	B > A	EII-2	.024
				No FQ−	.223
				WSum6	.002
				Critical contents	.001
				M−	.384
				GHR	.771
				PHR	.607
				DEPI	.617

(Continued on next page)

Table 1. (Continued)

Author(s)	Sample	Age	Comparison	Variable(s) that differentiate samples	p
			Stabilization of ED phase**		
			A > B	No FQ−	.741
				PHR	.561
				EII-2	.331
				WSum6	.193
			B > A	Critical contents	.435
				M−	.064
				GHR	.849
				DEPI	.954
Tibon, S., & Rothschild, L. (2009)	A) Anorexia, restricting subtype (29)	15.97	A > B	RFS-P	.572
	B) Anorexia binge eating/purging subtype or bulimia (32)	15.41		RFS-S	.006
				PTI	.293
				R	.089
				L	.593
				DEPI	.099
				EII-2	.119
Guinzbourg, M. (2011)	Control group: nonpatient (60)	22.4	Control > ED	R	.015
	ED patient group (106):	23.6		Blends/R	.002
	• Restrictive anorexia (25)			EA	.000
	• Bulimia (27)			FM	.001
	• EDNOS (54)			FM + m	.001
				C'	.001
				Y	.000
				FC	.000
				CF + C	.009
				H	.006
				COP	.000
				GHR	.000
				PHR	.000

(Continued on next page)

Table 1. (Continued)

Author(s)	Sample	Age	Comparison	Variable(s) that differentiate samples	p
			ED > Control	L	.000
				Fr + rF	.001
			Bulimia > Anorexia	Zd	.001
				Human Cont	.003
				Pure H	.001
				WDA%	.002
			Anorexia > Bulimia	2	.004
				Sum6	.024
				INC	.026
				MOR	.001
				DEPI	.022
				CDI	.000
				S-CON	.000
			Anorexia > EDNOS	W + D	.027
				DQv	.024
				F	.001
				2	.008
				INC	.002
				MOR	0
				L	.028
				Sum6	.028
				M−	.003
				DEPI	.001
				CDI	0
				S-CON	0
			EDNOS > Anorexia	Pure H	.001
				WDA%	.001
				XU%	.021
				Zd	.001

(Continued on next page)

Table 1. (Continued)

Author(s)	Sample	Age	Comparison	Variable(s) that differentiate samples	p
			Bulimia > EDNOS	D	.020
				F	.016
				C'F	.022
				CP	.013
				P > a + 1	.022
			EDNOS > Bulimia	FD	.005
Curiel-Levy, G., Canetti, L., Galili-Weisstub, E., Milun, M., Gur, E., & Bachar, E. (2012)	Anorexic group (35):	18.3	Psychiatric > Anorexic	AG	.002
	• Restrictive type (22)	18.4		PER	.012
	• Binge eating/purging type (13)			PHR	.028
	Control group of psychiatric patients (30):		Anorexic > Psychiatric	COP	.029
	• Depression (26)			GHR	ns
	• Dissociative disorder (2)				
	• Bipolar disorder (1)				
	• Anxiety disorder (1)				

Note. *Acute phase of illness at admission;
**Stabilization of eating disorders symptoms at discharge.

managing affective distress. Regarding contact with reality, both groups showed an improvement after treatment, with decreased distorted conceptions of human experience (M−) and increased reality testing (X+%). Disorganized thinking (WSum6) decreased in the B/P subgroup, while for the AN-R subgroup there was a minor change in the opposite direction. Introspective capacities (FD) increased in the AN-R subgroup, while it decreased in the B/P group.

The second hypothesis was partially confirmed in both groups. There was a decrease in distress and a significant reduction in anxiety and depression in self-report measures, but not with the Rorschach. These differences are attributable to the differing nature of the measurement methods; in both groups the conscious experience of reduction in depressive and anxious symptoms was accompanied by an increase in implicit dysphoric affective states (C') and by a significant elevation in the implicit stress overload index (D) at discharge.

These findings confirm that EDs act as a defense against suffering emotional pain. Results also indicate that these patients may be fearful of their emotions.

Rothschild et al. (2009) studied changes in implicit and explicit measures of patients with ED undergoing treatment. The aims were (1) to examine changes in ego functioning and mental distress in AN-R and AN (B/P) patients, after multimodal integrative treatment, and (2) to examine the relative contribution of the changes in ego functions and compare them with mental distress as a predictor of prognosis.

The sample included 56 patients, 31 of whom had restrictive anorexia and 25 were mixed (10 B/P and 15 BN), who were administered the Rorschach and self-report questionnaires (EAT-26, BDI, STAI-S, and the Eating Disorders Inventory-2 [EDI-2]; Garner, 1991) at admission after a stabilization period of no less than 2 weeks and at discharge.

When considering CS markers, all groups had unrealistic ideas about themselves and a confused or angry attitude, possibly related to a lack of impulse regulation or control (as shown in the critical contents for the Ego Impairment Index-2 [EII-2]; Viglione et al., 2003) and disorganized thinking (WSum6). The AN subgroup showed a serious thought disorder (11 < Wsum6 < 17), while the B/P patients presented severely disorganized thinking (WSum6 > 18). Both groups had potentially maladaptive relationships (PHR > GHR), with the only exception of the B/N subgroup during stabilization phase.

An increase in ego functioning was found on the Rorschach (EII-2, comprising the weighted sum of: no FQ−, indicating poor reality testing; WSum6, indicating thought disturbance; M−, indicating distortion in interpersonal perceptions; the critical contents of An, Bl, Ex, Fi, Fd, Sx, Xy, AG, and MOR, indicating poor ability to inhibit needs and urges; PHR and GHR, indicating poor and good object representations, respectively) but not on the self-report questionnaires. For both groups, the change in ego functions was due to an elevation in good human representations (GHR), whereas an improvement in impulse control (critical contents) was found only in the B/P group and not in the restrictive anorexic patients. Contradictory results were obtained in relation to distress, with a decrease found on self-report measures but not on Rorschach variables.

In patients with anorexia, the only predictor of reduction in eating symptoms was distress. By contrast, for the B/P group the change in EAT-26 was predicted by changes in measures of explicit and implicit distress as well as implicit aspects of ego functioning. This indicates that increased ego functioning is an important factor contributing to the reduction of symptoms in the B/P subgroup. While the change in ego functioning and mental distress was not related to improvement in BMI in the restrictive group, the improvement in implicit ego functioning contributed to a greater adequacy, although small, in the B/P group of patients regarding their BMI.

Tibon and Rothschild (2009) studied dissociative mechanisms in two samples of patients with anorexia (restrictive and B/P vomiting/purging forms) and bulimia (purging and non-purging). The Rorschach Reality Fantasy Scale (RFS; Smith, 1990), which stems from a psychoanalytic approach (Tibon et al., 2006) was used in addition to Rorschach CS variables. The RFS is based on Ogden's model (1985) and it provides an invitation to enter a transitional space between fantasy and reality. Each Rorschach response is located within a continuum, ranging from use of the inkblot's reality without any fantasy to a "fabulization" response where reality collapses into fantasy and the inkblot is experienced as real. Scores are given to each percept and the scale also assesses dissociative mechanisms. In this study, patients with AN B/P obtained higher scores compared with those with AN-R.

Regarding Rorschach CS protocols, a low number of responses (R < 20) was found in the AN subgroup, indicating defensiveness and struggles in looking at things from multiple perspectives, possibly due to emotional reasons. Patients from the AN subgroup seemed to observe and articulate the more sophisticated characteristics of their internal or external world and seemed able to engage in a meaningful way with the more complex and subtle characteristics of their experiences and relationships (30 < L < .99); by contrast, the B/P subgroup showed a coerced-avoidant approach, being unable to focus on the finer characteristics of their internal world or the environment that surrounds them, possibly as a defense against stress at the expense of a lack of awareness (L > .99).

The results suggest that bulimic processes and binge eating episodes are related to dissociative mechanisms between internal and external experiences. Patients with anorexia with purgative/vomiting forms are considered to show greater fluctuations between reality and fantasy. They tend to deny reality as a defense and to activate more addictive behavior to avoid becoming aware of conflict and to avoid the pain of evoking certain life experiences. Subjects with bulimia are described as better able to recognize affects but are more impulsive with difficulty in controlling and regulating their emotions.

Guinzbourg (2011) compared a control group of nonpatient young women (with no diagnosis of mental or physical illness and no evidence of an ED) with a group of patients with EDs, consisting of 23 patients with AN-R, 27 with BN, and 54 EDNOS (ED not otherwise specified) according to DSM-IV criteria. Differences were observed between the nonconsulting women and ED sample. The latter have an introversive coping style, avoid complexity when dealing with stimuli, have fewer resources, present less ability to process sensations and emotions, are less interested in people and social ties with limited expectations about human relationships, and present more self-centeredness.

Although the three subgroups shared some characteristics, they presented some different coping modalities. When comparing patients suffering from anorexia and bulimia, anorexic patients present a greater degree of introversion, a tendency to simplify their responses (W + D; H + DA%), less interest in social aspects (H and H Cont; M−), little confidence in their resources (DEPI), and considerable self-centeredness and self-focus (higher pairs). Patients with anorexia have fewer ways of dealing with sensations and emotions, not being able to register and express them appropriately. They are negligent in recognizing their own needs and experience greater distress and helplessness, denoting a poor integration of the self. Perceptual stereotypes, cognitive slips (INC and Sum6), and morbid contents (MOR) predominate, making them more vulnerable to confused emotional states that could involve them in self-harming behavior (S-CON). Their introspective ability is inefficient.

The same differences can be observed when comparing patients with AN-R and EDNOS. Comparing patients with bulimia and EDNOS, it is noted that these two groups have more traits in common. While patients with bulimia tend to be more passive and dependent and may lose control of their behavior, due to the effect of greater impulsivity, those with EDNOS have better control of their emotional expression (D and D Adj), experience less distress and anxiety (Y, m), tend to internalize their emotional expression (C'), and are more active in their attitudes and more introspective (FD) about their behaviors.

Curiel-Levy et al. (2012) examined the concept of self-centeredness in patients with anorexia, considering their tendency to fail to register their own needs and to serve the needs of others. Their sample of 35 patients with anorexia (22 AN-R and 13 B/P) was compared with 30 psychiatric patients (26 patients with depression, two with dissociative disorder, one with bipolar disorder, and one with anxiety disorder) using the Rorschach and the Wechsler Intelligence Scales.

Results show that patients with anorexia are less aggressive (AG) and give fewer personalized responses (PER) in relation to those in the psychiatric sample. They also have more cooperative movement (COP) and fewer poor human representations (PHR). Their willingness to adapt to the expectations of the environment might have made them less expressive of their feelings in relation to the psychiatric sample. Also, their higher activity level might be attributed to the fact that the psychiatric sample included a significant proportion of patients with depression.

Lis et al. (2011) followed up the case of a 17-year-old patient with anorexia. She was initially evaluated with the Rorschach and other instruments: the SRL-90-R (Derogatis & Lazarus, 1994), the Body Uneasiness Tests (BUT; Cuzzolaro, et al. 2006), a dynamic Operationalized Psychodynamic (OPD) interview (OPD Task Force, 2001) and the Projective Sheet Tests on Adult Attachment (APP; George & West, 2001). The Rorschach protocol was constricted and highly defensive (R = 17, Lambda = 1.86). Qualitatively, her responses rarely involved the management of affects, denoting an emotional block (FC:CF + C = 1:0) and severe control of her feelings (SumC':SumC = 4:0,5), low self-esteem (3r + (2)/(R) = 0,29), and inability for auto-representation realistically (H:(H) + Hd + (Hd) = 0:3), which predisposed her to adaptive difficulties in interpersonal relationships (CDI = 4; GHR: PHR = 1:2).

French School Studies

Research on EDs using the French School approach encompass small samples or single-case studies and aim to provide an in-depth analysis of personality organization. Analysis of the Rorschach is often combined with the Thematic Apperception Test (Verdon et al., 2014), because this combination can help to identify the psychological behaviors underlying symptoms and can reveal many subtleties of psychological functioning more easily and directly than clinical listening and observation at interview.

The findings show common functional characteristics associated with EDs, such as a lack of integration of the self, that distinguishes them from conventional neuroses and anaclitic depression. Furthermore, these studies show that the defense mechanisms and the expression of psychic conflicts in patients with ED are extremely varied and are not as stereotypical as the abnormal eating behaviors that define these disorders (Chabert & Vibert 2016; Vibert & Chabert 2009; Vibert & Cohen de Lara, 2011). While certain dynamic, topical, and economic aspects are regularly found in these patients, the analyses carried out with this methodology reveal modalities of psychic functioning organized according to singular and original configurations. Therefore, the presence of an ED does not allow us to prejudge any particular personality organization. On the contrary, the ED appears to be underpinned by various levels of psychopathological functioning ranging from neurosis to psychosis. The underlying psychopathological organizations, however, show a predominance of borderline personality functioning with narcissistic and depressive features.

Vibert and Chabert (2009) and Vibert and Cohen de Lara (2011) followed up 18 patients aged 15–21, who had a restrictive anorexia nervosa syndrome, with or without associated vomiting, and were hospitalized in the Adolescent and Young Adult Department of the Montsouris Mutualist Institute. From the Rorschach protocol, two patients had a neurotic organization (n = 2), characterized by solid sense of self-identity, contact with reality, presence of "observing-ego," and ability to manage boundaries between self and others (McWilliams, 2011). The other patients (n = 16) presented with borderline functioning, which means either defensive inhibition or overwhelmed defenses associated with excessive arousal. The Rorschach results showed two groups: anorexic restricting subtype (AN-R; n = 8) and anorexic–bulimic patients (AN-B; n = 8). Differences between these two groups concern fantasy expression, defensive processes, and relational dynamics. The AN-R patients are characterized by defensive inhibition and impoverished responses. *Thought*: These patients showed massive constriction of conflict expression and used reality as a medium to fill the internal void. *Narcissism*: They used narcissistic references (such as skinny clothes responses) to maintain their identity. *Relationships with others and object relationships*: They registered lack of relational percepts and impoverishment of object relations through the use of perceptual isolation of human or animal representations. In addition, their tendency to control everything coming from the other is an attempt to deny differences. Relationships, where they exist, are "mirrored relationships," where the other reflects the self and cannot be acknowledged as different from the self. *Impulse and affect*: Sensory and perceptual qualities are privileged over affect.

The AN-B patients presented massive projection, abundance of responses, and use of manic responses. Their functioning sometimes resembles a psychotic state, without reaching this level of profound disturbance, because repression of conflict is insufficient, and psychic stability appears precarious. *Thought*: Their self-representation boundaries appear porous and percepts are very often distorted and are regularly associated with identity impairment (e.g., raw anatomical or sexual content, or characters or animals that have lost their bodily integrity). *Narcissism*: Narcissistic defenses are regularly overwhelmed in these patients. Their attempt to control depressing thoughts and feelings appears to be ineffective, exemplifying an undifferentiated depressive narcissistic problem. *Relationships with others and object relationships*: Their massive projective identification undoes the differences between oneself and the other. *Impulse and affect*: They are overwhelmed by impulses that may be expressed in an overly excitable way. Confusion between self and object, and inside and outside, is common and the expression of destructive impulses threatens identity. Their greed for the object betrays the underlying narcissistic lack.

Vibert (2012) compared two patients hospitalized in the same ward using the Rorschach test, one with AN-R symptomatology, and the other with an AN-B symptomatology. The AN-R patient showed extreme inhibition as the principal trait. Instability of interpersonal boundaries and excessive impulses are common between AN-R and AN-B patients; however, the AN-R patient managed to ensure a sort of "waterproofing" of the boundaries and used inhibition as repression of impulses. *Thought*: The patient presents mental functioning impoverishment. *Narcissism*: The patient showed strong narcissistic structure, preserved by inhibition. *Relationships with others and object relationships*: She was not invested in object relationships and she had very tight limits between inside and outside, which protected the integrity of her identity. *Impulse and affect*: She controlled her impulses in a similar manner to her approach to object relations.

The AN-B patient showed massive projection as her main characteristic defense. *Thought*: she presented many slippages related to an excess of excitement that cannot be contained caused by the expression of fantasies, which testifies to a certain vitality of her psychic functioning. *Narcissism*: This patient invests in the object more heavily, but it threatens in return to invade her and harm her sense of her identity. *Relationships with others and object relationships*: The patient demonstrated a failure of boundaries through the leakage of impulses that are bound up with an investment of the object. *Impulse and affect*: The presence of excessive impulses that are not controlled.

Chabert and Vibert (2016) used projective tests (Rorschach and TAT) with 13 hospitalized girls suffering from anorexia with vomiting (AN-B) and bulimia (B) at the Montsouris Mutualist Institute in the Adolescent Psychiatry Service combined with the experience of psychotherapeutic treatment performed in the same service. The study shows a partial relationship between the functioning of these patients and perversion as defined by Freud (1927/1969) and Racamier (2012). According to this psychoanalytic formulation, in patients with a perverse structure, psychic functioning is firmly entrenched and supported by splitting and denial. Fantasy activity tends to be fixated in a repetitive mode and it maintains an intense libidinal investment, especially in its sadistic and masochistic forms. The perverse characteristics found in AN-B and B patients differ from the perverse organization itself. Instead of being rigidly fixated, they are characterized in particular by a greater narcissistic fragility, and by the more frequent appearance of depressive elements, especially when the symptomatology related to food disappears. In addition, as observed in the borderline states, the psychic functioning of these patients is very heterogeneous, fluid, and patchy, like a shifting mosaic.

Discussion

The findings from the CS and the French School are difficult to synthesize and they appear incompatible because the two approaches to the Rorschach are not comparable in terms of their methods of analysis and their underlying conceptual models; they explore very different dimensions in their attempts to reach an understanding of the personality traits associated with eating behavior that has become disturbed. Furthermore, the samples they employed vary quantitatively and the studies do not necessarily compare patients with similar symptomatology or in similar clinical settings. Hence, we will discuss the findings from both approaches in the light of Westen and Harnden-Fischer's (2001) conceptualization in order to compare them.

Comprehensive System and Westen and Harnden-Fischer

When considering Westen and Harnden-Fisher's conceptualization of EDs, results from CS studies do not offer a clear and uniform categorization.

From the analysis of protocols of anorexic groups among the different studies, those patients seem to be in a middle ground between the "constricted" and "emotionally dysregulated" categories. Connected to the latter, they seem to be characterized by high responsiveness to emotional stimuli (Afr), lack of impulse regulation/control (EII-2 critical contents), and difficulty in taking into account different perspectives (R). Being vulnerable to confused emotional states might also lead them to self-harming behavior (S-CON). On the constricted side of the description, they presented low introspective capacities (FD), linked to the presence of unrealistic ideas of themselves ((H) and (Hd)), and low capacity for expressing feelings and emotions (Lambda). Moreover, a similar frame can be observed in the BN and AN-BP subgroups.

When comparing the two subgroups during different phases of their EDs, BN and AN-B/P patients tend to improve some of their emotionally dysregulated features, such as lack of impulse control (EII-2 critical contents) and high responsiveness to emotional stimuli (Afr) and they tend to be more avoidant and self-centered (pairs) than the AN-R patients. These elements lead to a flexible categorization of these two groups, where AN-R patients tend to be more emotionally dysregulated and BN and AN-B/P patients seem to be more constricted. In fact, both AN-R and BN-AN-B/P subgroups do not completely fall into the "high functioning" categorization due to serious and severe disorganized thinking (WSum6). Only one study offered a description of EDNOS patients, which, when compared with AN-R and BN, showed similar characteristics of the high functioning profile: Those patients seem to have better control (Form %), to experience less distress and anxiety (C', Y, and m), and to be more active and introspective (FD).

French School and Westen and Harnden-Fischer

A clear classification of EDs emerges from the French School studies, which resembles the Westen and Harnden-Fischer (2001) conceptualization of EDs. According to the French School studies, patients with EDs can be divided into neurotic and borderline functioning. The first group is characterized by an integrated sense of self-identity, solid contact with reality, the presence of observing-ego, and the ability to manage boundaries between self and others; this is consistent with Westen and Harnden-Fischer's high functioning group, with the presence of consciousness, self-criticism, and integrated emotionality. Among the borderline group, a further division emerges between AN-R and AN-B.

The first is characterized by inhibition, disinvestment in relationships, and impulse control, which is consistent with Westen and Harnden-Fischer's constricted group. The AN-B showed massive use of projective identification, lack of boundaries between the self and the others, and no control of impulses, and this is consistent with Westen and Harnden-Fischer's emotionally dysregulated group.

Putting Together Two Rorschach Interpretations

Crucial areas to consider when analyzing Rorschach protocols through the lens of Westen and Harnden-Fisher's conceptualization are thought, interpersonal relationships, and emotionality. *Thought*: The two CS indices, FD and WSum6, seem to distinguish between high functioning profiles and the others, which are instead characterized by impoverished mental functioning and low introspectiveness. *Relationships*: The high functioning profile has good and multiple relationships with others, whereas the constricted group would struggle to have good relationships with others and the emotionally dysregulated group is able to establish interpersonal relationships but they are characterized by a lack of boundaries. *Emotionality*: The lack of impulse control/regulation and the higher responsiveness to stimuli seem to distinguish between the emotionally dysregulated group and the others, while between the high functioning and the constricted group the difference is the ability to express controlled emotions and the level of defensiveness.

Limitations

The low number of high functioning patients in the studies we reviewed does not allow us to make clear connections to Westen and Harnden-Fischer's high functioning profile, probably due to the hospital setting in which most of the studies were conducted. Furthermore, the limited number of studies means that we can only make some preliminary suggestions about the possible connections between findings in the two different systems and the theoretical, although empirically confirmed, model that posits links between EDs and personality.

Future Implications

We see two important issues. Firstly, EDs represent a serious concern in current clinical practice that appear to have increased in the last half century and we encourage further research into this area. Secondly, the integration between the symptomatology of the clinical disorders and personality functioning is an important issue (Connan et al., 2009; Lingiardi & McWilliams, 2017; Martinez & Craighead, 2015; McWilliams, 2011; Tasca et al., 2009), and we hope this article brings attention to this.

References

American Psychiatric Association (2013). *Diagnostic and statistical manual of mental disorders* (5th ed.).

Beck, A. T., Ward, C. H., Mendelson, M., Mock, J. E., & Erbaugh, J. K. (1961). An inventory for measuring depression. *Archives of General Psychiatry, 4*, 561–571.

Chabert, C. (1997). *Le Rorschach en Clinique adulte: Interprétation psychanalytique* [Rorschach Test in adults: A psychoanalytical interpretation] (2nd ed.). Dunod.

Chabert, C., & Vibert, S. (2016). Place des aménagements pervers chez des jeunes filles anorexiques et boulimiques: Étude clinique et projective [The role of perverse adjustments in young anorexic and bulimic women: A clinical and projective study]. *Psychologie clinique et projective, 22*, 91–110. https://doi.org/10.3917/pcp.022.0091

Connan, F., Dhokia, R., Haslam, M., Mordant, N., Morgan, G., Pandya, C., & Waller, G. (2009). Personality disorder cognitions in the eating disorders. *Behaviour Research and Therapy, 47*, 77–82. https://doi.org/10.1016/j.brat.2008.10.010

Curiel-Levy, G., Canetti, L., Galili-Weisstub, E., Milun, M., Gur, E., & Bachar, E. (2012). Selflessness in anorexia nervosa as reflected in the Rorschach Comprehensive System. *Rorschachiana, 33*(1), 78–93. https://doi.org/10.1027/1192-5604/a000028

Cuzzolaro, M. (2013). Disturbi dell'alimentazione e obesità. Trattamento multiprofessionale integrato? [Eating disorders and obesity. Multi-professional integrated treatment?]. *Psiche. Rivista Di Cultura Psicoanalitica, 1*, 1–13.

Cuzzolaro, M., Vetrone, G., Marano, G., & Garfinkel, R. E. (2006). The Body Uneasiness Test (BUT) development and validation of a new body image assessment scale. *Eating and Weight Disorders, 11*, 1–13. https://doi.org/10.1007/BF03327738

Day, J., Ternouth, A., & Collier, D. A. (2009). Eating disorders and obesity: Two sides of the same coin? *Epidemiologia e Psichiatria Sociale, 18*, 96–100.

Derogatis, L. R., & Lazarus, L. (1994). SCL-90 Brief Symptom Inventory and matching clinical rating scales. In M. E. Marnish (Ed.), *The use of psychological testing for treatment planning and outcome assessment* (pp. 217–248). Erlbaum.

de Traubenberg, N. R. (1970). *La pratique du Rorschach* [The practice of Rorschach]. Presses universitaires de France.

Exner, J. E. (2003). *The Rorschach: A comprehensive system: Vol. 1. Basic foundations* (4th ed.). John Wiley & Sons.

Fairburn, C. G., Cooper, Z., & Shafran, R. (2003). Cognitive behaviour therapy for eating disorders: A "transdiagnostic" theory and treatment. *Behaviour Research and Therapy, 41*(5), 509–528. https://doi.org/10.1016/S0005-7967(02)00088-8

Fairburn, C. G., & Harrison, P. J. (2003). Eating disorders. *Lancet, 361*, 407–416. https://doi.org/10.1016/S0140-6736(03)12378-1

Farstad, S. M., McGeown, L. M., & von Ranson, K. M. (2016). Eating disorders and personality, 2004–2016: A systematic review and meta-analysis. *Clinical Psychology Review, 46*, 91–105. https://doi.org/10.1016/j.cpr.2016.04.005

Freud, S. (1969). *La vie sexuelle* [The sexual life] (D. Berger, Trans.). PUF (Original work published in 1927).

Garner, D. M. (1991). *Eating Disorders Inventory-2, professional manual.* Psychological Assessment Resources.

Garner, D., Olmstead, M. P., Bohr, Y., & Garfinkel, P. (1982). The eating attitudes: Psychometric features and clinical correlates. *Psychological Medicine, 112,* 871–878.

George, C., & West, M. (2001). The development and preliminary validation of a new measure of adult attachment: The Adult Attachment Projective. *Attachment and Human Development, 3*(1), 30–61. https://doi.org/10.1080/14616730010024771

Gonzalez, A., Kohn, M. R., & Clarke, S. D. (2007). Eating disorders in adolescents. *Australian Family Physician, 36*(8), 614–619.

Guinzbourg, M. (2011). Eating disorders – a current concern: Similarities and differences among the anorexia, bulimia, and EDNOS categories. *Rorschachiana, 32*(1), 27–45. https://doi.org/10.1027/1192-5604/a000014

Hoek, H. W., & Van Hoeken, D. (2003). Review of the prevalence and incidence of eating disorders. *International Journal of Eating Disorders, 34*(4), 383–396. https://doi.org/10.1002/eat.10222

Lavender, J. M., Wonderlich, S. A., Crosby, R. D., Engel, S. G., Mitchell, J. E., Crow, S. J., Peterson, C. B., & Le Grange, D. (2013). Personality-based subtypes of anorexia nervosa: Examining validity and utility using baseline clinical variables and ecological momentary assessment. *Behaviour Research and Therapy, 51*(8), 512–517. https://doi.org/10.1016/j.brat.2013.05.007

Lingiardi, V. & McWilliams, N. (Eds.). (2017). *Psychodynamic diagnostic manual (2nd ed.): PDM-2.* Guilford Press.

Lis, A., Mazzeschi, C., Di Riso, D., & Salcuni, S. (2011). Attachment, assessment, and psychological intervention: A case study of anorexia. *Journal of Personality Assessment, 93*(5), 434–444. https://doi.org/10.1080/00223891.2011.594125

Martinez, M. A., & Craighead, L. W. (2015). Toward person(ality)-centered treatment: How consideration of personality and individual differences in anorexia nervosa may improve treatment outcome. *Clinical Psychology: Science and Practice, 22*(3), 296–314. https://doi.org/10.1111/cpsp.12111

McWilliams, N. (2011). *Psychoanalytic diagnosis: Understanding personality structure in the clinical process.* Guilford Press.

Meyer, G. J. (2004). The reliability and validity of the Rorschach and Thematic Apperception Test (TAT) compared to other psychological and medical procedures: An analysis of systematically gathered evidence. In M. J. Hilsenroth & D. L. Segal (Eds.), *Comprehensive handbook of psychological assessment, Vol. 2. Personality assessment* (pp. 315–342). John Wiley & Sons.

Mihura, J. L., Bombel, G., Dumitrascu, N., Roy, M., & Meadows, E. A. (2019). Why we need a formal systematic approach to validating psychological tests: The case of the Rorschach Comprehensive System. *Journal of Personality Assessment, 101*(4), 374–392. https://doi.org/10.1080/00223891.2018.1458315

Ogden, T. H. (1985). On potential space. *International Journal of Psychoanalysis, 65,* 129–140.

OPD Task Force (2001). *OPD–operationalized psychodynamic diagnosis: Foundations and manual.* Hogrefe and Huber Publishers.

Piotrowski, C. (2017). Rorschach research through the lens of bibliometric analysis: Mapping investigatory domain. *SIS Journal of Projective Psychology & Mental Health, 24*(1), 34–38.

Racamier, P. (2012). *Les perversions narcissiques* [Narcissistic perversions]. Payot.

Ritchie, H., & Roser, M. (2019). *Mental health* https://ourworldindata.org/mental-health

Rothschild, L., Lacoua, L., Eshel, Y., & Stein, D. (2008). Changes in defensiveness and in affective distress following inpatient treatment of eating disorders: Rorschach Comprehensive System and self-report measures. *Journal of Personality Assessment, 90*(4), 356–367. https://doi.org/10.1080/00223890802107982

Rothschild, L., Lacoua, L., & Stein, D. (2009). Changes in implicit and explicit measures of ego functions and distress among two eating disorder subgroups: Outcomes of integrative treatment. *Eating Disorders, 17*(3), 242–259. https://doi.org/10.1080/10640260902848592

Selvini-Palazzoli, M. (1965). *Anorexia nervosa*. Thieme.

Smith, B. (1990). Potential space and the Rorschach application of object scale relations theory. *Journal of Personality Assessment, 55*, 756–767. https://doi.org/10.1080/00223891.1990.9674110

Spielberger, C. D., Gorsuch, R. L., & Lushene, R. E. (1970). *STAI manual for the State-Trait Anxiety Inventory*. Consulting Clinical Press.

Steiger, H., Richardson, J., Schmitz, N., Israel, M., Bruce, K. R., & Gauvin, L. (2010). Trait-defined eating disorder subtypes and history of childhood abuse. *International Journal of Eating Disorders, 43*(5), 428–432.

Striegel-Moore, R. H., & Bulik, C. M. (2007). Risk factors for eating disorders. *American Psychologist, 62*(3), 181–198. https://doi.org/10.1037/0003-066X.62.3.181

Strober, M. (1983). An empirically derived typology of anorexia nervosa. In P. Darby, P. Garfinkel, D. M. Garner, & D. Coscina (Eds.), *Anorexia nervosa: Recent developments in research* (pp. 185–195). Alan R. Liss.

Tasca, G. A., Demidenko, N., Krysanski, V., Bissada, H., Illing, V., Gick, M., Weekes, K., & Balfour, L. (2009). Personality dimensions among women with an eating disorder: Towards reconceptualizing DSM. *European Eating Disorders Review, 17*, 281–289. https://doi.org/10.1002/erv.938

Thompson-Brenner, H., & Westen, D. (2005). Personality subtypes in eating disorders: Validation of a classification in a naturalistic sample. *The British Journal of Psychiatry, 186*(6), 516–524.

Thompson-Brenner, H., Eddy, K. T., Franko, D. L., Dorer, D. J., Vashchenko, M., Kass, A. E., & Herzog, D. B. (2008). A personality classification system for eating disorders: A longitudinal study. *Comprehensive Psychiatry, 49*, 551–560. https://doi.org/10.1016/j.comppsych.2008.04.002

Tibon, S., Handerzalts, J., & Weinberger, Y. (2006). Using the Rorschach for exploring the concept of Transitional space within the context of the Middle East. *International Journal of Applied Psychoanalytic Studies, 2*(1), 40–57. https://doi.org/10.1002/aps.30

Tibon, S., & Rothschild, L. (2009). Dissociative states in eating disorders: An empirical Rorschach study. *Psychoanalytic Psychology, 26*(1), 69–82. https://doi.org/10.1037/a0014675

Turner, B. J., Claes, L., Wilderjans, T. F., Pauwels, E., Dierckx, E., Chapman, A. L., & Schoevaerts, K. (2014). Personality profiles in eating disorders: Further evidence of the clinical utility of examining subtypes based on temperament. *Psychiatry Research, 219*, 157–165. https://doi.org/10.1016/j.psychres.2014.04.036

Verdon, B., Chabert, C., Azoulay, C., Emmanuelli, M., Neau, F., Louët, E., & Vibert, S. (2014). The dynamics of TAT processes: Psychoanalytical and psychopathological perspectives. *Rorschachiana, 35*(2), 103–133. https://doi.org/10.1027/1192-5604/a000056

Verdon, B., & Azoulay, C. (2020). *Psychoanalysis and projective methods in personality assessment: The French School*. Hogrefe Publishing.

Vibert, S., & Chabert, C. (2009). Anorexie mentale: Une traversée mélancolique de l'adolescence? Etude clinique et projective des processus identificatoires dans les troubles des conduites alimentaires [Anorexia nervosa: A melancholic voyage through adolescence? A clinical and projective study of identificatory processes in eating disorders]. *La Psychiatrie de l'Enfant, 2*(2), 339–372. https://doi.org/10.3917/psye.522.0339

Vibert, S., & Cohen de Lara, A. (2011). Anorexie mentale et fonctionnements limites à l'adolescence: Diversité des modalités d'expression des problématiques oedipiennes et de perte d'objet aux épreuves projectives [Anorexia nervosa and borderline functioning: Diversity of the psychic treatment of object loss and oedipal conflict at adolescence]. *L'Evolution psychiatrique, 76*(1), 55–74. https://doi.org/10.1016/j.evopsy.2010.11.008

Vibert, S. (2012). Inhibition défensive et fantasmes oedipiens: Approche psychanalytique et projective de deux cas d'anorexie mentale [Oedipal fantasies and defensive inhibition in anorexia in adolescence]. *Psychologie clinique et projective, 18*, 83–125. https://doi.org/10.3917/pcp.018.0083

Viglione, D. J., Perry, W., & Meyer, G. (2003). Refinements in the Rorschach ego impairment index incorporating the human representational variable. *Journal of Personality Assessment, 81*, 149–156.

Weiner, I. B. (1996). Some observations on the validity of the Rorschach inkblot method. *Psychological Assessment, 8*(2), 206–213. https://doi.org/10.1037/1040-3590.8.2.206

Westen, D., & Harnden-Fischer, J. (2001). Personality profiles in eating disorders: Rethinking the distinction between axis I and axis II. *American Journal of Psychiatry, 158*, 547–562. https://doi.org/10.1176/appi.ajp.158.4.547

Wildes, J. E., Marcus, M. D., Crosby, R. D., Ringham, R. M., Dapelo, M. M., Gaskill, J. A., & Forbush, K. T. (2011). The clinical utility of personality subtypes in patients with anorexia nervosa. *Journal of Consulting and Clinical Psychology, 79*, 665–674. https://doi.org/10.1037/a0024597

Wonderlich, S. A., Crosby, R. D., Joiner, T., Peterson, C. B., Bardone-Cone, A., Klein, M., Crow, S., Mitchell, J. E., Le Grange, D., Steiger, H., Kolden, G., Johnson, F., & Vrshek, S. (2005). Personality subtyping and bulimia nervosa: Psychopathological and genetic correlates. *Psychological Medicine, 35*, 649–657. https://doi.org/10.1017/S0033291704004234

History
Received June 26, 2020
Revision received October 28, 2020
Accepted November 19, 2020
Published online September 15, 2021

Sarah Vibert
Department of Psychology
Université Paris René Descartes
71 avenue Edouard Vaillant
92100 Boulogne-Billancourt
France
sarahvibert@parisdescartes.fr

Summary

Despite the abundance of studies devoted to eating disorders (EDs) in adolescence, few of them use the Rorschach methodology. Two types of studies are found in the literature, those using the Comprehensive System methodology and those using the French School methodology.

Several studies with Rorschach SC were performed with (ED) samples to detect their similarities and differences in relation to the nonconsulting population as well as between the subgroups. Other articles highlight the dissociative states of the anorexic group binge/purging type (AN B/P) and the selflessness of the anorexic restrictive group (AN-R).

Regarding the changes after an integrative treatment, two ED samples (AN-R and AN B/P and bulimia) were evaluated with the Rorschach and self-report scales at admission and discharge, analyzing explicit and implicit measures of defensiveness and affective distress.

Although both groups show improvement in ego functions, mental distress, and ED behaviors at discharge, they exhibit different configurations of change. In other clinical study of anorexia, based on Bowlby's theory and a related scale, the complementary tools were used to develop treatment planning and the role of the therapist. The conclusions of all these studies indicate that the different subgroups of EDs may require different treatment approaches.

Studies by the French School find a diversity of psychopathological organizations underlying EDs with a predominance of borderline personality disorders with a narcissistic and depressive register. Depending on whether or not driving involves attacks of bulimia vomiting, the defenses are very different: inhibition/rigidity (restricting type) or massiveness of projection/cleavage (purging type or bulimia).

Studies using the Comprehensive System and those using the French School method agree on the existence of a poverty of affects in restrictive anorexia and a defensive dissociation in purging and bulimia. In addition, the two types of studies show that secure attachment to the therapist seems to be a determinant in the psychological approach to restore a bond of confidence in oneself and in others.

Résumé

Malgré l'abondance des travaux consacrés aux troubles des conduites alimentaires à l'adolescence, peu d'entre eux utilisent la méthodologie du Rorschach. Deux types d'études sont retrouvées dans la littérature, celles utilisant la méthodologie Compréhensive System (Rorschach SC) et celles utilisant la méthodologie de l'École Française.

Plusieurs études utilisant le Rorschach SC ont été réalisées dans des échantillons de sujets présentant des troubles alimentaires pour détecter leurs similitudes et leurs différences par rapport à la population non consultante ainsi qu'entre les sous-groupes. Certains articles mettent en évidence les états dissociatifs du groupe anorexie avec frénésie alimentaire et conduites de purges (AN-B/P) et l'auto-centration du groupe anorexique restrictif (AN-R).

Concernant les changements après un traitement intégratif, deux échantillons de patients présentant des troubles alimentaires (AN-R et AN B / P et boulimiques) ont été évalués avec des échelles de Rorschach et d'auto-évaluation à l'admission et à la sortie, analysant des mesures explicites et implicites des modalités défensives et de la détresse affective. Bien que les deux groupes montrent une amélioration des fonctions de l'ego, des comportements de détresse mentale et de troubles de l'alimentation à la sortie, ils présentent différentes configurations de changement. Dans une autre étude clinique de l'anorexie, basée sur la théorie de Bowlby et une échelle connexe, les outils complémentaires ont été utilisés pour développer la planification du traitement et le rôle du thérapeute. Les conclusions de toutes ces études indiquent que les différents sous-groupes de troubles alimentaires peuvent nécessiter des approches plurielles de traitement.

Les études de l'École Française retrouvent une diversité des organisations psychopathologiques sous-jacentes aux troubles des conduites alimentaires avec une prédominance des troubles limites de la personnalité de registre narcissique et dépressif. Selon que la conduite associe ou non des crises de boulimie vomissement, les défenses sont très différentes : inhibition/rigidité (type restrictif) ou massivité de la projection/clivage (type avec purges ou boulimie).

Les études utilisant la méthode Comprehensive System et celles utilisant La méthode de l'École Française s'accordent sur l'existence d'une pauvreté des affects dans l'anorexie restrictive et d'une dissociation défensive dans le type avec conduites de purges et la boulimie. De plus, les deux types d'études montrent que l'attachement sécure au thérapeute semble très déterminant dans l'approche psychologique pour restaurer un lien de confiance en soi et dans les autres.

Resumen

A pesar de la cantidad de trabajos que abordan el tema de los trastornos alimenticios en la adolescencia, pocos de ellos utilizan el método Rorschach. Dos tipos de estudios son los que se encuentran en la literatura, aquellos que utilizan el Rorschach Sistema Comprehensivo y los que utilizan la metodología de la Escuela Francesa.

Diversos estudios fueron realizados con el Rorschach Sistema Comprehensivo en muestras de pacientes con Trastornos Alimenticios (ED) para detectar similitudes y diferencias entre una población no consultante y una poblacion con ED, así como en los distintos subgrupos entre sí . Otros artículos profundizaron en los estados disociativos de las anoréxicas del grupo bulimico purgativo (AN B/P) y la desmotivación propia de las pacientes anoréxicas de tipo restrictivo (AN-R).

Respecto a los cambios observados luego de un tratamiento integrativo, dos muestras de pacientes (AN-R y AN B/P y bulimicas) fueron estudiadas con Rorschach y cuestionarios de autollenado al momento de admisión y de alta del tratamiento, analizando mediciones de aspectos implícitos y explícitos de defensividad y distrés afectivo.

Aunque ambos grupos evidenciaron mejoría en funciones del yo, distrés mental y trastornos en la conducta alimenticia al alta, ambos grupos exhibieron diferentes configuraciones de cambio. En otro estudio clínico sobre anorexia, basado en la teoría de Bowlby, se utilizó además una escala relacionada con dicha teoría, La implementación de instrumentos complementarios fue utilizada para planificar el abordaje terapéutico y el rol del terapeuta. Las conclusiones de estos estudios indican que los diferentes subgrupos de Trastornos Alimenticios requieren de diferentes modelos de abordajes terapéuticos.

Estudios realizados por la Escuela Francesa encontraron una diversidad de organizaciones psicopatológicas subyacentes a los trastornos alimenticios con predominancia de los desórdenes borderline de personalidad, con rasgos narcisísticos y depresivos. Dependiendo de si la conducta implica o no los ataques de vómitos de las bulimicas, las defensas son muy diferentes inhibición/rigidez (en las formas restrictivas) o la proyección masiva/clivaje (en las de tipo purgativa o bulimias).

Los estudios que utilizan el Rorschach Sistema Comprehnsivo y los que utilizan la Escuela Francesa coinciden en la existencia de la pobreza afectiva de las anorexias restrictivas y la disociación defensiva de las formas purgativas y en las bulimias. Asimismo, los dos tipos de estudios muestran que el vínculo de apego seguro con el terapeuta parece ser determinante en el abordaje terapéutico para restaurar la confianza en si misma y en los otros.

要約

思春期の摂食障害（ED）に焦点を当てた研究が豊富にあるにも関わらず、ロールシャッハ法を用いた研究はほとんどない。過去の文献には、包括システムの方法論を用いた研究とパリ法を用いた研究の2種類があった。

包括システムを用いたいくつかの研究は、(ED)サンプルを用いて行われ、サブグループ間だけでなく、非コンサルテーション群との間の類似点と相違点を検出した（見出した）。他の論文では、拒食症グループの過食/パージングタイプ（AN B/P）の解離状態と拒食制限型グループ（AN-R）の無我状態が強調されている。

統合的治療後の変化については、2つのEDサンプル（AN-Rと AN B/P と過食症）について、入院時と退院時のロールシャッハ尺度と自記式尺度を用いて評価し、防衛と情動的苦痛の明示的・暗黙的尺度を分析した。

両群とも、退院時の自我状態、精神的苦痛、ED行動に改善が見られたが、変化の構成は異なっていた。他の拒食症の臨床研究では、Bowlby の理論と関連する尺度に基づいて、治療計画とセラピストの役割を開発するために補完的なツールが使用された。これらの研究の結論は、EDの異なるサブグループが異なる治療アプローチを必要とする可能性があることを示している。

フランス学派による研究では、自己愛性と抑うつ的な特徴を持つボーダーラインパーソナリティ障害が優勢なEDの基礎となる精神病理学的な仕組みの多様性が見出されている。欲動が過食症の嘔吐の発作を伴うかどうかに応じて、防衛は非常に異なってくる。（抑制／硬直：制限型、投影の大きさ／分離：パージングタイプまたは過食）

包括システムを使用した研究とフランス学派を使用した研究は、制限型アルキシアに感情の貧困、パージング及び過食では防衛的解離が存在するという点で一致している。さらに、2つのタイプの研究は、セラピストへの安全な愛着は、自分自身と他人との信頼の絆を回復するための心理学的アプローチの決定要因になっていることを示唆している。

A Commentary on "Eating Disorders and the Rorschach" (Guinzbourg de Braude et al., 2021)

Katarina Meskanen[1] and Massimiliano Pucci[2]

[1]Private Practice, Espoo, Finland
[2]Scuola di Psicoterapia Integrata, Massa, Italy

Eating disorders share a pathological core (viz., excessive preoccupation with weight, the body, and control of feeding; Fairburn et al., 2003) but the personality traits related to them are diverse (Vitousek & Manke, 1994; Wonderlich, 1995) and often overlooked. Yet, personality factors may explain several areas of functioning related to symptomatic expression (Farstad et al., 2016) and understanding the role of personality is important in the assessment and treatment of patients with eating disorders.

It is difficult to determine whether a certain personality trait reflects the cause or effect of an eating disorder. Behaviors related to eating disorders might be symptomatic expressions of personality pathology and thus part of a more general pattern of impulse and affect regulation (Westen & Harnden-Fischer, 2001). Premorbid personality pathology is thought to play a central role in the etiology of eating disorders, influencing the development of a specific subtype of eating disorder (Sohlberg & Strober, 1994; Vitousek & Manke, 1994; Wonderlich & Mitchell, 1992). Personality and eating disorders can also share common etiological factors (Lilenfeld et al., 2006). At the same time, personality traits may also be modified by eating disorders, as elevations in personality traits may be a complication or consequence of eating disorders (Wonderlich, 1995).

Personality variables are relevant in understanding the core psychological pathology in eating disorders and in treating them successfully. Focusing solely on changing the behavior of patients with eating disorder fails to address the role of their personality in generating and maintaining their symptoms, thus creating barriers to recovery. Personality dimensions can predict treatment outcome and symptom fluctuation (Farstad et al., 2016). As concurrent personality pathology may influence the course and treatment outcome of patients with eating disorders (Gartner et al., 1989; Lilenfeld et al., 2006; Wonderlich et al., 1994), its assessment and classification have value in more individualized treatment planning (Goldner et al., 1999; Rybicki et al., 1989). Being better able to identify the effect of personality on the core symptomatology is therefore crucial, and the examination of personality traits should not be limited to the boundaries of diagnostic eating disorder categories (Farstad et al., 2016).

Westen and Harnden-Fischer (2001) proposed three personality profiles in patients with eating disorders. This framework is applied in the article by Guinzbourg de Braude and colleagues (2021) in this issue. Their aim is to review previous research using the Rorschach with eating disorders and to consider the findings in the light of Westen and Harnden-Fischer's conceptualization to discover which characteristics in the Rorschach protocols are informative in the clinical context with patients suffering from eating disorders. The authors point out that the three different personality profiles may provide different Rorschach protocols in terms of thought, interpersonal relationships, and emotionality. The goal is to provide new insight and better define the functioning and personality of these patients.

However, there are some methodological issues. Firstly, this article reviews studies utilizing two very different approaches to the Rorschach: the Comprehensive System (CS) and the French School. The two approaches are not easily comparable in their underlying conceptual models. While the CS places greater importance on the perceptive aspect and is used as a performance-based instrument, the French school interprets the Rorschach as a projective instrument with reference to psychoanalytic theory. In the studies reviewed in the article, the Rorschach has also been used in different settings (treatment vs. diagnosis and understanding of personality functioning). Also, whereas the reviewed CS studies are more quantitative, the French school studies consider only small samples and case studies. The results obtained with these two approaches are thus difficult to synthesize.

The approach that one uses in interpreting the Rorschach seems to lead to different outcomes. Based on the article, results from the CS studies do not offer a uniform categorization of eating disorders that resembles Westen and Harnden-Fischer's conceptualization. Psychoanalytic theory and the French School provide a viewpoint that is more easily integrated with this conceptualization.

While reviewing the studies considered in the article, it is important to assess potential biases that can confound the conclusions. First, the samples can be biased. It is noteworthy that clinical patients typically show more comorbidity and increased psychopathology (Berkson's bias: the increased likelihood that an individual with two disorders, such as eating disorder and personality disorder, presents in the clinical setting as a function of seeking treatment for one or the other; see Vitousek & Stumpf, 2004). The second potential source of bias is the clinician, affecting conclusions at different stages and levels of assessment (Vitousek & Stumpf, 2004). We suspect this poses more of a potential problem for the French School for whom the Rorschach is a projective method, in contrast to the systematic scoring and norms of the CS.

Many of the studies are limited by the assessment of patients in an acute phase, in a state of starvation and malnourishment, and in a hospitalized setting. The discrimination of state and trait characteristics is difficult since starvation influences personality and behavior and the persistence of personality change after recovery is unclear (Keys et al., 1950; Vitousek & Stumpf, 2004). The influence of state variables such as depression or anxiety should also be carefully considered as this may influence the assessment (Farstad et al., 2016; Vitousek & Manke, 1994; Vitousek & Stumpf, 2004). Overall, assessing personality during an acute symptomatic episode may result in state effects in the assessment of personality and lead to an over-estimation of psychopathology (Pollice et al., 1997; Vitousek & Manke, 1994; Vitousek & Stumpf, 2004). Weight restoration and reversal of starvation may lead to changes that limit the reliability and applicability of personality assessment in an acute phase. Therefore, administering the Rorschach Test to patients in the acute phase of their disorder is another methodological issue.

The Rorschach relies on perceptual processes and executive functions, so neuropsychological factors play a role in the response process during testing. Neuropsychological changes have been described especially in anorexia (Tchanturia et al., 2005). For example, anorexic patients show deficits in tasks of attention and problem-solving (Lauer et al., 1999) and difficulties in abstraction and flexibility of thought along with an obsession for details (Jáuregui-Lobera, 2013). The low central coherence associated with anorexia may result in an excessive focus on details rather than the whole (Lang et al., 2014), which is likely to impact on performance when giving responses to the Rorschach Test. However, it remains unclear whether these neuropsychological deficits reflect a reversible state due to malnourishment or whether the deficit is related to a long-standing trait (Jáuregui-Lobera, 2013). Either way, it is likely that patients in an acute phase and in a condition of malnourishment will have difficulty with a performance-based test like the Rorschach, and thus administering the test in this phase could impact the reliability of results.

Another issue is the relatively young age of the patients (mainly adolescents or patients younger than 22 years) in the reviewed studies. The patients' even younger age at onset of the disorder adds to this confounding factor in drawing conclusions about their personality. At the typical age of onset of an eating disorder, especially anorexia, it is difficult to identify stable personality patterns and evaluate the independence of maladaptive patterns of a particular developmental period (Vitousek & Stumpf, 2004).

Future research should address these methodological challenges. Firstly, the possibility of assessing state effects rather than traits especially in an acute phase

 Rorschachiana (2021), *42*(2), 225–231

of psychological distress or physical malnutrition should be taken into consideration as a confounding factor. Making far-reaching conclusions of stable underlying
personality traits for individuals who are assessed in a hospitalized setting is
fraught with difficulty and requires caution. More research in more naturalistic
settings is needed to supplement results from the hospitalized setting. Also, more
research in the wider adult population is needed to improve on the generalizability
of the findings. Another issue affecting generalizability is the underrepresentation
of men and other gender identities in the eating disorder patient samples.

Current studies using the Rorschach and comparing patients with eating disorders with either other psychiatric patients or with individuals without mental or
physical illness are limited. Combining neuropsychological assessment with the
Rorschach could provide information on potential mediating or moderating neuropsychological effects.

Most of the previous research on the Rorschach and eating disorders has
focused on anorexia and bulimia. However, other forms of eating disorders such
as binge-eating disorder (BED), unspecified eating disorders, and other specified
feeding or eating disorders (OSFED) are the most common forms of eating disorders (e.g., Galmiche et al., 2019; Machado et al., 2007; Smink et al., 2012). This is
of particular importance as other forms of eating disorders may present themselves differently in a clinical setting. Furthermore, anorexic patients are overrep-
resented in the hospital due to the demanding treatment and life-threatening risks
of malnourishment. Future studies should make an attempt to focus on other eating disorders and should attempt to broaden the clinical setting in which personality is assessed.

The authors conclude that both sets of studies underline the self-centeredness
of anorexic patients with their difficulty in communicating their feelings and
thoughts. Anorexic patients are profoundly disconnected from their own emotions
and body sensations (Skårderud, 2007a, 2007b) and judge their own self-worth
based on their outer appearance (Fairburn et al., 2003), but labeling this as
self-centeredness might promote negative stereotyping and convey a problematic
attitude toward the patient (i.e., the image of self-centered as caring only about
oneself or one's own needs and feelings). In reaction to these patients, clinicians
may already experience troubling emotional responses; therefore, an empathetic
and understanding attitude toward these patients should be promoted. We recom-
mend the use of the term "self-involvement" or "self-absorbed" instead.

Despite the methodological and epistemological issues leading to low reliability
of the results, we recognize the article's strengths in promoting the need for clinicians to assess personality and enhance treatment outcome in patients with eating
disorder. The article offers one way to integrate the categorical diagnosis with the

evaluation of personality based on Westen and Harnden-Fischer's conceptualization. Identification of the personality profile could provide better understanding of the core psychopathology of these patients that is reflected in their Rorschach protocols. Identifying the different personality profiles can help predict the clinical course of the disorder, and focus treatment so that interventions are tailored to the individual patient's needs.

Thorough personality assessment helps the clinician to determine how problems are linked to the patient's personality. In general, psychiatric patients usually present with complex problems and symptoms are often pervasive, reflecting long-term difficulties and challenges in adjustment. These can be viewed as manifestations or consequences of underlying, enduring traits of personality (Harkness & Lilienfeld, 1997). Therefore, it is crucial that personality is carefully considered in treatment. Knowing about personality assists the clinician to plan and execute treatment in many ways, such as knowing where to focus effort, and where to expect change. Better targeted treatment leads to more realistic expectations about the treatment goals and gains of specific interventions. Furthermore, providing understanding about the effect of personality increases the patient's self-knowledge.

From the patient's point of view, developing an awareness of the connection between their personality and the clinical manifestation of their disorder can help in various ways. Firstly, patients might reach a higher level of self-coherence, which would in turn allow them to experience clinical symptoms as part of their inner reality and not as something alien to the self. Secondly, this could help patients to attribute a clearer and more personal meaning to their disorder, promoting acceptance and healing of painful affective states (e.g., underlying shame connected to the disorder). Finally, increased self-awareness promotes the therapeutic process toward a new integrated and functional self-representation and understanding of the disorder. The clinician also gains from a deeper understanding that can be applied to the therapy relationship. The benefit of increased mutual understanding between patient and clinician goes well beyond the diagnosis of a mental disorder.

References

Fairburn, C. G., Cooper, Z., & Shafran, R. (2003). Cognitive behaviour therapy for eating disorders: A "transdiagnostic" theory and treatment. *Behaviour Research and Therapy, 41*(5), 509–528. https://doi.org/10.1016/s0005-7967(02)00088-8

Farstad, S. M., McGeown, L. M., & von Ranson, K. M. (2016). Eating disorders and personality, 2004–2016: A systematic review and meta-analysis. *Clinical Psychology Review, 46*, 91–105. https://doi.org/10.1016/j.cpr.2016.04.005

Galmiche, M., Déchelotte, P., Lambert, G., & Tavolacci, M. P. (2019). Prevalence of eating disorders over the 2000–2018 period: A systematic literature review. *The American Journal of Clinical Nutrition, 109*(5), 1402–1413. https://doi.org/10.1093/ajcn/nqy342

Gartner, A. F., Marcus, R. N., Halmi, K., & Loranger, A. W. (1989). DSM-III-R personality disorders in patients with eating disorders. *American Journal of Psychiatry, 146*(12), 1585–1591. https://doi.org/10.1176/ajp.146.12.1585

Goldner, E. M., Srikameswaran, S., Schroeder, M. L., Livesley, W. J., & Birmingham, C. L. (1999). Dimensional assessment of personality pathology in patients with eating disorders. *Psychiatry Research, 85*(2), 151–159. https://doi.org/10.1016/s0165-1781(98)00145-0

Guinzbourg de Braude, S. M., Vibert, S., Righetti, T., & Antonelli, A. (2021). Eating disorders and the Rorschach: A research review from the French School and the Comprehensive System. *Rorschachiana, 42*(2), 202–224. https://doi.org/10.1027/1192-5604/a000136

Harkness, A. R., & Lilienfeld, S. O. (1997). Individual differences science for treatment planning: Personality traits. *Psychological Assessment, 9*(4), 349–360. https://doi.org/10.1037/1040-3590.9.4.349

Jáuregui-Lobera, I. (2013). Neuropsychology of eating disorders: 1995–2012. *Neuropsychiatric Disease and Treatment, 9*, 415–430. https://doi.org/10.2147/NDT.S42714

Keys, A., Brozek, J., Henschel, A., Michelsen, O., & Taylor, H. L. (1950). *The biology of human starvation.* University of Minnesota Press.

Lang, K., Lopez, C., Stahl, D., Tchanturia, K., & Treasure, J. (2014). Central coherence in eating disorders: An updated systematic review and meta-analysis. *The World Journal of Biological Psychiatry, 15*(8), 586–598. https://doi.org/10.3109/15622975.2014.909606

Lauer, C. J., Gorzewski, B., Gerlinghoff, M., Backmund, H., & Zihl, J. (1999). Neuropsychological assessments before and aftertreatment in patients with anorexia nervosa and bulimia nervosa. *Journal of Psychiatric Research, 33*(2), 129–138. https://doi.org/10.1016/s0022-3956(98)00020-x

Lilenfeld, L. R., Wonderlich, S., Riso, L. P., Crosby, R., & Mitchell, J. (2006). Eating disorders and personality: A methodological and empirical review. *Clinical Psychology Review, 26*, 299–320. https://doi.org/10.1016/j.cpr.2005.10.003

Machado, P. P., Machado, B. C., Gonçalves, S., & Hoek, H. W. (2007). The prevalence of eating disorders not otherwise specified. *International Journal of Eating Disorders, 40*(3), 212–217. https://doi.org/10.1002/eat.20358

Pollice, C., Kaye, W. H., Greeno, C. G., & Weltzin, T. E. (1997). Relationship of depression, anxiety, and obsessionality to state of illness in anorexia nervosa. *International Journal of Eating Disorders, 21*(4), 367–376. https://doi.org/10.1002/(sici)1098-108x(1997)21:4<367::aid-eat10>3.0.co;2-w

Rybicki, D. J., Lepkowsky, C. M., & Arndt, S. (1989). An empirical assessment of bulimic patients using multiple measures. *Addictive Behaviors, 14*(3), 249–260. https://doi.org/10.1016/0306-4603(89)90056-7

Skårderud, F. (2007a). Eating one's words, part I: "Concretised metaphors" and reflective function in anorexia nervosa – an interview study. *European Eating Disorders Review: The Professional Journal of the Eating Disorders Association, 15*(3), 163–174. https://doi.org/10.1002/erv.777

Skårderud, F. (2007b). Eating one's words, part II: The embodied mind and reflective function in anorexia nervosa – theory. *European Eating Disorders Review: The Professional Journal of the Eating Disorders Association, 15*(4), 243–252. https://doi.org/10.1002/erv.778

Smink, F. R., Van Hoeken, D., & Hoek, H. W. (2012). Epidemiology of eating disorders: incidence, prevalence and mortality rates. *Current Psychiatry Reports, 14*(4), 406–414. https://doi.org/10.1007/s11920-012-0282-y

Sohlberg, S., & Strober, M. (1994). Personality in anorexia nervosa: An update and a theoretical integration. *Acta Psychiatrica Scandinavica, 89*(Suppl. 378), 1–15. https://doi.org/10.1111/j.1600-0447.1994.tb05809.x

Tchanturia, K., Campbell, I. C., Morris, R., & Treasure, J. (2005). Neuropsychological studies in anorexia nervosa. *International Journal of Eating Disorders, S37*(1), S72–S76. https://doi.org/10.1002/eat.20119

Vitousek, K., & Manke, F. (1994). Personality variables and disorders in anorexia nervosa and bulimia nervosa. *Journal of Abnormal Psychology, 103*(1), 137–147. https://doi.org/10.1037/0021-843X.103.1.137

Vitousek, K. M., & Stumpf, R. E. (2004). Difficulties in the assessment of personality traits and disorders in eating-disordered individuals. *Eating Disorders, 13*(1), 37–60. https://doi.org/10.1080/10640260590893638

Westen, D., & Harnden-Fischer, J. (2001). Personality profiles in eating disorders: Rethinking the distinction between axis I and axis II. *American Journal of Psychiatry, 158*(4), 547–562. https://doi.org/10.1176/appi.ajp.158.4.547

Wonderlich, S. A. (1995). Personality and eating disorders. In K. D. Brownell & C. G. Fairburn (Eds.), *Eating disorders and obesity: A comprehensive handbook* (pp. 171–176). Guilford Press.

Wonderlich, S. A., Fullerton, D., Swift, W. J., & Klein, M. H. (1994). Five-year outcome from eating disorders: relevance of personality disorders. *International Journal of Eating Disorders, 15*(3), 233–243. https://doi.org/10.1002/1098-108x(199404)15:3<233::aid-eat2260150306>3.0.co;2-9

Wonderlich, S. A., & Mitchell, J. E. (1992). Eating disorders and personality disorders. In J. Yager, H. E. Gwirtsman, & C. K. Edelstein (Eds.), *Special problems in managing eating disorders* (pp. 51–86). American Psychiatric Association.

Published online September 15, 2021

Katarina Meskanen
Private Practice
Espoo
Finland
katarina.meskanen@psykat.fi

Special Issue: The Rorschach Test Today: An Update on the Research
Research Article

A Systematic Narrative Review of Evaluating Change in Psychotherapy With the Rorschach Test

Filippo Aschieri[1]◉ and Giulia Pascarella[2]

[1]European Center for Therapeutic Assessment, Università Cattolica del Sacro Cuore, Milan, Italy
[2]Private Practice, Brescia, Italy

Abstract: In 2004, Grønnerød conducted a meta-analysis on the use of the Rorschach Test to detect change in psychotherapy. Results showed which Rorschach variables were associated with change in clients, and to what extent. The purpose of this study was to update the picture from the year of publication of the previous meta-analysis until 2019. A systematic review of the literature was carried out, including 17 studies of relevance to this research. Results showed that the Rorschach Test captures the changes in patients after psychotherapy, particularly when treatment is tailored to the unique needs of clients. We describe the limitations of the studies included in this systematic review and propose strategies to increase the effectiveness of using the Rorschach to evaluate treatment outcome.

Keywords: treatment evaluation, treatment process, psychotherapy evaluation, Rorschach Test

Smith (2017) suggested that the most promising fields of development for personality assessment are forensic evaluations, Therapeutic Assessment (Finn, 2007), and monitoring of treatment progress. Over the years, a substantial number of studies have been conducted on the structure, validity, and use of the Rorschach Test in clinical practice and forensic psychology (Fontan et al., 2016; Meyer & Archer, 2001; Meyer et al., 2001; Mihura et al., 2013). However, since the validity of each test is conditional on the context of its specific use, the application of the Rorschach to the evaluation of change after treatment stands out as a specific area where more research is needed.

Grønnerød (2003, 2004, 2006) conducted a series of studies to address the value of the Rorschach in evaluating psychotherapy outcome. Since reliability is a prerequisite of validity, Grønnerød first explored the extent to which Rorschach results remain stable over time. In 2003 Grønnerød analyzed the test–retest reliability of the Rorschach and concluded that the test's temporal stability was moderate to high. Stability levels of variables depended on the length of retest intervals (longer intervals are associated with less stability) and on the number of participants (the larger the sample, the higher the stability). In addition, less stable variables were those that reflect personality states (i.e., features linked to transient conditions) that cannot, by definition, remain as stable as those related to personality traits. This suggested that the Rorschach could be an excellent tool for evaluating changes occurring during therapy. Grønnerød (2006) reanalyzed the same data set to address possible statistical confounds. He confirmed the strong influence of the retest period on stability levels and suggested that its impact was even stronger than initially thought. Results clearly showed that with sufficient attention to methodological rigor, the Rorschach method is as stable and as reliable as other assessment tools in capturing personality changes.

The suitability of the Rorschach to assess treatment outcome depends also on its general validity in assessing personality functioning. Meyer and Archer (2001) concluded that the Rorschach works neither better nor worse than other psychotherapy evaluation methods. Effect sizes for the validity of other methods fluctuated around $r = .30$, while for the Rorschach they were $.14 < r < .46$, with an average of $r = .34$ (Meyer & Archer, 2001). Hiller et al. (1999) compared the test with other tools, and found that it can achieve greater concurrent validity effect sizes compared with the Minnesota Multiphasic Personality Inventory (MMPI; Hathaway & McKinley, 1943) when objective criteria of behavior were used (such as hospitalization or discontinuation of therapy). The MMPI, on the other hand, seemed to provide greater effect sizes when compared with other self-report criteria. Hiller et al. (1999) suggested that the MMPI and other self-report tools provided information on how people present themselves, whereas the Rorschach shifted the focus onto what they actually do. Two further meta-analyses, focusing on the validity of specific variables, supported the Rorschach Prognostic Rating Scale (Meyer & Handler, 1997, 2000) and the Rorschach Oral Dependency Scale (Bornstein, 1999). These studies indirectly support the idea that the Rorschach Test can be a valid predictor of objective criteria such as the outcome of psychotherapy or addictive behaviors. Mihura and colleagues (2013) highlighted the validity of each Comprehensive System variable, differentiating among those with high, moderate, limited validity and with not enough empirical background to be reliably evaluated. With regard to the latter variables, Czopp and Zeligman (2016) advocated for their utility in clinical and forensic practice, especially when interpreted in the context of other conceptually related indicators. These studies point to the potential of the Rorschach as a valid measure of change after treatment.

In 2004, Grønnerød investigated through meta-analysis the relationship between Rorschach results and changes occurring in therapy. The author gathered all the studies in which the Rorschach was administered to the same participant at

Table 1. Summary of the results of Grønnerød (2004)

Magnitude of the effect size (r)	Rorschach variables
Low ($r < .20$)	a & p ($r = .17$); Miscellaneous Content ($r = .17$); Originals ($r = .16$); Special Scores ($r = .14$); Form Level ($r = .12$); SumC ($r = .10$); W & D ($r = .10$); Depth ($r = .09$); Object Relations ($r = .03$); A% ($r = .00$).
Middle ($.20 < r < .30$)	S ($r = .28$); Form ($r = .27$); R ($r = .26$); r & (2) ($r = .22$); Miscellaneous Variables ($r = .21$); EA & EB ($r = .20$).
High ($r > .30$)	SumShd > FM + m ($r = .58$); D Score ($r = .58$); Constructs ($r = .50$); FC ($r = .50$); Color Balance ($r = .49$); Organization ($r = .45$); Global ($r = .44$); Populars ($r = .38$); DEPI ($r = .37$); FM + m ($r = .36$); Afr ($r = .36$); CDI ($r = .36$); All H Content ($r = .34$); Shading ($r = .32$); AdjD ($r = .30$); M ($r = .30$).

least twice (i.e., before and after therapy). His work attempted to ascertain the effectiveness of the Rorschach in assessing progress in psychotherapy and to clarify whether poor interest in this method was justified in scientific research. Initially, the author conducted a literature search on PsycINFO focusing on all contributions on the topic published between 1921 and October 2003 concerning adult patients. He included articles, books, and dissertations using keywords such as *stabilit** or *retest** or (*consisten** and *time*), combined with (*therap** or *psychotherap** or *treat**) and (*outcom** or *contin** or *prognos** or *predict** or *improv** or *chang**; Grønnerød, 2004). Exclusion terms were: family rorschach*, joint rorschach*, consensus rorschach*, group rorschach*, ag = childhood, surgic*, brain damag*, brain lesion*, and case stud*. Overall, 24 studies were considered relevant and included in the analyses, involving a total of 1,202 participants. In total, the sensitivity to change of 32 variables was analyzed. The overall effect size was $r = .26$. Table 1 summarizes the main findings for each variable considered.

Grønnerød also assessed the influence of some moderators on the changes of the Rorschach variables, finding that the longer the interval between pretest and posttest, or the more intense the therapy (in terms of frequency of sessions), or the greater the attention paid to inter-rater agreement, the greater the ensuing effect size. Conversely, effect sizes decreased when levels of blind scoring were higher. This study showed a moderate sensitivity of the test in detecting changes induced by psychotherapy. In addition, it highlighted the highly individual character of changes, which are person-specific, and reflected in different ways by the Rorschach Test.

The present study aims to update this picture, considering how the Rorschach Test has been used to assess changes occurring during therapy through a systematic analysis of Rorschach literature in psychotherapy evaluation studies from 2004 to 2019. To facilitate the comparison between the results from the within-subjects studies identified in this systematic narrative review and Grønnerød's (2004) meta-analysis, we calculated all variables effect sizes (r) of statistically significant differences due to treatment (Table 5).

Method

First, a search was performed on PsycINFO using the same keywords and exclusion criteria used by Grønnerød (2004). We also adopted the following exclusion criteria from Grønnerød (2004): family Rorschach*, joint Rorschach*, consensus Rorschach*, group Rorschach*, ag = childhood, surgic*, brain damag*, and brain lesion*. Unlike Grønnerød (2004), we included only manuscripts in English, Italian, and French. In addition, we also extended our search to case studies. Only peer-reviewed papers were filtered in, and a time restriction with an interval from 2004 to 2019 was applied. At this point of the search, the material amounted to 472 articles (*identification* phase). Based on *abstracts*, 149 results were selected and 323 papers were excluded by the two authors, who reviewed the material together. In this phase, duplicates and studies in which the Rorschach Test had only very marginally significant effects or in which it was simply mentioned were discarded (*screening* phase).

The full text of the remaining articles was analyzed according to the following criteria:

- Studies conducted "with" the Rorschach Test, and not "on" the Rorschach. By studies with the Rorschach, we mean investigations in which the test is used as a tool to measure the changes in participants. By studies on the Rorschach, we mean studies aimed at demonstrating the validity and reliability of the test.
- Studies concerning exclusively research or case studies with an assessment before and after therapy (theoretical articles or other systematic reviews have been excluded).
- Studies including a pre- and a posttest phase, in which the test is used as a means of investigating changes occurred during therapy.
- Studies focusing exclusively on psychotherapy (works on pharmacotherapy or in the medical domain were not taken into account). This criterion led to the exclusion of the study by Keddy and Erdberg (2010), who mainly focused on the effect of the electroconvulsive therapy.
- No restrictions as regards the interpretation system of the Rorschach Test.

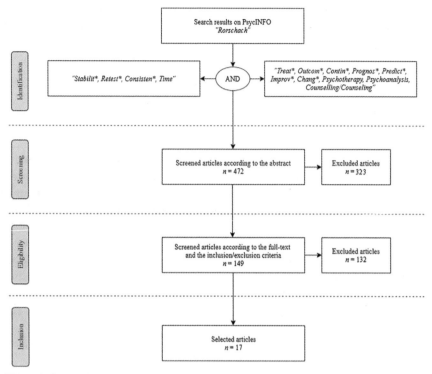

Figure 1. Research process.

At the end of this analysis, 132 articles were excluded based on the discussion between the authors and 17 were identified as useful for research purposes (*inclusion* phase; Figure 1).

Coding of Studies

The studies have been coded according to different features of their research design: (1) within-subjects or single-case research design. For comparison with Grønnerød's results, only within-subjects studies should be taken into consideration; (2) the use of an empirical or theoretical approach in the selection of the Rorschach variables (Table 2).

We selected 11 within-subjects studies and six single-case studies. Both types of research focused on certain variables and observed how they changed between the *baseline* and one or more *retests*. The studies have been divided according to the approach used in the choice of Rorschach variables. Two main approaches were followed in the selection of the Rorschach variables:

Table 2. Methodological characteristics of the selected studies

Record	Approach	Basic theory	Methodology
Blatt & Shahar (2004)	Empirical	Psychoanalysis and supportive-expressive therapy	Within-subject design
Fowler et al. (2004)	Empirical	Psychoanalysis	Within-subject design
Terlidou et al. (2004)	Empirical	Group analysis	Within-subject design
Gaudriault & Guilbaud (2005)	Mixed*	Psychoanalysis	Within-subject design
Blatt et al. (2007)	Empirical	Psychoanalysis	Within-subject design
Silverstein (2007)	Mixed	–	Single-case study
Benhaïjoub et al. (2008)	Theoretical	Psychoanalysis	Single-case study
Singh et al. (2008)	Empirical	–	Within-subject design
Berghout & Zevalkink (2009)	Empirical	Psychoanalysis	Within-subject design
Campo (2009)	Empirical	Psychoanalysis	Within-subject design
Inoue (2009)	Empirical	–	Single-case study
Gaudriault & Joly (2011)	Mixed	Psychoanalysis	Within-subject design
Yazigi et al. (2011)	Empirical	–	Within-subject design
Champagne & Léveillée (2012)	Mixed	Psychoanalysis	Single-case study
Berghout et al. (2013)	Empirical	Psychoanalysis	Within-subject design
Kaslow et al. (2014)	Empirical	Psychoanalysis	Single-case study
de Mattos Fiore et al. (2016)	Mixed	Psychoanalysis	Single-case study

Note. *Study uses variables both from the empirical and theoretical approaches.

- Empirical approach. In this approach, researchers analyze only the variables that are empirically supported and included in a Rorschach coding system. Psychological processes that researchers assume to be influenced by psychotherapy are operationalized through the variables already present in the systems. An example is the observation of the frequency and quality with which human figures are present in the protocol, the relationships between them or the activities they put in place as a means of evaluating empathy, interest toward others, and quality of internal representations (M, All H Content, MOA, etc.).
- Theoretical approach. In this approach, the Rorschach is used as a tool to measure theoretical processes assumed to be important in psychotherapy. Variables used to operationalize these processes in the Rorschach system are often not supported by normative data or studies regarding construct validity. The *osmotic responses* used in Gaudriault and Guilbaud (2005) are an example of this approach. They are responses of a fusional nature, in which duplication creates confusion about the uniqueness of the self or the duplicate. This is not true duplication but a state of symbiosis (e.g., Siamese

Table 3. Quality of quantitative studies

	(A)	(B)	(C)	(D)	(E)	(F)	Global rating
Fowler et al. (2004)	Poor	Fair	Poor	Fair	Good	Poor	Weak
Terlidou et al. (2004)	Fair	Fair	Fair	Fair	Good	Poor	Moderate
Gaudriault & Guilbaud (2005)	Fair	Fair	Poor	Poor	Poor	Fair	Weak
Blatt et. al (2007)	Fair	Fair	Good	Fair	Good	Fair	Strong
Singh et al. (2008)	Fair	Fair	Poor	Poor	Good	Poor	Weak
Berghout & Zevalkink (2009)	Fair	Fair	Good	Poor	Good	Fair	Strong
Campo (2009)	Poor	Fair	Poor	Poor	Good	Poor	Weak
Gaudriault & Joly (2011)	Fair	Fair	Poor	Poor	Poor	Poor	Weak
Yazigi et al. (2011)	Fair	Fair	Poor	Poor	Good	Poor	Weak
Berghout et al. (2013)	Fair	Fair	Good	Poor	Good	Poor	Moderate

Note. A = selection bias; B = study design; C = confounders; D = blinding; E = data collection method; F = withdrawal and drop-outs.

twins). Such responses, according to the authors, indicate narcissistic problems and should decrease with therapy.

However, this distinction does not cover the whole range of research on the subject. In some cases, in fact, both approaches are present. For example, Gaudriault and Joly (2011) used both osmotic responses (theoretical) and the egocentricity index (empirical).

Five categories of studies emerged from the combination of these aspects: within-subjects studies with an empirical approach ($n = 9$); within-subjects studies with a mixed approach ($n = 2$); single-case studies with an empirical approach ($n = 2$); and single-case studies with a theoretical approach ($n = 1$); single-case studies with a mixed approach ($n = 3$). As for the psychotherapy approach of the treatment used, Table 2 indicates that, in 13 cases out of 17, the theoretical orientation was psychodynamic.

Quality of the Studies

To assess the methodological quality of the selected quantitative studies, the Quality Assessment Tool for Quantitative Studies and the Quality Assessment Tool for Quantitative Studies Dictionary (Effective Public Health Practice Project [EPHPP], 2009) were used. The results of the evaluation are summarized in Table 3.

Out of a total of eight quantitative articles, three show strong or medium methodological precision whereas five articles are weak.

For single-case studies, on the other hand, seven criteria listed in the work of Shepherd et al. (2006) were used. Table 4 shows that the chosen studies, from the point of view of the investigated criteria, were of good quality. All manuscripts

Table 4. Quality of case studies according to Shepherd et al. (2006)

Case study	(1)	(2)	(3)	(4)	(5)	(6)	(7)
Blatt & Shahar (2004)	Yes	Yes	Yes	Yes	Yes	No	Yes
Silverstein (2007)	No	Yes	Yes	Yes	Yes	No	Yes
Benhaïjoub et al. (2008)	Yes	Yes	Yes	Yes	Yes	No	Yes
Inoue (2009)	Yes	Yes	Yes	Yes	Yes	Yes	Yes
Champagne & Léveillée (2012)	Yes	Yes	Yes	Yes	Yes	Yes	Yes
Kaslow et al. (2014)	Yes	Yes	Yes	Yes	Yes	No	Yes
de Mattos Fiore et al. (2016)	Yes	Yes	Yes	Yes	Yes	No	Yes

Note. 1 = explicit account of theoretical framework/literature review; 2 = clearly stated aims/objectives; 3 = clear description of the context/details; 4 = clear description of the sample; 5 = clear description of methodology/data collection methods; 6 = analysis of the data by more than one researcher; 7 = inclusion of sufficient original data to mediate between data and interpretation.

were rated independently by the authors. Ratings on each specific category of coding were compared and discussed until agreement was reached, even if the results of the global evaluation of the manuscript quality were quite similar between the two authors at the beginning of the process.

Results

Results of Within-Subjects Studies

The research we reviewed identified the same direction and degree of change for several variables as found by Grønnerød (2004; Table 5).

In general, after treatment, patients provide richer protocols with more responses (Singh et al., 2008). These protocols show more psychological involvement, more *Expressive Determinants* such as *animal* or *inanimate movement* and *Shadings* (Gaudriault & Guilbaud, 2005; Gaudriault & Joly, 2011; Yazigi et al., 2011) are present. Conversely, the number of *avoidant* protocols decreases after treatment (Berghout et al., 2013). Terlidou et al. (2004) found opposite trends of change for Diffuse Shading and Form determinants according to gender for their participants in group therapy. Males exhibited increased sensitivity to perceptual subtleties and reduced cognitive control, while females showed the opposite pattern. Authors interpreted this in relation to the specific goals in therapy for their male and female patients.

After treatment, Singh et al. (2008) found a significant and large increase in Human Contents. Also, human movements (M) increase to a moderate to large extent (Berghout et al., 2013; Singh et al., 2008).

Table 5. Summary of the results of the included within-subjects studies compared with Grønnerød (2004)

Rorschach variables	Effect size (r) (Grønnerød, 2004)	Results of the selected articles
SumShd > FM + m	.58	–
D Score	.58	Decreases after psychoanalytic psychotherapy (pre-/post-comparison: $r = -.20$; $p < .05$) (Yazigi et al., 2011).
		Decreases after psychoanalytic psychotherapy (pre-/post-comparison: $r = -.39$; $p < .05$) (Yazigi et al., 2011).
Constructs	.50	After treatment osmotic and fusional responses evolve into more differentiated and more interactive responses (Gaudriault & Guilbaud, 2005).
		Osmotic responses decrease their frequency in 77% of the protocols (Gaudriault & Joly, 2011).
FC/Color Balance	.50/.49	Increases after psychotherapy (pre-/post-comparison: $r = .79$; $p < .01$) (Singh et al., 2008).
		After treatment 40% of participants show a more controlled affective display as FC increases (Campo, 2009).
		CF + C decreases after psychoanalytic psychotherapy (pre-/post-comparison: $r = -.27$; $p < .05$) (Berghout et al., 2013).
Organization	.45	Zf decreases after psychoanalytic psychotherapy (pre-/post-comparison: $r = -.28$; $p < .05$) (Berghout et al., 2013).
		Zd+ and Zd– are not stable but there is not a clear pattern of change (Campo, 2009).
Global	.44	–
Populars	.38	Increase after psychoanalytic psychotherapy (pre-/post-comparison: $r = .49$; $p < .05$) (Yazigi et al., 2011).
		Increase after psychotherapy (pre-/post-comparison: $r = .85$: $p < .01$) (Singh et al., 2008).
		Increase after group analytic treatment (pre-/post-comparison: $r = .32$; $p < .01$). Additional analyses showed that at the end of the treatment, "the extent of maturity in the ability of perceptual integration as a whole (W), internalized representation of relationships (M), and good deal with common sense [...] (P)" is predicted by the values of these variables prior to treatment (Terlidou et al., 2004, p. 412).

(Continued on next page)

Table 5. (Continued)

Rorschach variables	Effect size (r) (Grønnerød, 2004)	Results of the selected articles
DEPI	.37	Decreases after treatment when the score is below 5. When the DEPI score is 5 or 6 it is less likely to change after treatment (Campo, 2009).
FM + m	.36	–
Afr	.36	Increases after psychotherapy (pre-/post-comparison: $r = .79$; $p < .01$). (Singh et al., 2008).
		Does not change in 63% of participants (Campo, 2009).
CDI	.36	Not stable but there is not a clear pattern of change (Campo, 2009).
All H content	.34	H and Hd increase after psychotherapy (pre-/post-comparison: $r = .47$; $p < .01$) (Singh et al., 2008).
Shading*	.32	SumShd increases after psychoanalytic psychotherapy (pre-/post-comparison: $r = .33$; $p < .05$) (Yazigi et al., 2011).
		SumT increases after psychoanalytic psychotherapy (pre-/post-comparison: $r = .28$; $p < .05$) (Yazigi et al., 2011).
		FV increases after psychoanalytic psychotherapy (pre-/post-comparison: $r = .24$; $p < .05$) (Yazigi et al., 2011).
		SumV increases after psychoanalytic psychotherapy (pre-/post-comparison: $r = .24$; $p < .05$) (Yazigi et al., 2011).
		SumY increases after psychoanalytic psychotherapy (pre-/post-comparison: $r = .26$; $p < .05$) (Yazigi et al., 2011).
		SumSh increases after psychoanalytic psychotherapy (pre-/follow-up comparison: $r = .30$; $p < .05$) (Berghout et al., 2013).
		Experienced Stimulation increases after psychoanalytic psychotherapy (pre-/post-comparison: $r = .24$; $p < .05$) (Yazigi et al., 2011).
AdjD	.30	D Score decreases after psychoanalytic psychotherapy (pre-/post-comparison: $r = -.20$; $p < .05$) (Yazigi et al., 2011).
		D Score decreases after psychoanalytic psychotherapy (pre-/post-comparison: $r = -.39$; $p < .05$) (Yazigi et al., 2011).

(Continued on next page)

Table 5. (Continued)

Rorschach variables	Effect size (r) (Grønnerød, 2004)	Results of the selected articles
M	.30	Increases after psychotherapy (pre-/post-comparison: $r = .42$; $p < .01$) (Singh et al., 2008).
		Ma increases after psychoanalytic psychotherapy (pre-/follow-up comparison: $r = .29$; $p < .05$) (Berghout et al., 2013).
S	.28	Very stable after 1 year of treatment (Campo, 2009).
Form	.27	F% and SumY are, taken together, indicative of two opposite trends of change for male and female participants to group therapy: male increase sensitivity to perceptual subtleties and reduce cognitive control, while females do the opposite (Terlidou et al., 2004).
		The frequency of Avoidant (High Lambda) patients decreases after psychoanalytic psychotherapy (pre-/follow-up comparison: $r = -.25$; $p < .05$) (Berghout et al., 2013).
R	.26	Increase after psychotherapy (pre-/post-comparison: $r = .42$; $p < .01$) (Singh et al., 2008).
Reflections + (2)	.22	Decrease after psychoanalytic psychotherapy (pre-/post-comparison: $r = -.20$; $p < .05$) (Yazigi et al., 2011).
		The score of 3r + (2)/R changes but no stable pattern emerges. Reflection response decrease in two out of three patients (Campo, 2009).
		In 15 out of 18 patients the score becomes closer to the expected range according to the Comprehensive System (Gaudriault & Guilbaud, 2005).
		In 18 out of 26 patients the score becomes closer to the expected range according to the Comprehensive System (Gaudriault & Joly, 2011).
Miscellaneous variables	.21	The percentage of patients with high score in PTI decreases from 16% to 5% after psychotherapy and to 4% in the follow-up (Berghout & Zevalkink, 2009).
		The average of OBS positive criteria increases after psychoanalysis (pre-/follow-up comparison: $r = .38$; $p < .01$) (Berghout et al., 2013).
		Expressive determinants (Ex: M, FM, m, T, V, FD) increase after therapy (Gaudriault & Guilbaud, 2005).
		Expressive determinants (Ex: M, FM, m, T, V, FD) increase after therapy in 88% of the sample (Gaudriault & Joly, 2011).

(Continued on next page)

Table 5. (Continued)

Rorschach variables	Effect size (r) (Grønnerød, 2004)	Results of the selected articles
		Cg increases after psychoanalytic psychotherapy (pre-/post-comparison: $r = .14$; $p < .05$) (Yazigi et al., 2011).
		An decreases after psychoanalytic psychotherapy (pre-/post-comparison: $r = -.26$; $p < .05$) (Yazigi et al., 2011).
		Xy decreases after psychoanalytic psychotherapy (pre-/post-comparison: $r = -.26$; $p < .05$) (Yazigi et al., 2011).
		Hx decreases after psychoanalytic psychotherapy (pre-/post-comparison: $r = -.35$; $p < .05$) (Yazigi et al., 2011).
EA & EB	.20	The frequency of Ambitent patients increases after psychoanalytic psychotherapy (pre-/follow-up comparison: $r = .26$; $p < .05$) (Berghout et al., 2013).
		EB style is very unstable. EA is stable in 60% of patients (Campo, 2009).
a & p	.17	a increases after psychoanalytic psychotherapy (pre-/follow-up comparison: $r = .34$; $p < .01$) (Berghout et al., 2013).
		FMp increases after psychoanalytic psychotherapy (pre-/post-comparison: $r = .31$; $p < .05$) (Yazigi et al., 2011).
Miscellaneous content	.17	–
Originals	.16	–
Special scores	.14	In introjective clients fabulized combinations decrease after psychoanalytic psychotherapy (pre-/post-comparison: $r = -.32$; $p < .01$) (Blatt et al., 2007).
		In anaclitic clients contaminations (pre-/post-comparison: $r = -.23$; $p < .01$) and confabulations (pre-/post-comparison: $r = -.26$; $p < .01$) decrease after psychoanalytic psychotherapy (Blatt et al., 2007).
		Sum6 increases after psychoanalysis (pre-/post-comparison: $r = .43$; $p < .01$) (Berghout et al., 2013).
		WSum6 increases after psychoanalysis (pre-/post-comparison: $r = .28$; $p < .05$) (Berghout et al., 2013).
		Lv2 special scores decrease after psychoanalytic psychotherapy (pre-/post-comparison: $r = -.15$; $p < .05$) (Yazigi et al., 2011).

(Continued on next page)

Table 5. (Continued)

Rorschach variables	Effect size (r) (Grønnerød, 2004)	Results of the selected articles
		The Boundary Disturbance and Thought Disorder Scale (BDS) decrease after (pre-/post-comparison: $r = -.19$; $p < .01$) (Fowler et al., 2004).
		DV1 increases after psychoanalytic psychotherapy (pre-/post-comparison: $r = .23$; $p < .05$) (Yazigi et al., 2011).
Form level	.12	F+ and F+% increase after psychotherapy (pre-/post-comparison: F+: $r = .92$; $p < .01$; F+%: $r = .80$; $p < .01$) (Singh et al., 2008).
		XA% remains stable in 50% of the clients. In the rest of the sample, it improves (Campo, 2009).
SumC	.10	–
W & D	.10	W increases after psychotherapy (pre-/post-comparison: $r = .42$; $p < .01$) (Singh et al., 2008).
		D increases after psychoanalytic psychotherapy (pre-/post-comparison: $r = .12$; $p < .05$) (Yazigi et al., 2011).
Depth	.09	–
Object relations	.03	HR and GHR increase after psychoanalytic psychotherapy (pre-/post-comparison: $r = .33$; $p < .05$) (Yazigi et al., 2011).
		The average MOA score decreases after treatment (pre-/post-comparison: $r = -.24$; $p < .01$) (Fowler et al., 2004).
		The average of pathological MOA categories decreases after treatment (pre-/post-comparison: $r = -.23$; $p < .01$) (Fowler et al., 2004).
		In introjective patients, psychoanalysis is more effective than supportive-expressive psychotherapy in reducing malevolent and destructive imagery in the MOA scale. The opposite is true for anaclitic patients (pre-/post-ANCOVA comparison: $r = .36$) (Blatt & Shahar, 2004).
A%	.00	A and A% decrease after psychotherapy (pre-/post-comparison: A: $r = -.88$; $p < .01$; A+%: $r = -.45$; $p < .01$) (Singh et al., 2008).

Note. *Grønnerød (2004) includes in the Shading category only T = 0 and T > 1.

Our results also confirm that the Rorschach allows for the identification of changes in conceptually relevant dimensions for individual patients (Constructs). Osmotic responses reported by Gaudriault and Guilbaud (2005) and Gaudriault and Joly (2011) move from total and undifferentiated fusion before therapy to more interactive and positive scenes.

The improvement found by Grønnerød (2004) in emotional regulation was also confirmed. According to Singh et al. (2008), emotional control (FC and Afr) increases significantly after treatment and unregulated emotional display (CF + C) decreases (Berghout et al., 2013).

Finally, Terlidou et al. (2004), Yazigi et al. (2011), and Singh et al. (2008) confirmed the improvement in Populars, namely, the ability to see reality in a socially shared way. This improvement is accompanied by less impairment in reality testing (Berghout & Zevalkink, 2009) and an increased level of perceptual accuracy after psychotherapy (F+% and XA%; Campo, 2009; Singh et al., 2008). Psychotherapy also facilitates more conventional perception with more global and common detail responses (Singh et al., 2008; Yazigi et al., 2011).

With reference to the phase model of psychotherapy outcome (Howard et al., 1993), the Rorschach Test can evaluate the different rhythms at which change in therapy occurs. Fowler et al. (2004) and Singh et al. (2008) carried out studies that confirmed the basic tenet of this model that behavioral change occurs more quickly than changes in the functioning of the personality.

Some Rorschach variables, which did not appear to change significantly after treatment in Grønnerød's studies, were actually impacted by treatment in the studies that we analyzed. For the Special Scores, Blatt et al. (2007) found a considerable change when considering the specificity of the client's psychopathology. In introjective patients, fabulized combinations decreased significantly, and in anaclitic patients, confabulations and contaminations decreased as well. Psychotherapy seems to impact thought processes, promoting a general improvement in the quality of the thinking, with decreasing occurrence of severe problems (BDS, Fowler et al., 2004; LV2 Special Scores, Yazigi et al., 2011), as well as promoting the ability to play "with ideas" (Berghout et al., 2013; Yazigi et al., 2011).

For Object Relations, Grønnerød found a very small effect size. However, Fowler et al. (2004) found, on average, an improvement of MOA scores and pathological representations after treatment. Blatt and Shahar (2004) found a significant change in the MOA scale in patients depending on the fit between the patients' features and type of treatment offered. In particular, they found that for introjective patients, psychoanalysis is more effective than supportive therapy in the reduction of malevolent and destructive imagery. The opposite is true for anaclitic patients. Of note, the significant effect size found in these studies could be explained by the intensity and quality of the treatment offered to patients (Fowler et al., 2004), and by tailoring the treatment modality to the particular features of each client (Blatt & Shahar, 2004).

Finally, the quality of human representations improves as well (Yazigi et al., 2011). Also, the overall variety of content increases, as suggested by the reduced frequency of animal contents (Singh et al., 2008).

Of note, two variables from the selected studies were diametrically divergent from Grønnerød's results. D Score decreased substantially after 1 and 2 years of psychoanalytic psychotherapy (Yazigi et al., 2011). Berghout and colleagues (2013) found less organizational activity after 4 years of psychoanalytic psychotherapy.

A final group of variables showed unclear or inconsistent patterns of change from the studies we surveyed. Campo (2009), who was interested in evaluating the stability of Rorschach variables after psychotherapy by counting how many protocols showed a difference in each indicator, found an inconsistent pattern of increase and decrease of EB & EA, Zd, DEPI, CDI, and Egocentricity Index in her sample. Unlike Grønnerød (2004), she did not find frequent changes in S. The Egocentricity Index has shown inconsistent changes in other studies as well. In the study by Yazigi et al. (2011), it decreased, whereas in the work of Gaudriault and Guilbaud (2005) and Gaudriault and Joly (2011) it tended to stay in the expected range according to the Comprehensive System. Finally, Yazigi et al. (2011) found, after 2 years of treatment, less Anatomy and X-ray contents and more Cg responses. Finally, Berghout et al. (2013) found an increase in active movements and Yazigi et al. (2011) found an increase in passive animal movements.

Results of Single-Case Studies

Silverstein (2007) analyzed changes in a patient with depression and somatic symptoms. He observed the changes in the client's protocols throughout treatment. Despite 2 years of treatment, the client's protocol still showed signs of anxiety and an ineffective coping style. According to Silverstein (2007), the first protocol, "represented [...] the picture of a man under siege. The second assessment, when [the client] was clinically stabilized, actually might reveal a more accurate picture of his premorbid personality, a personality characterized by ambivalence or unresourceful vacillation" (p. 137). In detail, some variables remained the same or similar in both protocols (Afr, CDI, AdjD, D Score, SumC). The human contents became more mature and $3r + (2)/R$ got closer to the expected range after psychotherapy. The inanimate movements (m) and form level (WDA%) increased. T increased from 1 to 2. In addition, the client's EB became Ambient (EB style). However, the WSumC score was very low, raising questions about the EB style's reliability.

Benhaïjoub et al. (2008) discussed the case of a woman suffering from postpartum depression. The authors focused on cards with maternal symbolism (Cards VII and IX). After about 7 months of brief psychoanalytically oriented psychotherapy (from the 6th month of pregnancy to 4 months after childbirth), the Rorschach responses indicated developments in the separation/individuation process. Moreover, after treatment, imagery became less fragmented and more organized. The patient still showed signs of struggling with managing impulse control and emotional regulation.

Inoue (2009) analyzed the case of a patient with posttraumatic stress disorder symptoms. The author considered the entire protocol and noticed a change in some variables after 10 months of EMDR treatment. Specifically, the frequency and the quality of human movement improved. The total number of M responses increased from 8 to 12. The quality of the movements changed from scary and dreadful to collaborative and open. Lambda decreased from .35 to .13. Color projection no longer appeared. 3r + (2)/R decreased from 0.48 to 0.39. HVI shifted from positive to negative. Blends (m, C', FD, V) increased by 44%. EA increased from 9.0 to 14.5. a:p responses remained passive (5:11). The Intellectualization Index increased from 0 to 5. XA% increased from 0.43 to 0.78. WDA% increased from 0.71 to 0.86. WSumC increased from 1.0 to 2.5. COP increased from 0 to 3. The GHR:PHR ratio changed, shifting from 4:9 to 7:6.

Champagne and Léveillée (2012) observed changes in a narcissistic patient, focusing on narcissism and the egocentricity index. After 1 year of psychotherapy, reflection responses [r & (2)] decreased from 3 to 1. After 2 years of treatment, 3r + (2)/R diminished from .86 to .50.

Kaslow et al. (2014) used the Rorschach Test to assess creativity in two writers. The authors used the Reality Fantasy Scale (RFS; Tibon et al., 2005). Treatment increased the awareness that reality and fantasy are different realms for one client, and improved access to potential space for both clients.

De Mattos Fiore et al. (2016) analyzed the case of a patient with a major depressive disorder (recurrent, severe, and with psychotic features), body dysmorphic disorder, bulimia, and borderline personality disorder. The authors focused on cards with relational distal properties (Cards II and III). The test was administered upon admission and in five annual retests, for a total of six protocols for each of the two cards considered. During the course of treatment, the client shifted from animal, inanimate, and aggressive movements toward human and collaborative movements. Reciprocity and autonomy were expressed by M rather than by FM. On Card II, aggressive animals turned into animals collaborating in the fifth retest (after 5 years). On Card III, there were disturbing scenes of unreal creatures associated with blood in the first protocol. In the fourth assessment (after 3 years) human contents were depicted in healthier interactions. Animal contents remained present in the retests. Only in the last assessment, after 5 years of therapy, did the responses involve distinct people, differentiated from one another, indicating autonomy and alterity.

Discussion

Grønnerød analyzed 24 studies from 1921 to 2003. We found 17 studies published from 2004 to 2019 in which researchers used the Rorschach to assess change in psychotherapy. There is therefore a base of research for the Rorschach to become a central tool in evaluating psychotherapy outcomes.

Within-subjects studies on the whole indicate an effect of psychotherapy on Rorschach variables related to how at ease patients are in unstructured contexts, how able they are to understand others, their capacity to mentalize their problems and others' needs, how socialized their perception of reality is, how effective and creative their thought process is, how sensitive they are to the clues in their environment, their capacity for assuming a differentiated identity, and how able they are to regulate their emotions. Many of the other variables that showed unclear patterns of change are among those for which the meta-analysis of Mihura et al. (2013) did not find sufficient empirical support. Future studies would benefit from measuring change in psychotherapy using those variables with the most solid empirical support in the Rorschach literature. Single-case studies illustrate the capacity of Rorschach results to provide rich, nuanced information about which goals were achieved by the treatment and which of them still needed work.

Few within-subjects studies have assessed change in psychotherapy while differentiating the sample based on specific psychological features and observing whether such features would have responded differently to different treatment modalities. This research approach is probably fruitful, since according to Blatt and Shahar (2004), some of the difficulty in identifying treatment differences arises from the assumption of homogeneity in which no attempt is made to differentiate among patients, assuming all patients are equivalent at the beginning of treatment. Thus, we could not address more complex questions such as whether certain treatments are more effective with certain kinds of patients, possibly resulting in different kinds of change (Blatt et al., 2002).

Limitations

Research on changes that occur in psychotherapy using the Rorschach Test has room for methodological improvement. Regarding quantitative studies, assessed recurring to the Quality Assessment Tool for Quantitative Studies (2009), the most common weaknesses are (see Table 3):

- The control of confounding variables, that is, taking into account additional non-research variables that may influence the results (e.g., gender, age, health, etc.). This aspect was considered in only four studies.
- Blinding, that is, the level of awareness of researchers and participants about the question of the research study. In no cases were the patients unaware of the reason why they were taking the test, and in only three cases did the researchers perform a blind scoring.
- In only three studies were data provided regarding patients who had dropped out of therapy or of the research project prior to completion.

The study design used – usually a before–after cohort study – is of good methodological quality for all quantitative research considered. Also selection *bias*, that is, errors made in recruiting subjects for the research study, is contained. Finally, the validity and reliability of the tools used for data collection are generally very high.

As for the case studies, indicated in Table 4, the criteria provided by Shepherd et al. (2006) were largely met, except for the analysis of the data by more than one researcher. Only in three out of six cases was the scoring of protocols carried out by different professionals, in order to assess inter-rater agreement and avoid distortions in the results.

Following the reading and analysis of all selected studies, however, other crucial questions have emerged regarding the methodological consistency of this type of research. Three problematic issues have essentially come to the fore (Table 6). The following shortcomings, besides being methodological weaknesses, make it difficult to identify what actually changes in the Rorschach in connection with the type of therapy carried out and the type of patients treated.

The first concerns the absence or presence of an evaluation of the effectiveness of the intervention through instruments other than the Rorschach. In other words, are the results of the test and of the retest somehow in line with those of other external sources? This is a crucial question, because it prevents possible biases such as the expectancy or Rosenthal effect, that is, the possible distortion of the results of an experiment due to the researcher's beliefs.

The second issue is whether or not the number of responses in the protocols has been taken into account. This raises two specific questions: Do the comparisons made by researchers between test and retest take into account the length of the protocols? Moreover, does the analysis of individual variables take into account their ratio to the total number of responses? The significance of a change, in fact, is relative since the ratio between the individual variable and the total

Table 6. Additional methodological problems of the included studies

Record	Evaluation of the effectiveness of the intervention through other instruments besides the Rorschach (yes/no, n)[a]	Computed the ratio between Rorschach variables and the total number of responses at protocol level, R (yes/no)	Integration of the literature (Grønnerød 2003, 2004)
Blatt & Shahar (2004)	no	no	no; n.a.[b]
Fowler et al. (2004)	yes (n = 1)	yes	no; n.a.[b]
Terlidou et al. (2004)	yes (n = 1)	yes (for some variables)	no; n.a.
Gaudriault & Guilbaud (2005)	no	no	no; no
Blatt et al. (2007)	no	no	no; no
Silverstein (2007)	no	no	no; no
Singh et al. (2008)	yes (n = 1)	no	no; yes
Benhaïjoub et al. (2008)	yes (n = 2)	no	no; no
Berghout & Zevalkink (2009)	yes (n = 4)	yes	no; no
Campo (2009)	no	no (except for 3r + (2)/R)	no; no
Inoue (2009)	yes (n = 1)	no	no; no
Gaudriault & Joly (2011)	no	no (except for 3r + (2)/R)	no; no
Yazigi et al. (2011)	no	no	no; no
Champagne & Léveillée (2012)	no	no (except for 3r + (2)/R)	yes; yes
Berghout et al. (2013)	no	yes	no; yes
Kaslow et al. (2014)	no	no	no; no
de Mattos Fiore et al. (2016)	no	no	no; no

Note. n[a] = number of instruments used besides the Rorschach; n.a.[b] = not applicable because these studies were published in the same year of Grønnerød (2004).

number of responses determines its frequency, and consequently its clinical relevance.

The third issue is the integration in the studies of the literature on psychotherapy and the use of the Rorschach to assess the changes due to treatment. In only three studies was Grønnerød's (2004) meta-analysis on the use of Rorschach for the evaluation of therapeutic change cited, and in only one was the author's 2003 study cited on the temporal stability of the test.

Clearly, inconsistencies between Grønnerød's meta-analysis that synthetizes 36 studies and our systematic narrative review should be considered with caution. Readers should refer to the fail-safe number reported in Grønnerød (2004) to evaluate how the results in this study are reliably indicating differences or should be considered as occasional drifts. As shown in Table 6, out of a total of 17 studies, only six confirmed the changes with an evaluation of treatment efficacy other than the Rorschach, only five compared the length of protocols before and after therapy, only two considered the relationship between the single variable and the total number of responses, and five did so for some variables only.

With regard to the need for specific expectations in terms of changes due to treatment, the study by Campo (2009) shows that it is more informative to observe changes on a case-by-case basis rather than looking for general rules (compare the general discussion [p. 115] with the conceptual-based discussion of results [p. 117]). The meaning and clinical relevance of a change, in fact, can only be understood in relation to the patient him- or herself, as it is tailored to his or her specific disorder and the type of treatment he or she is receiving. Evaluations should be individualized and the outcome of therapy should be observed on a case-by-case basis, as each patient possesses a unique set of personality characteristics and problems.

Studies included in this synthesis used diverging methodologies, mainly within-subjects and single-case studies, and Rorschach variables were selected either based on their empirical soundness or their suitability for measuring the specific construct under investigation. Study differentiation allows the results to be observed on a continuum ranging from the most rigorous, that is, those deriving from within-subjects researches with an empirical approach, to those more individualized and client-tailored, that is, the single-case studies with a theoretical approach, designed to address the individual patient and the type of therapy used. To close this gap, Persons (1991) emphasized the importance of assigning a subject to a treatment based on the results of his or her specific assessment, and not by reverting to standardized parameters related to the diagnosis (Nathan & Dotan, 2000). Each patient has his or her own ideal therapeutic path and the evaluation of psychotherapy itself will be more useful if conducted on a case-by-case basis. As such, one can assume that therapy activates different mechanisms in different types of patients. In addition to serving to assess change, the Rorschach could facilitate the construction of conceptually homogeneous groups of patients, enabling exploration of the effectiveness of specific typologies of treatment for their unique conditions.

Conclusion and Future Perspectives

To further enhance the use of the Rorschach as an instrument for evaluating change in psychotherapy, it will be important to pay more attention to confounding variables that may affect study results and to the use of blinding to prevent expectancy effects. Using other tools for the evaluation of treatment effectiveness alongside the Rorschach is recommended in order to validate results. In addition, more accuracy is required in sample selection and in reporting percentages and reasons for any abandonment of therapy or the research project, in order to perform more rigorous studies. References to the existing literature, both on the Rorschach and on psychotherapy itself, is also a key point for this specific area of investigation and should be strengthened. Finally, the analysis of the Rorschach itself should be improved. Many studies did not take into account the length of protocols before and after therapy and did not compare single variables with the total number of responses, reporting results that were often difficult to interpret.

Another important aspect involves consideration of the evaluation of psychotherapy with patients with homogeneous psychopathological patterns, beyond nosography. In other words, it is crucial to focus on personality components and on the patient's modes of adjustment, transcending mere diagnosis. The Rorschach is a test that captures the specific characteristics of the individual. For this reason, the Rorschach Test reaches its full potential when it is used each time, on a specific patient, to capture the unique functioning of his or her personality, taking into account his or her particular problem and the type of treatment provided.

In conclusion, what is even more important than symptom-based diagnosis is to understand the underlying structure of the observable phenomena by identifying broader and more patient-specific areas of functioning. Rorschach's test seems to be a preferential tool for this task, because through the analysis of responses we can infer the psychological processes that motivate actions in the daily life of the individual.

References

Benhaïjoub, S., Ladenburger, A., Lighezzolo, J., & De Tichey, C. (2008). Dépression maternelle et prévention: Approche clinique et projective [Maternal depression and prevention: Clinical and projective approach]. *L'évolution psychiatrique, 73*, 331–352. https://doi.org/10.1016/j.evopsy.2008.02.012

Berghout, C. C., & Zevalkink, J. (2009). Clinical significance of long-term psychoanalytic treatment. *Bulletin of the Menninger Clinic, 73*(1), 7–28. https://doi.org/10.1521/bumc.2009.73.1.7

Berghout, C. C., Zevalkink, J., Pieters, A. N. J., & Meyer, G. J. (2013). Rorschach-CS scores of six groups of patients evaluated before, after, and two years after long-term psychoanalytic psychotherapy and psychoanalysis. *Rorschachiana, 34*(1), 24–55. https://doi.org/10.1027/1192-5604/a000039

Blatt, S. J., Besser, A., & Ford, R. Q. (2007). Two primary configurations of psychopatology and change in thought disorder in long-term intensive inpatient treatment of seriously disturbed young adults. *American Journal of Psychiatry, 164*(10), 1561–1567. https://doi.org/10.1176/appi.ajp 2007.05111853

Blatt, S. J., & Shahar, G. (2004). Stability of the patient-by-treatment interaction in the Menninger Psychotherapy Research Project. *Bulletin of the Menninger Clinic, 68*(1), 23–38. https://doi.org/10.1521/bumc.68.1.23.27733

Blatt, S. J., Shahar, G., & Zuroff, D. C. (2002). Anaclitic/sociotropic and introjective/autonomous dimensions. In J. C. Norcross (Ed.), *Psychotherapy relationships that work: Therapist contributions and responsiveness to patients* (pp. 315–333). Oxford University Press.

Bornstein, R. F. (1999). Criterion validity of objective and projective dependency tests: A meta-analytic assessment of behavioral prediction. *Psychological Assessment, 11*(1), 48–57. https://doi.org/10.1037/1040-3590.11.1.48

Campo, V. (2009). Variations of Rorschach variables in therapeutic follow-up. *Rorschachiana, 30*(2), 101–128. https://doi.org/10.1027/1192-5604.30.2.101

Champagne, A., & Léveillée, S. (2012). Évaluation des enjoux narcissiques à partir du test de Rorschach au terme d'une psychothérapie [Evaluation of narcissism with the Rorschach Test after psychotherapy]. *Pratiques Psychologiques, 18*(4), 385–399. https://doi.org/10.1016/j.prps.2011.01.004

Czopp, T. S., & Zeligman, R. (2016). The Rorschach Comprehensive System (CS) psychometric validity of individual variables. *Journal of Personality Assessment, 98*(4), 335–342. https://doi.org/10.1080/00223891.2015.1131162

de Mattos Fiore, M. L., Lottenberg Semer, N., & Yazigi, L. (2016). From the "imperfect illness" to the possibility of developing good internal objects. *Rorschachiana, 37*(2), 166–181. https://doi.org/10.1027/1192-5604/a000081

Effective Public Health Practice Project. (2009). *Quality assessment tool for quantitative studies dictionary.* http://www.ephpp.ca/tools.html

Finn, S. E. (2007). *In our client's shoes: Theory and techniques of therapeutic assessment.* Erlbaum.

Fontan, P., Andronikof, A., Mattlar, C., & Mormont, C. (2016). Dimensions of the Rorschach comprehensive system: Parallel analysis and principal component analysis of a European adult nonpatient sample. *Rorschachiana, 37*(2), 114–146. https://doi.org/10.1027/1192-5604/a000079

Fowler, J. C., Ackerman, S. J., Speanburg, S., Bailey, A., Blagys, M., & Conklin, A. C. (2004). Personality and symptom change in treatment-refractory inpatients: Evaluation of the phase model of change using Rorschach, TAT, and DSM-IV Axis V. *Journal of Personality Assessment, 83*(3), 306–322. https://doi.org/10.1207/s15327752jpa8303_12

Gaudriault, P., & Guilbaud, C. (2005). Évolution des boulimiques en psychothérapie dans le test de Rorschach [Evolution of bulimics in psychotherapy in the Rorschach Test]. *L'évolution Psychiatrique, 70*(3), 577–593. https://doi.org/10.1016/j.evopsy.2004.07.007

Gaudriault, P., & Joly, V. (2011). Psychothérapie des boulimiques et Rorschach [Bulimic and Rorschach psychotherapy]. *Médicine & Hygiène – Psychothérapies, 31*(2), 119–129. https://doi.org/10.1037/t03306-000

Grønnerød, C. (2003). Temporal stability in the Rorschach method: A meta-analytic review. *Journal of Personality Assessment, 80*(3), 272–293. https://doi.org/10.1207/S15327752JPA8003_06

Grønnerød, C. (2004). Rorschach assessment of changes following psychotherapy: A meta-analytic review. *Journal of Personality Assessment, 83*(3), 256–276. https://doi.org/10.1207/s15327752jpa8303_09

Grønnerød, C. (2006). Reanalysis of the Grønnerød (2003) Rorschach temporal stability meta-analysis data set. *Journal of Personality Assessment, 86*(2), 222–225. https://doi.org/10.1207/s15327752jpa8602_12

Hathaway, S. R., & McKinley, J. C. (1943). *The Minnesota Multiphasic Personality Inventory*. University of Minnesota Press.

Hiller, J. B., Rosenthal, R., Bornstein, R. F., Berry, D. T. R., & Brunell-Neuleib, S. (1999). A comparative meta-analysis of Rorschach and MMPI validity. *Psychological Assessment, 11*(3), 278–296. https://doi.org/10.1037/1040-3590.11.3.278

Howard, K. I., Lueger, R. J., Maling, M. S., & Martinovich, Z. (1993). A phase model of psychotherapy outcome: Causal mediation of change. *Journal of Consulting & Clinical Psychology, 61*(4), 678–685. https://doi.org/10.1037/0022-006X.61.4.678

Inoue, N. (2009). Evaluation of an EMDR treatment outcome using the Rorschach, the TAT, and the IES-R. A case study of a human-caused trauma survivor. *Rorschachiana, 30*(2), 180–218. https://doi.org/10.1027/1192-5604.30.2.180

Kaslow, N. J., Flanagan, P. D., Carlin, E. R., Harris, R., Hickman, E. E., & Reviere, S. L. (2014). Empirically-supported case studies of creativity in writers in psychoanalysis. *SIS Journal of Projective Psychology & Mental Health, 21*, 11–24.

Keddy, P., & Erdberg, P. (2010). Changes in the Rorschach and MMPI-2 after Electroconvulsive Therapy (ECT): A collaborative assessment case study. *Journal of Personality Assessment, 92*(4), 279–295. https://doi.org/10.1080/00223891.2010.481982

Meyer, G. J., & Archer, R. P. (2001). The hard science of Rorschach research: What do we know and where do we go. *Psychological Assessment, 13*(4), 486–502. https://doi.org/10.1037/1040-3590.13.4.486

Meyer, G. J., & Handler, L. (1997). The ability of the Rorschach to predict subsequent outcome: A meta-analysis of the Rorschach Prognostic Rating Scale. *Journal of Personality Assessment, 69*(1), 1–38. https://doi.org/10.1207/s15327752jpa6901_1

Meyer, G. J., & Handler, L. (2000). Correction to Meyer and Handler (1997). *Journal of Personality Assessment, 74*(3), 504–506. https://doi.org/10.1207/S15327752JPA7403_12

Meyer, G. J., Finn, S. E., Eyde, L. D., Kay, G. G., Moreland, K. L., Dies, R. R., et al. (2001). Psychological testing and psychological assessment: A review of evidence and issues. *American Psychologist, 56*(2), 128–165. https://doi.org/10.1037/0003-066X.56.2.128

Mihura, J. L., Meyer, G. J., Dumitrascu, N., & Bombel, G. (2013). The validity of individual Rorschach variables: Systematic reviews and meta-analyses of the Comprehensive System. *Psychological Bulletin, 139*(3), 548–605. https://doi.org/10.1037/a0029406

Nathan, P. E., & Dotan, S. L. (2000). Research on psychotherapy efficacy and effectiveness: Between Scylla and Charybdis? *Psychological Bulletin, 126*(6), 964–981. https://doi.org/10.1037/0033-2909.126.6.964

Persons, J. B. (1991). Psychotherapy outcome studies do not accurately represent current models of psychotherapy: A proposed remedy. *American Psychologist, 46*, 99–106.

Shepherd, J., Harden, A., Rees, R., Brunton, G., Garcia, J., Oliver, S., & Oakley, A. (2006). Young people and healthy eating: A systematic review of research on barriers and facilitators. *Health Education Research – Theory & Practice, 21*(2), 239–257. https://doi.org/10.1093/her/cyh060

Silverstein, M. L. (2007). Rorschach Test findings at the beginning of treatment and 2 years later, with a 30-year follow-up. *Journal of Personality Assessment, 88*(2), 131–143. https://doi.org/10.1080/00223890701267944

Singh, D. K., Majhi, G., Prakash, J., & Singh, A. R. (2008). Changes in Rorschach indices: Pre and post treatment assessment. *SIS Journal of Projective Psychology & Mental Health, 15,* 42–47.

Smith, B. L. (2017). Can this marriage be saved? Personality assessment and clinical psychology in the 21st century. *Psihološka Istraživanja, 20*(2), 311–318. https://doi.org/10.5937/Pslstra1702311S

Terlidou, C., Moschonas, D., Kakitsis, P., Manthouli, M., Moschona, T., & Tsegos, I. K. (2004). Personality changes after completion of long-term group-analytic psychotherapy. *Group Analysis, 37*(3), 401–418. https://doi.org/10.1177/533316404045524

Tibon, S., Handelzalts, J., & Weinberger, Y. (2005). Using the Rorschach for exploring the concept of transition space within the political context of the Middle East. *International Journal of Applied Psychoanalytic Studies, 2*(1), 40–57. https://doi.org/10.1002/aps.30

Yazigi, L., Lottenberg Semer, N., Amaro, T. C., de Mattos Fiore, M. L., Silva, J. F. R., & Botelho, N. (2011). Rorschach and the WAIS-III after one and two years of psychotherapy. *Psicologia: Reflexão e Crítica, 24*(1), 10–18. https://doi.org/10.1590/S0102-79722011000100003

History
Received August 8, 2020
Revision received November 30, 2020
Accepted December 17, 2020
Published online September 15, 2021

ORCID
Filippo Aschieri
 https://orcid.org/0000-0002-1164-5926

Filippo Aschieri
European Center for Therapeutic Assessment
Università Cattolica del Sacro Cuore
L.go Gemelli 1
20123 Milan
Italy
filippo.aschieri@unicatt.it

Summary

In 2004, Grønnerød conducted a meta-analysis on the use of the Rorschach test to detect changes due to psychotherapy. The results showed which Rorschach variables were associated with the change in clients and to what extent. The present study aims to update this picture from the year of publication of the previous meta-analysis to 2019. A systematic review of the literature was conducted and 17 studies relevant to the research were included. The results show that the Rorschach test captures changes in clients after psychotherapy, especially when treatment is adapted to their specific needs. Within-subjects studies on the whole indicate an effect of psychotherapy on Rorschach variables related to how at ease clients are in unstructured contexts, how able they are to understand others, their capacity to mentalize their problems and others' needs, how socialized their perception of reality is, how effective and creative their thought process is, how sensitive they are to the clues in their environment, their capacity for assuming a differentiated identity, and how able they are to regulate their emotions. Many of the variables that showed unclear patterns of change have limited empirical support. In the future, research should focus on personality components and on the patient's modes of adjustment, transcending mere diagnosis. The Rorschach test seems to be a preferential tool for this task, because through the analysis of responses we can infer the psychological processes that motivate actions in the daily life of the individual.

Riassunto

Nel 2004, Grønnerød ha condotto una meta-analisi sull'utilizzo del test di Rorschach per rilevare i cambiamenti dovuti alla psicoterapia. I risultati hanno mostrato quali variabili Rorschach erano associate al cambiamento nei clienti e in che misura. Lo scopo di questo studio è aggiornare il quadro dall'anno di pubblicazione della precedente meta-analisi fino al 2019. È stata condotta una revisione sistematica della letteratura e sono stati inclusi 17 studi rilevanti per la ricerca. I risultati mostrano che il test di Rorschach cattura i cambiamenti nei pazienti dopo la psicoterapia, in particolare quando il trattamento è adattato alle esigenze specifiche dei clienti. Gli studi nel complesso indicano un effetto della psicoterapia sulle variabili Rorschach relative a quanto i pazienti si sentano a loro agio in contesti non strutturati, quanto sono capaci di capire gli altri, alla loro capacità di mentalizzare i problemi e le esigenze degli altri, quanto è socializzata la loro percezione della realtà, quanto è efficace e creativo il loro processo di pensiero, quanto sono sensibili agli stimoli nel loro ambiente, la loro capacità di assumere un'identità differenziata e quanto sono in grado di regolare le proprie emozioni. Molte delle variabili che hanno mostrato pattern di cambiamento poco chiari hanno un supporto empirico limitato. In futuro, è fondamentale concentrarsi sulle componenti della personalità e sulle modalità di adattamento del paziente, trascendendo la semplice diagnosi. Il test di Rorschach sembra essere uno strumento preferenziale per questo compito, perché attraverso l'analisi delle risposte possiamo inferire i processi psicologici che motivano le azioni nella vita quotidiana dell'individuo.

Résumé

En 2004, Grønnerød a mené une méta-analyse sur l'utilisation du test de Rorschach pour détecter les changements dans la psychothérapie. Les résultats ont montré quelles variables de Rorschach étaient associées au changement chez les clients et dans quelle mesure. Le but de cette étude est d'effectuer une mise à jour entre l'année de publication de la méta-analyse précédente et 2019. Une revue systématique de la littérature a été réalisée, incluant 17 études pertinentes pour cette recherche. Les résultats ont également montré que le test de Rorschach capture les changements chez les patients après la psychothérapie, en particulier lorsque le traitement est adapté aux besoins spécifiques des clients. Les études intra-sujets sur l'ensemble montrent un effet de la psychothérapie dans les variables de Rorschach liées à la facilité avec laquelle les patients sont dans des contextes non structurés, à leur capacité à comprendre les autres, à leur capacité à mentaliser leurs problèmes et les besoins des autres, à comment socialiser leur perception de la réalité est, à quel point leur processus de pensée est efficace et créatif, à quel point ils sont sensibles aux indices dans leur environnement, à leur capacité à assumer une identité différenciée et à leur capacité à réguler leurs émotions. Une grande quantité des variables qui montraient des schémas de changement peu clairs ont en fait un soutien empirique limité. À l'avenir, il est crucial de se concentrer sur les composantes de la personnalité et sur les modes d'ajustement du patient, au-delà du simple diagnostic. Le test de Rorschach semble être un outil privilégié pour cette tâche, car grâce à l'analyse des réponses, nous pouvons déduire les processus psychologiques qui motivent les actions dans la vie quotidienne de l'individu.

Resumen

En 2004, Grønnerød realizó un metanálisis sobre el uso del Test de Rorschach para detectar cambios en la psicoterapia. Los resultados mostraron las variables de Rorschach que se relacionaron con cambios en los pacientey la medida de esa relación. El propósito de este estudio es actualizar el estado del arte desde el año de publicación del metaanálisis anterior hasta 2019. Se realizó una revisión sistemática de la literatura, incluyendo 17 estudios de relevancia para esta investigación. Los resultados también mostraron que el Test de Rorschach refleja los cambios en los pacientes después de la psicoterapia, particularmente cuando el tratamiento se orienta a las necesidades únicas de los pacientes Los estudios intra-sujetos en general apuntan a los efectos de la psicoterapia en las variables de Rorschach relacionadas con la comodidad de los pacientes en contextos no estructurados, que tan capaces son de comprender a los demás, la capacidad para mentalizar sus problemas y las necesidades de los demás, qué tan convencional es su percepción de la realidad, cuán efectivo y creativo es su proceso de pensamiento, qué tan sensibles son a los indicios de su entorno, su capacidad para asumir una identidad diferenciada y qué tan capaces son de regular sus emociones. Muchas de las variables que mostraron patrones de cambio poco claros tienen un apoyo empírico limitado. A futuro, es fundamental centrarse en los componentes de la personalidad y en los modos de adaptación del paciente, trascendiendo el mero diagnóstico. El Test de Rorschach parece ser una herramienta privilegiada para esta tarea, pues a través del análisis de respuestas podemos inferir los procesos psicológicos que motivan acciones en la vida cotidiana de la persona.

要約

Grønnerødは2004年に、心理療法における変化を検証するため、ロールシャッハ・テストの使用に関するメタ分析を行った。その結果、どのロールシャッハ変数がクライエントの変化とどれくらい関連しているかが示された。本研究は、前回のメタアナリシスの発表さから2019年までの状況を加え、さらにデータを更新することを目的としている。文献のシステマティックレビューを実施し、本研究に関連する17の研究を新たに含めた。その結果、ロールシャッハ・テストは、心理療法後のクライエントの変化を捉えていた。そして、治療がクライエントの特定のニーズに合っていた場合には、特にその変化を捉えていることが示された。全体的に対象者内の研究では、以下のことに関連するロールシャッハ変数に対して心理療法の効果が示されている。構造化されていない状況でクライエントがどれだけ安心しているか、他者を理解する能力、自分の問題や他者のニーズを思い浮かべる能力、現実の認識がどれだけ社会化されているか、思考プロセスがどれだけ効果的で創造的か、環境の手がかりにどれだけ敏感か、分化したアイデンティティを担う能力、感情をコントロールする能力である。変化のパターンが不明瞭な変数の多くは、実証的な裏付けが限られている。今後は、単なる診断を超えて、パーソナリティの構成要素と患者の適応様式に焦点を当てた研究が必要である。ロールシャッハ・テストは、この課題に適したツールであるように思われる。なぜならば、反応の分析を通じて個人の日常生活における行動の動機付けとなる心理的プロセスを推察できるからである。

A Commentary on "A Systematic Narrative Review of Evaluating Change in Psychotherapy" (Aschieri & Pascarella, 2021)

More Rigor Is Needed in Research on the Rorschach and Treatment Change

Christopher J. Hopwood[1], Mathew M. Yalch[2], and Xiaochen Luo[3]

[1]Department of Psychology, University of California, Davis, CA, USA
[2]Department of Psychology, Palo Alto University, CA, USA
[3]Department of Education and Counseling Psychology, Santa Clara University, CA, USA

The Rorschach inkblots are one of the most widely used sets of test stimuli in the history of psychology, and a substantial body of evidence supports the construct validity of a number of variables, particularly from the Comprehensive and Performance Assessment systems (Mihura et al., 2013; for review see Meyer et al., 2016). As Aschieri and Pascarella (this issue) point out, the instrument has significant potential for the examination of treatment change, and is often used for this purpose (Aschieri & Pascarella, 2021). In particular, as a performance-based test, Rorschach scores are relatively independent of biases associated with questionnaires, which likely explains the relatively strong performance of the Rorschach for predicting behavioral outcomes in previous research (Hiller et al., 1999). In this sense, the Rorschach has the potential to communicate whether or not a patient has actually improved, somewhat independent of their desire to communicate that they have improved, as a function of treatment.

Initial evidence by Grønnerød (2004) supported the use of some Rorschach variables for this purpose, and the results of the follow-up study by Aschieri and Pascarella generally support those conclusions. However, a more general conclusion is that a lot more research, and a lot more rigorous research, is needed to determine whether and how to use the Rorschach to evaluate treatment change. Aschieri and Pascarella raised this issue in the discussion, and noted that many of the studies they reviewed had mixed evidence for overall design quality. In this commentary, we build upon their recommendations by offering several specific

Rorschachiana (2021), *42*(2), 258–264
https://doi.org/10.1027/1192-5604/a000146

ideas for how to improve research on the Rorschach as a measure of treatment outcome. We note that in the past, methodological critiques played a catalyzing role in strengthening evidence for the Rorschach, which has by and large held up against pointed challenge. We hope that our critique has a similar effect.

How Do You Know If the Patient Really Got Better?

Nearly all of the studies in the publications by both Grønnerød (2004) and Aschieri and Pascarella (this issue) used a pre–post design. The implicit assumption of this approach is that all of the patients in a given treatment improved. However, we know from the psychotherapy literature that many patients do not improve (Barth et al., 2013). As such, it seems likely that the results of these reviews mixed together evidence of changes in patients who got better with evidence of changes in patients who did not get better – one can change, after all, in ways that cannot be described as improvement.

Several design features could help deal with this issue. The first would be to compare groups of people who were in therapy and who were not in therapy. This would help determine which Rorschach changes are associated with treatment, specifically. However, it would not distinguish those patients who truly benefited from therapy from those who did not. Thus, the second design feature would be to compare Rorschach changes among psychotherapy patients who did or did not improve, based on other indicators. The use of other relatively objective indicators to reliably depict variation in treatment effects would provide a strong anchor for elucidating which Rorschach variables are associated with genuine clinical gains.

A third would be to use longitudinal data analytic techniques to triangulate within-person changes on Rorschach variables to within-person changes on other variables that signify therapeutic improvement. Such designs provide relatively specific information about individual differences in within-person patterns (Grimm et al., 2016). Moreover, elaborations of these designs can point to lagged and even causal mechanisms of change (Robins & Richardson, 2010). However, a limitation of such designs for the Rorschach is that they typically require multiple assessments, which is difficult for time-consuming assessment procedures, and may introduce unwelcome practice effects or interfere with therapy, depending on the patient's experience of being assessed many times with the Rorschach and other measures.

A fourth would be to preregister what variables are expected to change, and constrain analyses to those variables. Preregistration and direct replication are the only ways researchers can test hypotheses in a confirmatory way that lends maximum confidence to the results (Nosek et al., 2018). With respect to the

Rorschachiana (2021), *42*(2), 258–264

Rorschach specifically, preregistration of hypothesized effects presents a way to constrain the large universe of Rorschach variables that may be sensitive to treatment and helps eliminate the temptation for post hoc hypothesizing (Kerr, 1998).

How Do We Interpret the Results of Rorschach Protocol Changes When the Assessor Was Not Blind?

Aschieri and Pascarella noted that sensitivity to change tends to decrease when Rorschach scoring is blind. This suggests that the scorer – that is, the clinician – will tend to score the Rorschach in a way that is more suggestive of clinical improvement. Without meaning to cast aspersions on the motivations of clinicians, which we do not question, we see this kind of effect as entirely expectable. We all generally want to believe that we do a good job, and we want to see the best in our patients. There are also clinical or ethical issues at play here, insofar as asking a person who does not know the patient or have a sense of the case history to administer the Rorschach can potentially have negative effects on the treatment and therapeutic relationship. But from a research design perspective, should we even be considering the results of studies with non-blind scoring? The results of such studies likely reflect the implicit biases of the clinicians administering and scoring the instrument, and of the authors writing the papers. This poses a significant challenge for Rorschach research, which may be somewhat specific to the instrument insofar as a Rorschach administration is, itself, an intense interpersonal experience (Schafer, 1954). Nevertheless, much less can be made of studies that include Rorschach protocols generated by people who were not blind than studies with blind scoring, and, as such, including studies with non-blind Rorschach protocols in reviews serves to weaken the overall evidence base.

Should We Expect Everyone to Change in the Same Ways?

Aschieri and Pascarella note that we do not necessarily expect all patients to change in the same ways, and thus a different pattern of changes on the Rorschach may be indicative of clinical improvement across patients. Yet, meta-analytic and narrative literature reviews average changes across studies, which implicitly assumes that everyone does, indeed, change in the same ways. If some clinical changes are person-specific, group designs would not be optimal for determining the sensitivity of the Rorschach to those changes. Idiographic methods capable of dealing with this problem are gaining popularity in clinical research, in part because this problem emerges throughout the field (Wright & Woods, 2020). However, such designs typically require multiple assessments over time. An aforementioned alternative would be to preregister hypotheses one patient at a time, so that different hypotheses would be made about pre–post changes across patients. Such results could not be aggregated across patients to provide an overall summary of the sensitivity of Rorschach variables to treatment outcome (this is the nature of idiographic models), but they could speak to the validity of the Rorschach for this purpose, in general.

Is There a Difference Between Improvements in Patient Functioning and Improvements in the Therapeutic Relationship?

Psychotherapy researchers typically distinguish between clinical improvements outside of therapy, and improvements in the therapeutic relationship, which are often viewed as mechanisms of change (Najavits & Strupp, 1994). This distinction appears to be muddied in most Rorschach studies of treatment change (and this issue is compounded when the therapist also administers the instrument). In some sense, this reflects a strength of the instrument in that it suggests that the Rorschach very likely has indicators sensitive to both process and outcome. But to draw conclusions about what Rorschach variable changes are communicating, this distinction is critical.

To be more specific, our review of Aschieri and Pascarella's results seem to indicate that the Rorschach may be especially good at detecting improvements in interpersonal relations (e.g., changes in H, M, GHR, MAH). How can we tell if these results indicate improvement in the therapeutic relationship, or improvements in social functioning more generally? One approach would be to correlate changes in Rorschach scores with changes in instruments that have been previously validated to distinguish between clinical improvement and therapeutic alliance. Another would be to use research designs to distinguish these domains, such as associating Rorschach changes with within-dyad variation in the alliance, and comparing those associations with changes according to reports from informants who know the patient but do not have access to what has been happening in psychotherapy.

Do Changes Last?

As therapists, we typically want to help the patient change in a way that will last beyond treatment termination. High quality psychotherapy studies typically include follow-up data collected several months or years following termination (Steinert et al., 2016). Such data are absent in the current Rorschach literature, and thus no conclusions can be made about whether any pre-post changes on the instrument reflect the enduring impacts of treatment.

Should We Treat All Rorschach Variables the Same Way?

Hundreds of variables have been developed to score the Rorschach, and validity support for those variables varies substantially (Mihura et al., 2013). Aschieri and Pascarella use the term "theoretical" to describe variables that are not supported by empirical evidence. In construct validation theory (Loevinger, 1957), theory and data go hand in hand; we would not interpret variables that lack support as theoretical, but rather as of questionable value, pending further research. As the authors also say, "Many of the other variables which showed unclear patterns of change are among those for which the meta-analysis of Mihura et al. (2013) did not find sufficient empirical support." We would suggest that it would be better, all things being equal, to focus on variables with evidence for construct validity, unless there is truly a strong theoretical reason to expect a specific variable to do something, coupled with pre-registered tests of that hypothesis in well-designed studies.

Are the Findings Available in the Current Literature Representative?

A well-known problem with meta-analyses and narrative reviews is that they can only review the literature that is available. This literature is often biased, often because there are various incentives to publish positive findings and disincentives to publish non-positive findings (the so-called file drawer problem; Rosenthal, 1979). It seems likely that this is an even bigger problem in case studies, in which clinicians are much more likely to publish cases that went well than cases that went poorly. This speaks to the tremendous importance of doing well-designed studies at the outset.

Does Theoretical Orientation Matter?

By and large, the Rorschach is used in psychodynamic and psychoanalytic therapy. As such, it is difficult to know whether the instrument is sensitive to clinical improvement in general, or just within that orientation. There are historical reasons and potentially valid clinical reasons for this (like psychoanalysis, the Rorschach aims to assess features of the individual that are "deeper" than is the case with some other instruments). We are not sure whether this is a problem or not, but so long as this literature is largely restricted to one orientation, perhaps it is better to ask whether the Rorschach is sensitive to changes in *psychoanalytic* psychotherapy, than to changes in psychotherapy in general.

Is the Rorschach an Economical Way to Evaluate Treatment Change?

A natural critique might be that there are more efficient methods than the Rorschach for evaluating treatment change, even if it is valid for that purpose. Here, we have mentioned several times that longitudinal data would help solve various methodological issues, but also that this is particularly difficult with the Rorschach. Ultimately, evidence is needed that the instrument can do something other methods cannot so as to make a strong case for its unique value. This issue does not appear to have been addressed in the literature on treatment change.

Overall, while we agree that there is tremendous promise in the unique potential of the Rorschach to pick up on psychotherapeutic improvement, we conclude that it is premature, in light of limitations in the existing literature reviewed herein, to claim that, "There is therefore a base of research for the Rorschach to become a central tool in evaluating psychotherapy outcomes" (Aschieri & Pascarella, this issue). Research in this area can best be described as scattered, and in general it is not well connected to the complementary lines of work on psychotherapy and change process. In this context, Aschieri and Pascarella did a tremendous service both by hinting at some of the ways that the Rorschach could turn out to be useful for assessing treatment outcomes, but also by exposing the work that needs to be done, and highlighting the need for greater rigor in this area, toward more robust conclusions.

References

Aschieri, F., & Pascarella, G. (2021). A systematic narrative review of evaluating change in psychotherapy with the Rorschach Test. *Rorschachiana, 42*(2), 232–257. https://doi.org/10.1027/1192-5604/a000142

Barth, J., Munder, T., Gerger, H., Nüesch, E., Trelle, S., Znoj, H., Jüni, P., & Cuijpers, P. (2013). Comparative efficacy of seven psychotherapeutic interventions for patients with depression: A network meta-analysis. *PLoS Medicine, 10*(5), Article e1001454. https://doi.org/10.1371/journal.pmed.1001454

Grimm, K. J., Ram, N., & Estabrook, R. (2016). *Growth modeling: Structural equation and multilevel modeling approaches*. Guilford Publications.

Grønnerød, C. (2004). Rorschach assessment of changes following psychotherapy: A meta-analytic review. *Journal of Personality Assessment, 83*(3), 256–276. https://doi.org/10.1207/s15327752jpa8303_09

Hiller, J. B., Rosenthal, R., Bornstein, R. F., Berry, D. T. R., & Brunell-Neuleib, S. (1999). A comparative meta-analysis of Rorschach and MMPI validity. *Psychological Assessment, 11*(3), 278–296. https://doi.org/10.1037/1040-3590.11.3.278

Kerr, N. L. (1998). HARKing: Hypothesizing after the results are known. *Personality and Social Psychology Review, 2*(3), 196–217. https://doi.org/10.1207/s15327957pspr0203_4

Loevinger, J. (1957). Objective tests as instruments of psychological theory. *Psychological Reports, 3*(3), 635–694. https://doi.org/10.2466/pr0.1957.3.3.635

Meyer, G. J., Viglione, D. J., & Mihura, J. L. (2016). Psychometric foundations of the Rorschach Performance Assessment System (R-PAS). In R. E. Erard & F. B. Evans (Eds.), *The Rorschach in multimethod forensic assessment: Conceptual foundations and practical applications* (pp. 23–91). Routledge.

Mihura, J. L., Meyer, G. J., Dumitrascu, N., & Bombel, G. (2013). The validity of individual Rorschach variables: Systematic reviews and meta-analyses of the Comprehensive System. *Psychological Bulletin, 139*(3), 548–605. https://doi.org/10.1037/a0029406

Najavits, L. M., & Strupp, H. H. (1994). Differences in the effectiveness of psychodynamic therapists: A process-outcome study. *Psychotherapy: Theory, Research, Practice, Training, 31*(1), 114–123. https://doi.org/10.1037/0033-3204.31.1.114

Nosek, B. A., Ebersole, C. R., DeHaven, A. C., & Mellor, D. T. (2018). The preregistration revolution. *Proceedings of the National Academy of Sciences, 115*(11), 2600–2606. https://doi.org/10.1073/pnas.1708274114

Robins, J. M., & Richardson, T. S. (2010). Alternative graphical causal models and the identification of direct effects. In P. Shrout, K. Keyes, & K. Ornstein (Eds.), *Causality and psychopathology: Finding the determinants of disorders and their cures* (pp. 103–158). Oxford University Press.

Rosenthal, R. (1979). The file drawer problem and tolerance for null results. *Psychological Bulletin, 86*(3), 638–641. https://doi.org/10.1037/0033-2909.86.3.638

Schafer, R. (1954). *Psychoanalytic interpretation in Rorschach testing: Theory and application*. Grune & Stratton.

Steinert, C., Kruse, J., & Leichsenring, F. (2016). Long-term outcome and non-response in psychotherapy. *Psychotherapy and Psychosomatics, 85*, 235–237. https://doi.org/10.1159/000442262

Wright, A. G. C., & Woods, W. C. (2020). Personalized models of psychopathology. *Annual Review of Clinical Psychology, 16*, 49–74. https://doi.org/10.1146/annurev-clinpsy-102419-125032

Published online September 15, 2021

Christopher J. Hopwood
Department of Psychology
University of California
Davis, CA
USA
chopwoodmsu@gmail.com

Special Issue: The Rorschach Test Today: An Update on the Research
Original Article

Developments in the Rorschach Assessment of Disordered Thinking and Communication

James H. Kleiger[1] ⓘ and Joni L. Mihura[2]

[1]Private Practice, Bethesda, MD, USA
[2]Department of Psychology, University of Toledo, OH, USA

Abstract: In its first 100 years, the Rorschach has been heralded as a valuable method for investigating disturbances in thought organization and reasoning. It has survived periods of intense scrutiny and criticism, as contemporary researchers continued to demonstrate the empirical validity of the Rorschach as a measure of disordered thinking (Mihura et al., 2013). It is fitting to mark the centenary of Rorschach's "experiment" by summarizing contemporary contributions of the Rorschach Performance Assessment System (R-PAS) and reviewing the empirical and conceptual bases for using the inkblots to assess disordered thinking and communication.

Keywords: disordered thinking, thought disorder, psychosis assessment, Rorschach

As we approach the centennial for the publication of Hermann Rorschach's *Psychodiagnostics* (1921), it is appropriate to reflect on some of the more enduring contributions of Rorschach's original experiment. Chief among Rorschach's legacy has been the discovery that his inkblot method was sensitive to the fault lines in thinking (Kleiger, 2015). Rorschach's finding that certain types of responses and unusual details (e.g., "oligophrenic detail") reflected thought disturbances and a vulnerability to schizophrenia were amplified by Rapaport (Rapaport et al., 1946), Holt (Holt, 2009; Holt & Havel, 1960), Margaret Singer (Singer & Wynne, 1966) and Johnston and Holzman (Holzman et al., 2005; Johnston, 1975; Johnston & Holzman, 1979).

Foundations

Rapaport and colleagues' (1946) contribution to labeling and conceptualizing forms of what they referred to as "deviant verbalizations" were foundational to all efforts with subsequent systems to identify disturbed response patterns on the Rorschach. Holt and Havel (1960) took Rapaport's deviant verbalizations and developed the psychoanalytically rooted PRIPRO Scoring System, with nearly

Rorschachiana (2021), 42(2), 265–280
https://doi.org/10.1027/1192-5604/a000132

100 scoring variables, to link primary process thinking to deviant verbalizations in Rorschach responses.

Johnston and Holzman (Johnston, 1975; Johnston & Holzman, 1979) used the scores of Rapaport et al. (1946) to create the Thought Disorder Index (TDI) as a Rorschach-based measure of levels of pathological thinking.[1] The TDI, with 23 scoring categories, became an internationally accepted research metric for a broad range of studies into the differential diagnosis of psychotic-spectrum individuals, thought disorder in biological relatives, identifying children at risk for psychosis, thought disorder associated with cortical damage, brain morphology, neurophysiology, and genetic linkage of disordered thinking (see Holzman et al., 2005). Like Holt's PRIPRO, the TDI requires numerous scoring decisions per Rorschach response and lacks reference norms and, therefore, it is primarily a research instrument with limited clinical utility.

Contemporary clinical application of Rorschach assessment of disordered thinking was a result of Exner's Rorschach Comprehensive System (CS), the most widely used approach in the United States from the mid-1970s through the first decade of the 21st century (Meyer et al., 2013; Ritzler & Alter, 1986). The CS encompassed a leaner set of scores than the TDI that included unusual verbalizations, incongruous combinations of images, and inappropriate logic and indices for identifying pathological thinking and perception (Exner et al., 1976). The most recent CS edition (Exner, 2003) had six different types of scores, four with two severity levels, that were combined into a weighted sum (*WSum6*). But, importantly, to be used as a clinical measure, the CS provided normative reference samples.

Support for Assessment of Psychotic Phenomena Amid Criticism of Rorschach Validity

In the mid-1990s, a series of criticisms against the CS were initiated regarding the test's interrater reliability, validity of interpretations of individual variables, the nature of Exner's research database (Wood et al., 1996), and differences between the CS norms and norms of other samples (Shaffer et al., 1999; Wood et al., 2001). To address the norms, researchers began a project of international scope to

---

1   The TDI was based on the Delta Index (Watkins & Stauffacher, 1952), which was developed as a method to quantify the Rapaport categories of deviant verbalization.

collect contemporary normative data from the United States and other countries (Meyer et al., 2007), which showed that the previous CS norms were over-pathologizing.

Other researchers mounted widespread criticism against the validity of a broad range of variables, which reached its apex when one researcher called for a "moratorium" on the clinical and forensic use of the Rorschach until the validity of each individual score was better established (Garb, 1999). Despite this provocative proclamation, consistent with earlier reviews (Jørgensen et al., 2000, 2001; Viglione, 1999), the critics continued to voice support for the validity of Rorschach scores that assess thought disorder and psychotic phenomena (Wood et al., 2003).

To address the criticism of the validity of individual Rorschach scores, Mihura and colleagues (2013) responded by conducting an exhaustive meta-analytic review of the published peer-reviewed validity literature for 65 CS variables, published in the premiere psychology journal for systematic reviews and meta-analyses, *Psychological Bulletin*. Consistent with the previously mentioned reviews and endorsement by the harshest of critics, they found robust validity for the scores assessing thought disorder and psychotic phenomena. In response, the Rorschach critics stated that they could find no bias in the researchers' decisions and lifted their all-out call for a moratorium on the Rorschach (Wood et al., 2015; also see Mihura et al., 2015). Notably, scores related to disordered thinking and reality testing scores defined the top tier of valid test variables.

R-PAS Contributions to Assessing Disordered Thinking

Many years before Exner's death in 2006, he and his CS Rorschach Research Council were working on several research projects to improve test validity and utility, such as revised administration guidelines to optimize the number of responses and how to address problems with constricted protocols (Exner, 2000). However, following Exner's death and the decision of his heirs 2 years later not to continue the development of the CS, four members of the research council and a forensic psychologist transferred their research to creating the Rorschach Performance Assessment System (R-PAS; Meyer et al., 2011), designed as a replacement, not a competitor or alternative, to the CS (Meyer et al., 2017). The R-PAS developers used results from an early draft, under review by the journal, of Mihura and colleagues' (2013) Rorschach validity meta-analyses to choose variables for the new system, which naturally included the strongly supported thought disorder variables.

          Rorschachiana (2021), 42(2), 265–280

Cognitive Codes

The first edition of R-PAS retained the same six individual disordered thinking scores and their weightings as in the CS. Five of the Cognitive Codes have the same names as in the CS (*DV, DR, INC, FAB,* and *CON*). Four Cognitive Codes are designated as Level 1 or Level 2, according to degree of severity, with Level 1 responses reflecting more benign, playful, or immature expressions of language or logic, and Level 2 scores representing more flagrant departures in language and logic, reflective of psychotic phenomena, such as perceptual distortions, disorganized speech, illogical and bizarre reasoning, and conceptual confusion.

DV (Deviant Verbalization) reflects the examinee's use of a mistaken or inappropriate word or phrase that disrupts communication. For example, the respondent may say, "He's all *clowned up* in some kind of suit" (*DV1*) or give a more incomprehensible response like, "*An ancillarian vestige pig*" (*DV2*).[2]

DR (Deviant Response) is scored when the examinee's response becomes loosely related to or divergent from the task. *DR1s* reflect a minor loss of set (e.g., "Looks like a bat. My uncle shot one in the backyard"), while DR2s represent a more disorganized and fluid commentary (e.g., "Something hiding. If you tell the truth, you won't get in trouble. But if you're sneaky and something like these people, you'll realize it").

INC (Incongruous Combination) and *FAB* (Fabulized Combinations), generically referred to as "combinative" or "combinatory" responses, involve unrealistic perceptual combinations or merging of two or more blot details. *INC1s* reflect mild incongruities, such as "A butterfly with hands," whereas *INC2* responses depict a more bizarre combination of incompatible elements (e.g., "Looks like a bat with missiles and landing gears").

Like *INCs*, *FAB1* and *FAB2* codes reflect implausible or impossible/bizarre combinations between two or more distinct response objects. "Two bears giving each other hi-fives" (*FAB1*) is a milder combination than the more bizarre synthesis, "Two people and between them are their hearts joined together" (*FAB2*).

CON (Contamination) is a rare code but is considered the most severe form of combinatory or perceptually based codes. *CONs* reflect a perceptual merging of incompatible blot elements, where one image is superimposed on another (e.g., "The whole thing looks like people eating fried chicken" where the whole blot is simultaneously seen as the fried chicken and the people).

The sixth code, *ALOG* (Autistic Logic), used for illogical reasoning, was renamed as *PEC* (Peculiar Logic). The strained logic, offered spontaneously in the response phase, must be used to justify the response. For example, "It must be a man and

---

2   Cognitive Code examples taken from the R-PAS manual (Meyer et al., 2011).

woman in love because they are next to each other" is an explicit conclusion based on incidental details.

Each Cognitive Code receives a score from 1 to 7 to compute the Weighted Sum of the Six Cognitive Codes (*WSumCog*),[3] representing a continuum of disordered thinking ranging from milder lapses in reasoning, linguistic anomalies, or ordering of thoughts to more severe impairment in reasoning and thought organization. *SevCog* (*DV2 + DR2 + INC2 + FAB2 + PEC + CON*) denotes the most severe forms of cognitive disorganization and illogicality.

Conceptual Issues

As potent as these scoring signs are in their diagnostic utility, efforts to develop conceptually coherent and clinically nuanced understanding of the scores themselves have lagged behind. Some clinicians overlook or fail to grasp the connection between these codes and the disturbances in thinking that they represent. Other clinicians are too quick to view these scores narrowly as "thought disorder scores," which often leads to circular reasoning that the examinee or patient must have a thought disorder (Kleiger, 2016). But what is thought disorder anyway?

Terminological Problems

A precise definition of the term "thought disorder" has been elusive (Hart & Lewine, 2017; Kleiger, 1999, 2017; Roche et al., 2015). To mark this ambiguity, we refer to the term "thought disorder" in quotes. Questions about the nature of the term – whether we are measuring speech, communication, or underlying thought, and whether "thought disorder" is unitary, multivariate, categorical, or dimensional – have blurred our understanding and reduced our ability to communicate effectively about what we are observing and assessing (Kleiger, 1999, 2017).

Some challenged the assumption that equates speech with underlying thought and argued that it is not thought, but speech, that is disordered (e.g., Chaika, 1990). However, substituting the label "speech or language disorder" for "thought disorder" further confuses the issue by ignoring the underlying cognitive functions associated with disturbances in concept formation and reasoning.

In developing her Scale for Thought, Language, and Communication (TLC), Andreasen (1986) advocated a new terminology to replace "thought disorder."

---

3   Referred to as *WSum6* in the CS.

She later recommended the terms "communication disorder," "dysphasia," or "dyslogia" be used instead (Andreasen, 1982b) which, for better or worse, did not gain traction. However, the ideas behind these terms were clear: What we call "thought disorder" includes (a) disturbances in generating speech, selecting, and coherently linking words (a cognitive–linguistic element) and/or (b) expressing ideas due to faulty inference-making or logic (a cognitive–reasoning or logic component).

The cognitive–linguistic component reflects attentional and executive functions as well as language semantics, fluency, and coherence. Phenomenologically, difficulties in these functions are observed in odd word usage, distracted, tangential, derailed, and incoherent speech. Traditionally, the cognitive–linguistic element forms the basis of the concept of thought disorders of form (Fish, 1967) or formal thought disorder (FTD).

The cognitive–reasoning component reflects errors in inference-making, logic, and reasoning. Reasoning, a broader cognitive function that subsumes inference-making and logic, involves making sense of one's experiences and observations. Inferences are the mental steps in the reasoning process, and logic is a form of reasoning that involves clearly defined rules for reaching conclusions. Historically, some employed the term "cognitive slippage" to refer to lapses in logic; however, the vague and imprecise meaning of this term has made this less useful clinically.

However, even this broader definition of "thought disorder" still implies the existence of a categorical phenomenon, suggesting that an individual either has a "thought disorder" or does not. Categorical use of the term ignores the dimensionality of disturbances in speaking and reasoning. Movement away from categorical models of the psychopathology of psychosis to dimensionality is represented in the work of Barch et al. (2013), which contributed significantly to DSM-5 (American Psychiatric Association, 2013) by placing the symptom dimension, disorganized speech, along a continuum of severity. Even Bleuler (1911) maintained that there is no sharp separation between disordered and ordinary thinking. Instead, he wrote that people demonstrate varying degrees of disturbed or what he termed "autistic thinking."

Use of the term "thought disorder" also implies psychopathology of psychotic severity. In DSM-5, the term "disorganized speech" is included as one of the diagnostic features of several syndromes within the Schizophrenia Spectrum and Other Psychotic Disorders section. Previously regarded as diagnostically specific to schizophrenia, it is currently accepted that disturbances in thinking are both dimensional and cross-diagnostic phenomena (Hart & Lewine, 2017).

In addressing the categorical problem with the term "thought disorder," Harrow and Quinlan (1977) proposed the term "disordered thinking," which implies dimensionality, as opposed to a fixed category of psychopathology. We suggest that this term be widened to include language and communication difficulties. Thus, the term "disordered thinking and communication" frees us from focusing only on thinking or speech. It moves away from a categorical mindset and the pathognomonic diagnostic pigeonholing that often follows, placing problems with speech and reasoning along a continuum and avoiding the diagnostic trap of concluding that "the patient has a thought disorder, so they must be psychotic." At the more severe end of the continuum is FTD and impaired reasoning that may well be symptomatic of psychotic spectrum disorders, whereas milder disruptions in fluency, filtering, and focus, and reasoning errors reflective of immaturity, magical thinking, and superstition, occur in nonpsychotic conditions as well as in nonclinical individuals.

Conceptualizing Disordered Thinking and Communication on the Rorschach

A more precise understanding of the functions we are assessing frees diagnosticians from using names of test scores to describe an examinee's problems in thinking and language, conceptualizing beyond the score-names themselves and organizing Rorschach categories in terms of the cognitive and linguistic functions that underlie these scores.

For Rorschach purposes, disordered thinking and communication can be grouped into three categories: (a) problems with language and speech organization; (b) errors in reasoning, inference-making, or logic; and (c) impoverishment in speech, thinking, and perception.

Problems With Language and Speech Organization

The first category includes anomalies in language semantics and coherence, as well as disturbances in cognitive focusing, filtering, and self-monitoring, which listeners find confusing. Rorschach codes that capture disorganized speech and linguistic anomalies are *DVs* and *DRs*. But, in general, listening to subtle breaks in cadence, rate, rhythm, linkage, and the cohesion and coherence provides clues to underlying fragmentation or disorganization. For example, Husain pointed out that in conventional verbal communication, sentences usually require a subject, verb, and object, whereas sentences spoken by more disorganized individuals may lack these elements leading to fragmented verbal communication (Husain, Personal communication, March 11, 2016).

Errors in Reasoning, Inference-Making, and Logic

Examinees demonstrate conceptual difficulties by various types of errors in reasoning or mistaken beliefs about causality. Fallacious reasoning may occur when individuals base conclusions on incidental factors, when they assume relationships between logically unrelated events, or when they make inferences that extend well beyond observable data.

Illogicality is implicit in Rorschach variables such as *PEC*, where conclusions are based on incidental or concrete elements in the inkblots; formal characteristics include immediacy, reductionism, selectivity, and certainty (Kleiger, 1999). Such qualities are also found in a form of data-gathering bias referred to as "jumping to conclusions" or JTC (Garety & Freeman, 2013), which overlaps conceptually with formal qualities of reasoning found in *PEC* responses, in which people form conclusions quickly, focusing narrowly on selective information, and expressing a high degree of certainty.

Although it has not been studied empirically, the link between JTC and *PEC* is interesting because JTC has been associated with delusional thinking (Garety & Freeman, 2013; McLean et al., 2017). Bleuler's (1911) use of the term "autistic thinking" is intriguing to describe illogical reasoning in schizophrenia and he noted that it has an "irrefutable quality," meaning that individuals who reason in this manner cannot be dissuaded from their beliefs. The principle of irrefutability bridges the reasoning process underlying *PEC* responses and the cognitive bias of JTC in terms of immediacy and certainty. The psychological and psychodynamic underpinnings of *PEC* and its link to JTC have been addressed by Kleiger (Kleiger, 1999, 2017; Kleiger & Weiner, 2019).

Rorschach responses with blot elements combined or condensed in incongruous, improbable, or impossible ways receive codes of *INC, FAB,* and *CON.* Blatt and Ritzler (1974) furthered the relationship between ego psychological and object relational approaches by conceptualizing Cognitive Codes as different degrees of disruption in psychological boundaries (e.g., between self and others or between internal and external experience). Whereas *INC* and *FAB* are based on inferring an inappropriate relationship between unrelated events, objects, or experiences, *CON* is a loss of boundaries between independent objects, concepts, images, or frames of reference. *INCs* and *FABs* have also been found more commonly in the manic form of thought disturbance, where these responses are often presented with humor, flippancy, and playfulness (Holzman et al., 2005).

Although the CS originally included the score CONFAB for perceptual over-generalizations (also referred to as a "DW response"), neither the CS nor R-PAS had a specific code for reasoning errors that involve excessive or inappropriate inferences, embellishments, narratives, or attribution of meaning to the inkblot (Kleiger & Peebles-Kleiger, 1993). Referred to as "confabulatory thinking" in the TDI and Rapaport and Holt systems, these responses contain inappropriate degrees of embellishment or specificity consistent with Rapaport's original concept of "increased distance from the inkblot" (Rapaport et al., 1946).

In addition to formal codes for disorganized and illogical thinking, elevated Critical Contents (e.g., blood, aggression, sex) may reflect the emergence of primitive ideation. R-PAS codes Critical Content separately; however, Holt's PRIPRO system (Holt, 2009; Holt & Havel, 1960) incorporated a set of content variables to reflect the emergence of primary process thinking into the response.

Impoverished Speech, Thinking, and Perception
Derived from the term "poverty," impoverishment relates to the quality, quantity, diversity, or complexity of speech, thinking, and perception. Impoverishment describes speech that is sparse, repetitive, halting, and lacking in detail. Connections between thoughts are weak; ideas are repeated and unelaborated; conceptual underpinnings are often concrete and bound closely to the properties of the stimulus item or environment. Outwardly, elements of speech may be simple, meager, and repetitive, lacking in details, elaboration, or diversity of expression. The ability to symbolize is limited or absent, leaving the impoverished thinker unable to abstract meaning from literal features of objects or the environment. Others termed this prerequisite symbolizing capacity "interpretation awareness" (Bohm, 1958) and viewed the Rorschach task as one of modifying the reality of the inkblots (Peterson & Schilling, 2010).

There are currently no CS or R-PAS scores designed to target this impoverishment of thinking. R-PAS variables relating to response productivity, complexity, engagement, and synthetic functioning may relate to impoverishment. However, these scores are nonspecific and can occur for a variety of reasons, such as defenses against open engagement with the task or neurocognitive deficits. Nonetheless, impoverishment in the presence of illogical reasoning or disorganized thinking may represent what Andreasen (1982a) referred to as "negative thought disorder," characterized by peculiar and restricted thought processes, illogicality, neologisms, and poverty of speech.

Contemporary Research Contributions

The Rorschach validity meta-analyses (Mihura, et al., 2013), described earlier, showed that the Rorschach disordered thinking scores clearly differentiated between psychotic and nonpsychotic patients. These scores were also related to other mental processes associated with psychosis, such as attentional functioning via pupillary dilation (Minassian et al., 2004) and prepulse inhibition (Perry et al., 1999) in schizophrenic patients. However, none of the studies during the span of years in which the meta-analytic literature search was conducted (i.e., 1974 to 2011) used clinical ratings of disordered thinking as the validity criterion for these scores. In fact, only in recent years has the broader psychosis literature begun to deconstruct the psychosis construct into its constituent parts.

For example, Biagiarelli and colleagues (2015) found strong associations between the CS disordered thinking scale (*WSum6*) and clinical ratings on the PANSS (Positive and Negative Syndrome Scale; Kay et al., 1987) Conceptual Disorganization scale. More recently, Eblin and colleagues (2018) found a strong association between the R-PAS disordered thinking scale (*WSumCog*) and clinical ratings on a composite scale of disordered thought processes comprising TLC positive thought disorder items, the Scale for the Assessment of Positive Symptoms (Andreasen, 1984), and the Magical Ideation Scale (Eckblad & Chapman, 1983). In addition, Buckingham and colleagues (Buckingham et al., 2020) found a strong association between the R-PAS disordered thinking scale (*WSumCog*) and clinical ratings on a composite measure of the Brief Psychiatric Rating Scale (Overall & Gorham, 1988) Conceptual Disorganization scale and SCID-P (Structured Clinical Interview for DSM Disorders-Psychotic Screen; Spitzer et al., 1990) Loose Associations and Incoherence items.

Future Directions

Dimensionalizing Rorschach Measures of Disordered Thinking and Communication?

Increasingly, categorical models have been strongly challenged (Kotov et al., 2017) with continued support for the dimensional nature of psychopathology (Clark et al., 1995). Rorschach measures of disordered thinking have historically used different strategies to denote the range of benign versus pathological scores. The TDI grouped different categories of thinking processes within four levels of severity referred to as .25, .50, .75, and 1.0 levels. The lowest level (.25) contained flippant comments and playful combinations of ideas whereas the highest level (1.0) contained the categories most specific to psychotic levels of formal thought disorder, including incoherence and neologisms. R-PAS currently uses a similar system, except that it also weights some scores for two levels of severity, such as whether a respondent deviates from the task of answering the question, "What might this be?" only moderately (Level 1) or significantly (Level 2). The R-PAS developers have been working on a measure of disordered thinking and communication that fully dimensionalizes the Cognitive Scores (Meyer et al., 2020).

Short-Form R-PAS Measure of Psychosis

Capitalizing on the strength of the Rorschach for identifying disordered thinking and perceptual aberrations, R-PAS researchers have started to study the viability of a scaled-down version of the Rorschach, called the Thought and Perception Assessment System (TPAS) focused only on these variables. The major shortening of R-PAS to derive TPAS is to code only the psychosis variables, which also significantly shortens the time required to learn how to administer the test. A second option with TPAS is to use a shortened card set. True score theory (Allen & Yen, 1979/2002) and the principle of aggregation (Rushton et al., 1983) predict lower reliability values when reducing the number of cards. However, initial research (Eblin et al., 2018) found negligible differences in reliability for a reduced card set compared with the standard 10-card set. Specifically, the full set resulted in interrater reliability (ICC) of .94, and the 5, 4, and 3 card sets in .89, .88, .90, respectively. Future research is planned to replicate these findings and determine whether revised administration procedures that do not require examiners to ask specific clarification questions about irrelevant scores (e.g., Determinants) provides equivalent results.

References

Allen, M. J., & Yen, W. M. (2002). *Introduction to measurement theory.* Waveland Press (Original work published 1979, Brooks/Cole)

American Psychiatric Association (2013). *Diagnostic and statistical manual of mental disorders (DSM-5).*

Andreasen, N. C. (1982a). Negative v positive schizophrenia – definition and validation. *Archives of General Psychiatry, 39*(7), 789–794.

Andreasen, N. C. (1982b). Should the term "thought disorder" be revised? *Comprehensive Psychiatry, 23*(4), 291–299. https://doi.org/10.1016/0010-440X(82)90079-7

Andreasen, N. C. (1984). *The Scale for the Assessment of Positive Symptoms (SAPS).* The University of Iowa.

Andreasen, N. C. (1986). Scale for the Assessment of Thought, Language, and Communication (TLC). *Schizophrenia Bulletin, 12*(3), 473–482. https://doi.org/10.1093/schbul/12.3.473

Barch, D. M., Bustillo, J., Gaebel, W., Gur, R., Heckers, S., Malaspina, D., Owen, M. J., Schultz, S., Tandon, R., Tsuang, M., Van Os, J., & Carpenter, W. (2013). Logic and justification for dimensional assessment of symptoms and related clinical phenomena in psychosis: Relevance to DSM-5. *Schizophrenia Research, 150*(1), 15–20. https://doi.org/10.1016/j.schres.2013.04.027

Biagiarelli, M., Roma, P., Comparelli, A., Andraos, M. P., Di Pomponio, I., Corigliano, V., Curto, M., Masters, G. A., & Ferracuti, S. (2015). Relationship between the Rorschach Perceptual Thinking Index (PTI) and the Positive and Negative Syndrome Scale (PANSS) in psychotic patients: A validity study. *Psychiatry Research, 225*(3), 315–321. https://doi. org/10.1016/j.psychres.2014.12.018

Blatt, S. J., & Ritzler, B. A. (1974). Thought disorder and boundary disturbances in psychosis. *Journal of Consulting and Clinical Psychology, 42*(3), 370–381. https://doi.org/ 10.1037/h0036688

Bleuler, E. (1911). *Dementia praecox or the group of schizophrenias (1951–03305-000).* International Universities Press.

Bohm, E. (1958). *A textbook in Rorschach test diagnosis.* Grune & Stratton.

Buckingham, K. N., Meyer, G. J., O'Gorman, E. T., & Mihura, J. L. (2020). Deconstructing psychosis and cross-validating the R-PAS variables targeting its constructs [Abstract]. *Schizophrenia Bulletin, 46*(S1), S180. https://doi.org/10.1093/schbul/sbaa030.431

Chaika, E. O. (1990). *Understanding psychotic speech: Beyond Freud and Chomsky.* Charles C. Thomas.

Clark, L. A., Watson, D., & Reynolds, S. (1995). Diagnosis and classification of psychopathology: Challenges to the current system and future directions. *Annual Review of Psychology, 46*, 121–153. https://doi.org/10.1146/annurev.ps.46.020195.001005

Eblin, J. J., Meyer, G. J., Mihura, J. L., Viglione, D. J., & O'Gorman, E. T. (2018). Development and preliminary validation of a brief behavioral measure of psychotic propensity. *Psychiatry Research, 268*, 340–347. https://doi.org/10.1016/j.psychres.2018.08.006

Eckblad, M., & Chapman, L. J. (1983). Magical ideation as an indicator of schizotypy. *Journal of Consulting and Clinical Psychology, 51*(2), 215–225. https://doi.org/10.1037/ 0022-006X.51.2.215

Exner, J. E. (2000). *2000 Alumni newsletter.* Rorschach Workshops.

Exner, J. E. (2003). *The Rorschach: A comprehensive system* (4th ed.). John Wiley & Sons.

Exner, J. E., Weiner, I. B., & Schuyler, W. (1976). *A Rorschach workbook for the Comprehensive System.* Rorschach Workshops.

Fish, F. (1967). *Fish's clinical psychopathology.* John Wright & Sons.

Garb, H. N. (1999). Call for a moratorium on the use of the Rorschach Inkblot Test in clinical and forensic settings. *Assessment, 6*(4), 313–317. https://doi.org/10.1177/ 107319119900600402

Garety, P. A., & Freeman, D. (2013). The past and future of delusions research: From the inexplicable to the treatable. *The British Journal of Psychiatry, 203*(5), 327–333. https://doi.org/10.1192/bjp.bp 113.126953

Harrow, M., & Quinlan, D. (1977). Is disordered thinking unique to schizophrenia? *Archives of General Psychiatry, 34*(1), 15–21. https://doi.org/10.1001/archpsyc.1977. 01770130017001

Hart, M., & Lewine, R. R. J. (2017). Rethinking thought disorder. *Schizophrenia Bulletin, 43*(3), 514–522. https://doi.org/10.1093/schbul/sbx003

Holt, R. R. (2009). *Primary process thinking: Theory, measurement, and research (2009– 06164-000).* Jason Aronson.

Holt, R. R., & Havel, J. (1960). A method for assessing primary and secondary process in the Rorschach. In *Rorschach psychology* (pp. 263–318). Wiley.

Holzman, P. S., Levy, D. L., & Johnston, M. H. (2005). The use of the Rorschach technique for assessing formal thought disorder. In R. F. Bornstein & J. M. Masling (Eds.), *Scoring the Rorschach: Seven validated systems* (pp. 55–95). Lawrence Erlbaum Associates.

Johnston, M. H. (1975). *Thought disorder in schizophrenic patients and their relatives (1977–06000-001)*. ProQuest Information & Learning.

Johnston, M. H., & Holzman, P. S. (1979). *Assessing schizophrenic thinking: A clinical and research instrument for measuring thought disorder* (1st ed.). Jossey-Bass.

Jørgensen, K., Andersen, T. J., & Dam, H. (2000). The diagnostic efficiency of the Rorschach Depression Index and the Schizophrenia Index: A review. *Assessment, 7*(3), 259–280. https://doi.org/10.1177/107319110000700306

Jørgensen, K., Andersen, T. J., & Dam, H. (2001). The diagnostic efficiency of the Rorschach depression index and the schizophrenia index: A review. *Assessment, 8*(3), 355–355.

Kay, S. R., Fiszbein, A., & Opfer, L. A. (1987). The Positive and Negative Syndrome Scale (PANSS) for Schizophrenia. *Schizophrenia Bulletin, 13*(2), 261–276. https://doi.org/10.1093/schbul/13.2.261

Kleiger, J. H. (1999). *Disordered thinking and the Rorschach: Theory, research, and differential diagnosis*. Analytic Press.

Kleiger, J. H. (2015). An open letter to Hermann Rorschach: What has become of your experiment? *Rorschachiana, 36*(2), 221–241 https://doi.org/10.1027/1192-5604/a000071

Kleiger, J. H. (2016). Thinking about thought disorder. *Rorschach Training Programs Newsletter*, 1–2.

Kleiger, J. H. (2017). *Rorschach assessment of psychotic phenomena: Clinical, conceptual, and empirical developments*. Routledge/Taylor & Francis Group.

Kleiger, J. H., & Peebles-Kleiger, M. J. (1993). Toward a conceptual understanding of the deviant response in the Comprehensive Rorschach System. *Journal of Personality Assessment, 60*, 74–90.

Kleiger, J. H., & Weiner, I. B. (2019). Autistic thinking: Conceptual understanding and Rorschach assessment. *Rorschachiana, 40*(2), 130–151. https://doi.org/10.1027/1192-5604/a000117

Kotov, R., Krueger, R. F., Watson, D., Achenbach, T. M., Althoff, R. R., Bagby, R. M., Brown, T. A., Carpenter, W. T., Caspi, A., Clark, L. A., Eaton, N. R., Forbes, M. K., Forbush, K. T., Goldberg, D., Hasin, D., Hyman, S. E., Ivanova, M. Y., Lynam, D. R., Markon, K., ... Zimmerman, M. (2017). The Hierarchical Taxonomy of Psychopathology (HiTOP): A dimensional alternative to traditional nosologies. *Journal of Abnormal Psychology, 126*(4), 454–477. https://doi.org/10.1037/abn0000258

McLean, B. F., Mattiske, J. K., & Balzan, R. P. (2017). Association of the jumping to conclusions and evidence integration biases with delusions in psychosis: A detailed meta-analysis. *Schizophrenia Bulletin, 43*(2), 344–354.

Meyer, G. J., Erdberg, P., & Shaffer, T. W. (2007). Toward international normative reference data for the Comprehensive System. *Journal of Personality Assessment, 89*, S201–S216. https://doi.org/10.1080/00223890701629342

Meyer, G. J., Hsiao, W.-C., Viglione, D. J., Mihura, J. L., & Abraham, L. M. (2013). Rorschach scores in applied clinical practice: A survey of perceived validity by experienced clinicians. *Journal of Personality Assessment, 95*(4), 351–365. https://doi.org/10.1080/00223891.2013.770399

Meyer, G. J., O'Gorman, E. T., Mihura, J. L., Viglione, D. J., & Vanhoyland, M. (2020). *Scales of Problematic Communication and Thinking*. Department of Psychology, University of Toledo Manuscript-in-progress.

Meyer, G. J., Viglione, D. J., & Mihura, J. L. (2017). Psychometric foundations of the Rorschach Performance Assessment System (R-PAS). In R. E. Erard & F. B. Evans (Eds.), *The Rorschach in multimethod forensic assessment: Conceptual foundations and practical applications* (pp. 23–91). Routledge/Taylor & Francis Group.

Meyer, G. J., Viglione, D. J., Mihura, J. L., Erard, R. E., & Erdberg, P. (2011). *Rorschach Performance Assessment System: Administration, coding, interpretation, and technical manual*. Rorschach Performance Assessment System, LLC.

Mihura, J. L., Meyer, G. J., Bombel, G., & Dumitrascu, N. (2015). Standards, accuracy, and questions of bias in Rorschach meta-analyses: Reply to Wood, Garb, Nezworski, Lilienfeld, and Duke (2015). *Psychological Bulletin, 141*(1), 250–260. https://doi.org/10.1037/a0038445

Mihura, J. L., Meyer, G. J., Dumitrascu, N., & Bombel, G. (2013). The validity of individual Rorschach variables: Systematic reviews and meta-analyses of the comprehensive system. *Psychological Bulletin, 139*(3), 548–605. https://doi.org/10.1037/a0029406

Minassian, A., Granholm, E., Verney, S., & Perry, W. (2004). Pupillary dilation to simple vs. Complex tasks and its relationship to thought disturbance in schizophrenia patients. *International Journal of Psychophysiology, 52*(1), 53–62. https://doi.org/10.1016/j.ijpsycho.2003.12.008

Overall, J. E., & Gorham, D. R. (1988). The Brief Psychiatric Rating Scale (BPRS): Recent developments in ascertainment and scaling. *Psychopharmacology Bulletin, 24*(1), 97–99.

Perry, W., Geyer, M. A., & Braff, D. L. (1999). Sensorimotor gating and thought disturbance measured in close temporal proximity in schizophrenic patients. *Archives of General Psychiatry, 56*(3), 277–281. https://doi.org/10.1001/archpsyc.56.3.277

Peterson, C. A., & Schilling, K. M. (2010). Card pull in projective testing. *Journal of Personality Assessment, 47*(3), 267–275. https://doi.org/10.1207/s15327752jpa4703_7

Rapaport, D., Gill, M., & Schafer, R. (1946). *Diagnostic psychological testing: The theory, statistical evaluation, and diagnostic application of a battery of tests: Volume II*. The Year Book Publishers.

Ritzler, B., & Alter, B. (1986). Rorschach teaching in APA-approved clinical graduate programs 10 years later. *Journal of Personality Assessment, 50*(1), 44–49. https://doi.org/10.1207/s15327752jpa5001_6

Rushton, J. P., Brainerd, C. J., & Pressley, M. (1983). Behavioral development and construct validity: The principle of aggregation. *Psychological Bulletin, 94*(1), 18–38. https://doi.org/10.1037/0033-2909.94.1.18

Roche, E., Creed, L., MacMahon, D., Brennan, D., & Clarke, M. (2015). The epidemiology and associated phenomenology of formal thought disorder: A systematic review. *Schizophrenia Bulletin, 41*(4), 951–962. https://doi.org/10.1093/schbul/sbu129

Shaffer, T. W., Erdberg, P., & Haroian, J. (1999). Current nonpatient data for the Rorschach, WAIS-R, and MMPI-2. *Journal of Personality Assessment, 73*(2), 305–316. https://doi.org/10.1207/S15327752JPA7302_8

Singer, M. T., & Wynne, L. C. (1966). Principles for scoring communication defects and deviances in parents of schizophrenics: Rorschach and TAT scoring manuals. *Psychiatry, 29*(3), 260–288. https://doi.org/10.1080/00332747.1966.11023470

Spitzer, R. L., Williams, J. B. W., Gibbon, M., & First, M. B. (1990). *User's guide for the structured clinical interview for DSM-III-R: SCID*. American Psychiatric Association.

Viglione, D. J. (1999). A review of recent research addressing the utility of the Rorschach. *Psychological Assessment, 11*(3), 251–265. https://doi.org/10.1037/1040-3590.11.3.251

Watkins, J. G., & Stauffacher, J. C. (1952). An index of pathological thinking in the Rorschach. *Journal of Projective Techniques, 16*, 276–286. https://doi.org/10.1080/08853126.1952.10380431

Wood, J. M., Garb, H. N., Nezworski, M. T., Lilienfeld, S. O., & Duke, M. C. (2015). A second look at the validity of widely used Rorschach indices: Comment on Mihura, Meyer,

Dumitrascu, and Bombel (2013). *Psychological Bulletin, 141*(1), 236–249. https://doi.org/10.1037/a0036005

Wood, J. M., Nezworski, M. T., & Garb, H. N. (2003). What's right with the Rorschach? *The Scientific Review of Mental Health Practice, 2*(2), 142–146.

Wood, J. M., Nezworski, M. T., Garb, H. N., & Lilienfeld, S. O. (2001). The misperception of psychopathology: Problems with the norms of the Comprehensive System for the Rorschach. *Clinical Psychology: Science and Practice, 8*(3), 350–373. https://doi.org/10.1093/clipsy/8.3.350

Wood, J. M., Nezworski, M. T., & Stejskal, W. J. (1996). The Comprehensive System for the Rorschach: A critical examination. *Psychological Science, 7*(1), 3–10. https://doi.org/10.1111/j.1467-9280.1996.tb00658.x

History
Received May 5, 2020
Revision received August 24, 2020
Accepted September 29, 2020
Published online September 15, 2021

ORCID
James Kleiger
ⓘ https://orcid.org/0000-0002-5738-4311

James H. Kleiger
6320 Democracy Blvd
Bethesda, MD 20817
USA
james.kleiger@gmail.com

Summary

Despite years of criticism about its empirical underpinnings and clinical benefits, even the staunchest critics never wavered in their endorsement of the Rorschach as a scientifically valid method for assessing disordered thinking and psychotic phenomena. Following a review of recent meta-analyses, which firmly established Comprehensive Rorschach System variables as robust measures of disorder thinking and perception, the authors describe the development of a revised set of variables in the Rorschach Performance Assessment system (R-PAS) and review research establishing their validity. Scoring variables and their empirical association with disordered thinking are strengthened when clinicians broaden their perspectives to the conceptual underpinnings of what these scores mean. Questioning the nature of the term "thought disorder," the authors suggest a more inclusive definition and describe ways of organizing our understanding about the Rorschach assessment of disordered thinking and communication. The authors close with a discussion of directions for future research into the Rorschach assessment of disordered thinking and communication.

Résumé

Malgré des années de critiques sur ses fondements empiriques et ses avantages cliniques, même les critiques les plus fervents n'ont jamais hésité dans leur approbation du Rorschach en tant que méthode scientifiquement valide pour évaluer la pensée désordonnée et les phénomènes psychotiques. À la suite d'une revue des méta-analyses récentes, qui ont fermement établi les variables du système intégré du Rorschach en tant que mesures robustes de la pensée et de la perception des troubles, les auteurs décrivent le développement d'un ensemble révisé de variables dans le système d'évaluation des performances de Rorschach (R-PAS) et examinent la recherche afin d'établir leur validité. Les variables de notation et leur association empirique avec la pensée désordonnée sont renforcées lorsque les cliniciens élargissent leurs perspectives aux fondements conceptuels de la signification de ces scores. Remettant en question la nature du terme « trouble de la pensée », les auteurs suggèrent une définition plus inclusive et décrivent des moyens d'organiser notre compréhension de l'évaluation de Rorschach des troubles de la pensée et de la communication. Les auteurs concluent par une discussion des directions possible pour les futures recherches sur l'évaluation du Rorschach pour les troubles de la pensée et de la communication.

Resumen

A pesar de años de críticas sobre sus fundamentos empíricos y beneficios clínicos, incluso los críticos más acérrimos nunca dudaron en respaldar al Rorschach como un método científicamente válido para evaluar el trastorno del pensamiento y los fenómenos psicóticos. Tras una revisión de metanálisis recientes que establecieron firmemente las variables del Sistema Comprensivo de Rorschach como medidas sólidas del trastorno del pensamiento y la percepción, los autores describen el desarrollo de un conjunto revisado de variables en el Protocolo de Evaluación del Rorschach (R-PAS) y revisan la investigación estableciendo su validez. Las variables de puntuación y su asociación empírica con el trstorno de pensamiento se fortalecen cuando los clínicos amplían sus perspectivas a los fundamentos conceptuales de lo que significan estas puntuaciones. Al cuestionar la naturaleza del término "trastorno del pensamiento", los autores sugieren una definición más inclusiva y describen formas de organizar nuestra comprensión sobre la evaluación de Rorschach de los trastornos del pensamiento y la comunicación. Los autores finalizan con una discusión sobre las direcciones para futuras investigaciones sobre la evaluación de los trastornos del pensamiento y la comunicación en el Rorschach.

要約

思考とコミュニケーションにおける実証的基盤と臨床的有用性についての長年の批判にも関わらず、最も頑固な批評家でさえ、思考の障害と精神病の現象を評価するための科学的に有効な方法としてロールシャッハを支持するという意見で揺らぐことはなかった。最近のメタアナリシスのレビューでは、包括的システムの変数が思考と知覚の障害を評価する強力な方法として確立されている。著者らは、R-PASの変数の改訂版の開発について述べ、その妥当性を立証する研究をレビューしている。臨床家がこれらのスコアの意味の概念的裏付けのための見通しを広げると、変数をスコアすること思考障害との経験的な関連性は強化される。著者らは、「思考障害」という言葉の性質に疑問を持ち、よりインクルーシブな定義を提案し、思考障害とコミュニケーションのロールシャッハ評価についての理解を整理する方法を述べている。著者らは、思考障害とコミュニケーションのロールシャッハ評価に関する将来の研究の方向性についての議論で締めくくられている。

A Commentary on "Developments in the Rorschach Assessment of Disordered Thinking and Communication" (Kleiger & Mihura, 2021)

Lindy-Lou Boyette and Arjen Noordhof

Department of Clinical Psychology, University of Amsterdam, The Netherlands

"Why on earth would one use the Rorschach to assess disordered thinking?" was the almost Pavlovian reaction of the second author to the request to write this commentary. This uninformed response was markedly changed after reading the excellent contribution by Kleiger and Mihura (2021), as well as the research they cite. The authors convincingly argue for the reliability and validity of a set of Rorschach scales that assess thought disorder. Hence, we see no reason why one shouldn't use these scales for this purpose.

Apart from reliability and validity, the question "why use the Rorschach?" encompasses utility. This deserves attention if one wishes to convince new researchers and clinicians to start using the instrument. We will review current instruments for disordered thinking and communication and discuss the hypothetical (incremental) utility of the Rorschach in research and in clinical practice.

Other Research Instruments

We concur with the authors that the Rorschach is at the moment (unfortunately!) not valid for the assessment of the negative dimension of thought disorder and therefore will focus only on the assessment of the positive dimension. Four different methods of assessment have been used for this purpose: (1) clinician ratings of free-speech, (2) semistructured interviews, (3) questionnaires, and (4) performance-based or projective tasks, such as the Rorschach itself.

The standard research instrument for disordered thinking and communication is the Scale for the Assessment of Thought, Language and Communication (TLC; Andreasen, 1986). The TLC is most commonly used in research and is generally included in the assessment of convergent validity of other instruments.

The TLC consists of 18 clinician-rated items concerning *communication disorders* (e.g., tangentiality, perseveration), *language disorder* (e.g., word approximations, neologisms) and *thought disorder* (e.g., poverty of speech and illogicality). Clinicians base their assessment on observations of spontaneous speech, for instance a standard psychiatric interview. The TLC has been critiqued for being less sensitive to subtle, subclinical gradations of disturbance as found in the speech of non-affected relatives of patients with psychotic disorders and individuals without a psychiatric disorder (Docherty et al., 1997).

An interesting alternative to the TLC is the Thought and Language Disorder (TALD) scale (Kircher et al., 2014). Just like the TLC it uses clinician ratings of spontaneous speech (25 items based on a 50-minute unstructured interview). Additionally, the TALD assesses the patient's own perspective through a semistructured interview concerning five more internal and subtle symptoms. Clinician-rated symptoms had strong convergence with other clinician-rated scales and clear divergence from ratings of depression and mania. Correlations between self-reported and clinician-rated positive symptoms were either non-significant (TALD, SAPS/SANS) or low ($r = .22$ with TLC linguistic control).[1]

An alternative attempt at assessing the patient's perspective is the Formal Thought Disorder Scale (FTD; Barrera et al., 2008), which is the only questionnaire we are aware of that is specifically directed at disordered thinking and communication.[2] Both a self-report and an informant version are available. Both showed adequate reliability. Total scores showed moderate convergence ($r = .30$ for self-report and $r = .52$ for informant-report) with clinician-rated symptoms assessed by the Comprehensive Assessment of Symptoms and History (CASH) (Andreasen et al., 1992), while self-report and informant-report were uncorrelated.

The final class of instruments use performance-based or projective tasks to elicit speech from subjects, which is then rated by an observer. The Thought Disorder Index (TDI) (Solovay et al., 1986) is based on verbatim scripts of responses to the Rorschach inkblots (Rorschach, 1942) and, potentially, any observed deviant verbalizations as noted by the observer during completion of the verbal subtests of the Wechsler Adult Intelligence Scale (WAIS-R; Wechsler, 1981). The Thought and Language Index (TLI; Liddle et al., 2002) uses either the Rorschach or

---

1   Another clinician-rated interview is the CLANG (Chen et al., 1997) which we
    have omitted due to space constraints. The currently discussed instruments all
    follow a definition of disordered thinking and communication broadly compa-
    rable to Andreasen (1986). The CLANG is based on a highly different
    conceptualization, namely psycholinguistic concepts.
2   There are also several self-report omnibus tests that include scales related to
    these phenomena, but we omit these for lack of space.

Thematic Apperception Test (TAT; Murray, 1943) cards to elicit speech but is much briefer than the TDI, collecting eight 1-minute speech samples. The Bizarre-Idiosyncratic Thinking Scale (BIT; Marengo et al., 1986) is also quite quick to administer, as it employs only the WAIS Comprehension subtest and a 12-item proverb test.

Of the performance-based or projective instruments, the Rorschach is the only instrument with meta-analytic support for reliability and validity. In regard to its most recent version, the Rorschach Performance Assessment System (R-PAS; Meyer et al., 2011), a second strong and unique quality is the inclusion of age-based norms. This is important as the frequency and severity of disordered thinking and communication is higher in children and adolescents (Roche et al., 2015). The most notable limitation to the Rorschach/R-PAS is the time and effort needed to learn how to administer, score, and interpret the instrument. It is therefore positive that the R-PAS team is working on shortened versions and further simplified, perhaps automated coding.

Research Utility

First some thoughts on research utility of the Rorschach. In general, we believe multimethod to be preferable to monomethod assessment. A major disadvantage of the latter is the conflation of phenomena with their measurement. If one attempts to assess the same phenomenon with different methods, there are likely to be substantial divergences between methods. This is clearly demonstrated by the aforementioned covariance patterns of the perspectives of clinicians, informants, and patients. This does not necessarily indicate a lack of validity as different informants (self, clinician, carer) have different perspectives and contexts and hence should not necessarily converge (Noordhof et al., 2008). Performance-based tests like the Rorschach add another source of divergence to this puzzle. For research, such divergent findings are crucially important. They may indicate that one or both methods are unreliable or invalid, but often they instead point towards the fact that the phenomena under consideration are complex, multifaceted, and not yet fully understood. Such acknowledgement is extremely important for any genuinely scientific project.

So why add a performance-based task? One advantage of performance-based tasks is that they do not rely on introspection or outside observation. Hence, they may tap into domains that are not easily captured by observation or introspection and which may otherwise remain unknown or dynamically unconscious (Finn, 1996). A second possible advantage of performance-based tasks is that they can have demonstrable incremental predictive utility (Shedler et al., 1993). We are not aware of any research demonstrating incremental predictive utility with the Rorschach scales reviewed here, for instance in regard to transition to clinical disorder or psychotic relapse or remission, and this would be a fruitful line for future research. Third, as performance-based tests are less transparent, they can add value to the assessment of malingering. There is an historic interest in the Rorschach as a measure of malingering psychosis and although there is support for this use (Kleiger, 2017), a specific malingering pattern has not yet established (Perry & Kinder, 1990). The R-PAS, which is more standardized than older versions of the Rorschach in terms of number of responses, could be of interest for this topic.

Furthermore, as mentioned, the TLC has been critiqued for not capturing the more subtle aspects of disordered thinking and communication. The Rorschach is a likely candidate to improve on this as the sumscale (WSumCog) is based on the frequency of both mild and more severe indications. The TALD and FTD may be used for the same purpose. We do not know of any research comparing these approaches in terms of their utility for capturing mild disturbances but would certainly be very interested in the outcomes.

Clinical Utility

The Rorschach is not only a research instrument. It is also promoted very much as a clinical tool. Hence, we wondered what clinical utility might be obtained if nonusers learn to use the test. Utility is very dependent on the context and goals of use (Kamphuis et al., 2020), so we will discuss possible uses in three contexts that we deem most relevant: the clinic for psychotic disorders, assessment of personality (disorder), and psychoanalytically oriented structural diagnosis.

Based on our personal experience (LLB conducted assessment for a psychosis department for over 10 years), none of the aforementioned instruments – including the Rorschach – are currently routinely used in the clinical care of patients with psychotic disorders or individuals with at-risk mental states. Eblin et al. (2018) argue that the Rorschach may have incremental validity for (1) assessing psychosis when used in conjunction with neuropsychological and neuroimaging tasks, (2) for identifying individuals at risk for psychosis, and (3) for assessing social and functional deficits. In the psychosis clinic, assessment of functioning is currently generally limited to cognitive functioning, for which purpose neuropsychological test batteries are conducted. Neuropsychological and neuroimaging tasks are not utilized for identifying or assessing psychosis. Instead, semistructured interviews containing multiple symptom dimensions of psychosis, such as the CASH (Andreasen et al., 1992) and PANSS (Kay et al., 1989) or the CAARMS for at-risk states (Yung et al., 2003), are standard. These interviews all contain a few observational, clinician-rated items of disordered thinking and communication (in case of the CASH, this is a small subset of TLC items). By definition, these items will not capture the full range of disordered thinking and communication. However, in order to convince clinicians to include the Rorschach, empirical evidence on its incremental validity for assessing factors relevant for the clinical care of patients with psychotic disorders or individuals with at-risk mental states, of which several have been discussed, is needed.

Current use of the Rorschach is more frequent in care settings that are not specific to psychosis. In these contexts, it could very well be of help in detecting subtle forms of disordered thinking and communication, which are commonly encountered in patients with a diverse range of primary diagnoses (Van Os & Reininghaus, 2016). At the core of the alternative model for personality disorders (AMPD) in section 3 of DSM-5 (APA, 2013), there is a hierarchical structure of personality traits consisting of five broad domains and disordered thinking and communication pertain to the broad domain of psychoticism. The Rorschach might be used in a multimethod approach to the assessment of facets in the domain of psychoticism. The AMPD cannot only be applied to severe personality disorders, but also to mildly problematic features of personality in many other patients. This potentially opens up a vast area of possible uses of the Rorschach, although, on a more skeptical note, we have not encountered evidence that this would result in substantial treatment utility (nor did we find evidence to the contrary).

Finally, the processes Kleiger and Mihura (2021) discuss are often inscribed in a psychoanalytic orientation towards how the mind works. From this perspective it can be argued that *primary process thinking* is not an exclusive property of overtly psychotic people but is generally *repressed* in neurotic subjects leading to compromise formations like dreams, slips, and symptoms. Such formations and secondary defense mechanisms are the typical result of neurotic resolutions to the Oedipus complex. Primary processes become mainly unconscious, and their libidinal force expresses or erupts in, for example, jokes or permitted transgressions. If these defenses are strongly developed, one would expect Rorschach responses that are reflective of specific secondary defenses (e.g., isolation of affect or humor) rather than primary process responses. In psychotic structures (Kernberg, 1984) the oedipal constellation is not resolved by general repression, and primary process thinking and primary defenses are thus much more prominent and overt, which would presumably result in primary process (or uncensored) responses on the Rorschach. This would certainly be the case in manifest psychosis, but people with psychotic structures are often capable of adapting to neurotic expectations and thereby appearing rather "normal." It stands to reason, and is an interesting hypothesis for research, that especially for the group that is not manifestly psychotic the Rorschach would be useful. Furthermore, in people who have mainly developed neurotic compromises primary process thinking may still be present in a way that is not easily detectable and for which the Rorschach might be a useful diagnostic tool. Likewise, primary process thinking in people diagnosed as *borderline* (Kernberg, 1967) seems like an area for which the Rorschach can also be useful. For example, it could help to distinguish between people with borderline disorder characterized by mainly neurotic structure but much traumatic reactivity, acting out, and unmitigated transference on the one hand, and people with borderline disorder for whom primary process thinking is a rather important feature of the general structure of their personality on the other. Such distinctions have important clinical implications for how analytically informed therapies should proceed (e.g., McWilliams, 2011). However, as a cautionary note: In order to have incremental utility, the Rorschach should outperform clinical judgment on the basis of the development of speech and transference, which remains to be demonstrated.

Conclusion

Kleiger and Mihura have convinced us that the Rorschach is valid and reliable for the assessment of disordered thinking and communication, and we do now think that the instrument deserves a more prominent place in research. We have made some recommendations for further areas of study. We have also presented ideas for how its use in clinical practice may be helpful. The Rorschach should no longer be harshly judged on criteria that are not typically met by alternatives. Nevertheless, solid evidence for utility is the royal road towards broader adoption of the instrument.

References

American Psychiatric Association (2013). *Diagnostic and statistical manual of mental disorders* (DSM-5).

Andreasen, N. C. (1986). Scale for the Assessment of Thought, Language, and Communication (TLC). *Schizophrenia Bulletin, 12*(3), 473–482. https://doi.org/10.1093/schbul/12.3.473

Andreasen, N. C., Flaum, M., & Arndt, S. (1992). The Comprehensive Assessment of Symptoms and History (CASH): An instrument for assessing diagnosis and psychopathology. *Archives of General Psychiatry, 49*(8), 615–623. https://doi.org/10.1001/archpsyc.1992.01820080023004

Barrera, A., McKenna, P. J., & Berrios, G. E. (2008). Two new scales of formal thought disorder in schizophrenia. *Psychiatry Research, 157*(1–3), 225–234. https://doi.org/10.1016/j.psychres.2006.09.017

Chen, E. Y. H., Lam, L. C. W., Kan, C. S., Chan, C. K. Y., Kwok, C. L., Nguyen, D. G. H., & Chen, R. Y. L. (1997). Language disorganization in schizophrenia: Validation and assessment with a new clinical rating instrument. *Hong Kong Journal of Psychiatry, 6*(1), 4–13.

Docherty, N. M., Miller, T. N., & Lewis, M. A. (1997). Communication disturbances in the natural speech of schizophrenic patients and non-schizophrenic parents of patients. *Acta Psychiatrica Scandinavica, 95*(6), 500–507. https://doi.org/10.1111/j.1600-0447.1997.tb10138.x

Eblin, J. J., Meyer, G. J., Mihura, J. L., Viglione, D. J., & O'Gorman, E. T. (2018). Development and preliminary validation of a brief behavioral measure of psychotic propensity. *Psychiatry Research, 268*, 340–347. https://doi.org/10.1016/j.psychres.2018.08.006

Finn, S. (1996). Assessment feedback integrating MMPI-2 and Rorschach findings. *Journal of Personality Assessment, 67*(3), 543–557. https://doi.org/10.1207/s15327752jpa6703_10

Kamphuis, J. H., Noordhof, A., & Hopwood, C. J. (2020). When and how assessment matters: An update on the Treatment Utility of Clinical Assessment (TUCA). *Psychological Assessment, 33*(2), 122–132. https://doi.org/10.1037/pas0000966

Kay, S. R., Opler, L. A., & Lindenmayer, J. P. (1989). The Positive and Negative Syndrome Scale (PANSS): Rationale and standardisation. *The British Journal of Psychiatry: Supplement, 13*(7), 59–67.

Kernberg, O. F. (1967). Borderline personality organization. *Journal of the American Psychoanalytic Organization, 15*, 641–685.

Kernberg, O. F. (1984). *Severe personality disorders, psychotherapeutic strategie.* Yale University Press.

Kircher, T., Krug, A., Stratmann, M., Ghazi, S., Schales, C., Frauenheim, M., Turner, L., Fährmann, P., Hornig, T., Katzev, M., Grosvald, M., Müller-Isberner, R., & Nagels, A. (2014). A rating scale for the assessment of objective and subjective formal thought and language disorder (TALD). *Schizophrenia Research, 160*(1–3), 216–221. https://doi.org/10.1016/j.schres.2014.10.024

Kleiger, J. H. (2017). *Rorschach assessment of psychotic phenomena: Clinical, conceptual, and empirical developments.* Routledge/Taylor & Francis.

Kleiger, J. H., & Mihura, J. L. (2021). Developments in the Rorschach assessment of disordered thinking and communication. *Rorschachiana, 42*(2), 265–280. https://doi.org/10.1027/1192-5604/a000132

Liddle, P. F., Ngan, E. T. C., Caissie, S. L., Anderson, C. M., Bates, A. T., Quested, D. J., White, R., & Weg, R. (2002). Thought and language index: An instrument for assessing thought and language in schizophrenia. *British Journal of Psychiatry, 181*(4), 326–330. https://doi.org/10.1192/bjp.181.4.326

Marengo, J. T., Harrow, M., Lanin-Kettering, I., & Wilson, A. (1986). Evaluating bizarre-idiosyncratic thinking: A comprehensive index of positive thought disorder. *Schizophrenia Bulletin, 12*(3), 497–511. https://doi.org/10.1093/schbul/12.3.497

McWilliams, N. (2011). *Psychoanalytic diagnosis. Understanding personality structure in the clinical process* (2nd ed.). The Guilford Press.

Meyer, G. J., Viglione, D. J., Mihura, J. L., Erard, R. E., & Erdberg, P. (2011). *Rorschach performance assessment system: Administration, coding, interpretation, and technical manual.* Rorschach Performance Assessment System, LLC.

Murray, H. A. (1943). *The Thematic Apperception Test manual*. Harvard University Press.

Noordhof, A., Oldehinkel, A. J., Verhulst, F. C., & Ormel, J. (2008). Optimal use of multi-informant data on co-occurrence of internalizing and externalizing problems: The TRAILS study. *International Journal of Methods in Psychiatric Research, 17*(3), 174–183. https://doi.org/10.1002/mpr.258

Perry, G. G., & Kinder, B. N. (1990). The susceptibility of the Rorschach to malingering: A critical review. *Journal of Personality Assessment, 54*(1–2), 47–57. https://doi.org/10.1207/s15327752jpa5401&2_5

Roche, E., Creed, L., Macmahon, D., Brennan, D., & Clarke, M. (2015). The epidemiology and associated phenomenology of formal thought disorder: A systematic review. *Schizophrenia Bulletin, 41*(4), 951–962. https://doi.org/10.1093/schbul/sbu129

Rorschach, H. (1942). Lemkau P., & Kronenberg B. (1942). *Psychodiagnostics: A diagnostic test based on perception*. Hans Huber.

Shedler, J., Mayman, M., & Manis, M. (1993). The illusion of mental health. *American Psychologist, 48*(11), 1117–1131. https://doi.org/10.1037/0003-066X.48.11.1117

Solovay, M. R., Shenton, M. E., Gasperetti, C., Coleman, M., Kestnbaum, E., Carpenter, J. T., & Holzman, P. S. (1986). Scoring manual for the thought disorder index. *Schizophrenia Bulletin, 12*(3), 483–496. https://doi.org/10.1093/schbul/12.3.483

Wechsler, D. (1981). *Wechsler Adult Intelligence Scale manual: Revised form*. Psychological Corp.

Van Os, J., & Reininghaus, U. (2016). Psychosis as a transdiagnostic and extended phenotype in the general population. *World Psychiatry, 15*(2), 118–124. https://doi.org/10.1002/wps.20310

Yung, A. R., Yuen, H. P., Phillips, L. J., Francey, S., & McGorry, P. D. (2003). Mapping the onset of psychosis: The Comprehensive Assessment of At Risk Mental States (CAARMS). *Schizophrenia Research, 60*(1), 30–31.

Published online September 15, 2021

Lindy-Lou Boyette
Department of Clinical Psychology
University of Amsterdam
Nieuwe Achtergracht 129D
1001 NK Amsterdam
The Netherlands
l.l.n.j.boyette@uva.nl

Instructions to Authors

Rorschachiana is the scientific publication of the International Society for the Rorschach. The journal is interested in advancing theory and clinical applications of the Rorschach and other projective techniques, and research work that can enhance and promote projective methods.

***Rorschachiana* publishes the following types of articles:** Original Articles, Research Articles, and Case Studies.

Manuscript Submission: Manuscripts should be submitted online at
https://www.editorialmanager.com/ror
Detailed instructions to authors are provided at **http://www.hgf.io/ror**

Copyright Agreement: By submitting an article, the author confirms and guarantees on behalf of themselves and any coauthors that they hold all copyright in and titles to the submitted contribution, including any figures, photographs, line drawings, plans, maps, sketches and tables, and that the article and its contents do not infringe in any way on the rights of third parties. The author indemnifies and holds harmless the publisher from any third-party claims. The author agrees, upon acceptance of the article for publication, to transfer to the publisher on behalf of themselves and any coauthors the exclusive right to reproduce and distribute the article and its contents, both physically and in nonphysical, electronic, and other form, in the journal to which it has been submitted and in other independent publications, with no limits on the number of copies or on the form or the extent of the distribution. These rights are transferred for the duration of copyright as defined by international law. Furthermore, the author transfers to the publisher the following exclusive rights to the article and its contents:

1. The rights to produce advance copies, reprints, or offprints of the article, in full or in part, to undertake or allow translations into other languages, to distribute other forms or modified versions of the article, and to produce and distribute summaries or abstracts.
2. The rights to microfilm and microfiche editions or similar, to the use of the article and its contents in videotext, teletext, and similar systems, to recordings or reproduction using other media, digital or analog, including electronic, magnetic, and optical media, and in multimedia form, as well as for public broadcasting in radio, television, or other forms of broadcast.
3. The rights to store the article and its content in machine-readable or electronic form on all media (such as computer disks, compact disks, magnetic tape), to store the article and its contents in online databases belonging to the publisher or third parties for viewing or downloading by third parties, and to present or reproduce the article or its contents on visual display screens, monitors, and similar devices, either directly or via data transmission.
4. The rights to reproduce and distribute the article and its contents by all other means, including photomechanical and similar processes (such as photocopying or facsimile), and as part of so-called document delivery services.
5. The right to transfer any or all rights mentioned in this agreement, as well as rights retained by the relevant copyright clearing centers, including royalty rights to third parties.

Online Rights for Journal Articles: Guidelines on authors' rights to archive electronic version of their manuscripts online are given in the document "Guidelines on sharing and use of articles in Hogrefe journals" on the journal's web page at http://www.hgf.io/ror

September 2021

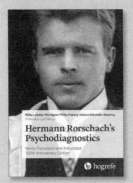
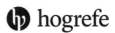